Running Injuries

Editors

MICHAEL FREDERICSON
ADAM S. TENFORDE

PHYSICAL MEDICINE AND REHABILITATION CLINICS OF NORTH AMERICA

www.pmr.theclinics.com

Consulting Editor
SANTOS F. MARTINEZ

February 2016 • Volume 27 • Number 1

ELSEVIER

1600 John F. Kennedy Boulevard • Suite 1800 • Philadelphia, Pennsylvania, 19103-2899

http://www.theclinics.com

PHYSICAL MEDICINE AND REHABILITATION CLINICS OF NORTH AMERICA Volume 27, Number 1
February 2016 ISSN 1047-9651, ISBN 978-0-323-41710-5

Editor: Jennifer Flynn-Briggs
Developmental Editor: Donald Mumford

Reprints. For copies of 100 or more of articles in this publication, please contact the Commercial Reprints Department, Elsevier Inc., 360 Park Avenue South, New York, NY 10010-1710. Tel.: 212-633-3874; Fax: 212-633-3820; E-mail: reprints@elsevier.com.

Physical Medicine and Rehabilitation Clinics of North America (ISSN 1047-9651) is published quarterly by Elsevier Inc., 360 Park Avenue South, New York, NY 10010-1710. Months of issue are February, May, August, and November. Business and Editorial Offices: 1600 John F. Kennedy Blvd., Suite 1800, Philadelphia, PA 19103-2899. Customer Service Office: 3251 Riverport Lane, Maryland Heights, MO 63043. Periodicals postage paid at New York, NY and additional mailing offices. Subscription price per year is $280.00 (US individuals), $538.00 (US institutions), $100.00 (US students), $335.00 (Canadian individuals), $709.00 (Canadian institutions), $210.00 (Canadian students), $415.00 (foreign individuals), $709.00 (foreign institutions), and $210.00 (foreign students). Foreign air speed delivery is included in all *Clinics* subscription prices. All prices are subject to change without notice. **POSTMASTER:** Send address changes to *Physical Medicine and Rehabilitation Clinics of North America*, Customer Service Office: Elsevier Health Sciences Division, Subscription Customer Service, 3251 Riverport Lane, Maryland Heights, MO 63043. **Customer Service: 1-800-654-2452 (US). From outside of the United States, call 314-447-8871. Fax: 314-447-8029. E-mail: JournalsCustomer Service-usa@elsevier.com (for print support); JournalsOnlineSupport-usa@elsevier.com (for online support).**

Physical Medicine and Rehabilitation Clinics of North America is indexed in *Excerpta Medica, MEDLINE/ PubMed (Index Medicus), Cinahl,* and *Cumulative Index to Nursing and Allied Health Literature.*

Contributors

CONSULTING EDITOR

SANTOS F. MARTINEZ, MD, MS
Diplomate, American Board of Physical Medicine and Rehabilitation, Certificate of Added Qualification Sports Medicine, Campbell Clinic Orthopaedics, Memphis, Tennessee

EDITORS

MICHAEL FREDERICSON, MD, FACSM
Director of Physical Medicine and Rehabilitation Sports Medicine, Division of Physical Medicine and Rehabilitation; Professor, Department of Orthopaedic Surgery; Head Physician, Stanford Track and Field, Stanford University, Redwood City, California

ADAM S. TENFORDE, MD
Department of Physical Medicine and Rehabilitation, Harvard Medical School, Spaulding Rehabilitation Hospital, Spaulding National Running Center, Cambridge, Massachusetts

AUTHORS

ROBERT L. BAKER, BS, MBA
Doctoral Candidate; Emeryville Sports Physical Therapy, Emeryville, California

IRENE S. DAVIS, PhD, PT, FAPTA, FACSM, FASB
Department of Physical Medicine and Rehabilitation, Spaulding National Running Center, Spaulding-Cambridge Outpatient Center, Harvard Medical School, Cambridge, Massachusetts

REBECCA A. DUTTON, MD
Sports Medicine Fellow, Division of Physical Medicine and Rehabilitation, Department of Orthopaedic Surgery, Stanford University, Redwood City, California

JONATHAN T. FINNOFF, DO
Consultant, Associate Professor, Department of Physical Medicine and Rehabilitation, Mayo Clinic School of Medicine, Rochester, Minnesota; Clinical Professor, Department of Physical Medicine and Rehabilitation, University of California Davis School of Medicine, Sacramento, California; Mayo Clinic Sports Medicine Center, Mayo Clinic Square, Minneapolis, Minnesota

MICHAEL FREDERICSON, MD, FACSM
Director of Physical Medicine and Rehabilitation Sports Medicine, Division of Physical Medicine and Rehabilitation; Professor, Department of Orthopaedic Surgery; Head Physician, Stanford Track and Field, Stanford University, Redwood City, California

ERIN FUTRELL, PT, OCS
Center for Interprofessional Studies and Innovation, MGH Institute of Health Professions, Charlestown, Massachusetts

BRYAN HEIDERSCHEIT, PT, PhD
Professor, Departments of Orthopedics and Rehabilitation and Biomedical Engineering; Director, UW Runners' Clinic; Director, Badger Athletic Performance Research, University of Wisconsin-Madison, Madison, Wisconsin

MARTIN D. HOFFMAN, MD
Professor of Physical Medicine and Rehabilitation, University of California Davis; and Chief of Physical Medicine and Rehabilitation, VA Northern California Health Care System, Sacramento, California

KENNETH J. HUNT, MD
Department of Orthopaedic Surgery, Stanford University, Redwood City, California

MICHAEL J. KHADAVI, MD
Director of Physical Medicine and Rehabilitation Sports Medicine, Carondelet Orthopaedic Surgeons, Overland Park, Kansas

BRIAN Y. KIM, MD, MS
Clinical Instructor, Division of Sports Medicine and Non-Operative Orthopaedics, Department of Family Medicine, David Geffen School of Medicine at University of California Los Angeles; Primary Care Sports Medicine Fellow, Department of Intercollegiate Athletics, University of California Los Angeles, Los Angeles, California

BRIAN J. KRABAK, MD, MBA, FACSM
Clinical Professor, Rehabilitation, Orthopedics and Sports Medicine, Seattle Children's Sports Medicine, Team Physician, University of Washington; Team Physician, Seattle University, Seattle, Washington

EMILY KRAUS, MD
Division of Physical Medicine and Rehabilitation, Department of Orthopaedic Surgery, Stanford University, Redwood City, California

SHANE McCLINTON, DPT, OCS, FAAOMPT, CSCS
Assistant Professor, Doctor of Physical Therapy Program; Coordinator, Des Moines University Running and Cycling Clinic, Des Moines University, Des Moines, Iowa

JENNY McCONNELL, AM, FACP, DPT, B App Sci(Phty), Grad Dip Man Ther, M Biomed Eng
Director, McConnell Physiotherapy Group; Visiting Fellow, Centre for Sports Medicine Research and Education, University of Melbourne, Melbourne, Victoria, Australia

CARLO J.E. MILANI, MD, MBA
Resident, Physical Medicine and Rehabilitation, University of Washington, Seattle, Washington

AURELIA NATTIV, MD
Professor, Division of Sports Medicine and Non-Operative Orthopaedics, Departments of Family Medicine and Orthopaedic Surgery, David Geffen School of Medicine at UCLA; Team Physician, Department of Intercollegiate Athletics, UCLA, Los Angeles, California

SATHISH RAJASEKARAN, MD
Fellow, Department of Orthopaedics and Rehabilitation, University of Iowa Sports Medicine, Iowa City, Iowa; Clinical Assistant Professor, Division of Physical Medicine and Rehabilitation, University of Alberta, Edmonton, Alberta, Canada

CARLOS E. RIVERA, MD
Staff Physician, Campbell Clinic Orthopaedics, Memphis, Tennessee

WOLF SCHAMBERGER, MD, FRCPC, Dip Sports Med, Dip Electrodiagnosis
Clinical Associate Professor, Division of Physical Medicine and Rehabilitation, Faculty of Medicine, University of British Columbia, Vancouver, Canada

BRIAN SNITILY, MD
Resident, Physical Medicine and Rehabilitation, University of Washington, Seattle, Washington

RICHARD B. SOUZA, PT, PhD, ATC, CSCS
Associate Professor, Departments of Physical Therapy and Rehabilitation Science, Radiology and Biomedical Imaging, and Orthopaedic Surgery, University of California, San Francisco, San Francisco, California

ADAM S. TENFORDE, MD
Department of Physical Medicine and Rehabilitation, Harvard Medical School, Spaulding Rehabilitation Hospital, Spaulding National Running Center, Cambridge, Massachusetts

AMY YIN, MD
Division of Physical Medicine and Rehabilitation, Department of Orthopaedic Surgery, Stanford University, Redwood City, California

Contents

Injuries to the hip and pelvis among runners can be among the most challenging to treat. Advances in the understanding of running biomechanics as it pertains to the lumbopelvic and hip regions have improved the management of these conditions. Conservative management with an emphasis on activity modification and neuromuscular exercises should comprise the initial plan of care, with injection therapies used in a supportive manner.

Patellofemoral pain is characterized by insidious onset anterior knee pain that is exaggerated under conditions of increased patellofemoral joint stress. A variety of risk factors may contribute to the development of patellofemoral pain. It is critical that the history and physical examination elucidate those risk factors specific to an individual in order to prescribe an appropriate and customized treatment plan. This article aims to review the epidemiology, risk factors, diagnosis, and management of patellofemoral pain.

Iliotibial band syndrome (ITBS) has known biomechanical factors with an unclear explanation based on only strength and flexibility deficits. Neuromuscular coordination has emerged as a likely reason for kinematic faults guiding research toward motor control. This article discusses ITBS in relation to muscle performance factors, fascial considerations, epidemiology, functional anatomy, strength deficits, kinematics, iliotibial strain and strain rate, and biomechanical considerations. Evidence-based exercise approaches are reviewed for ITBS, including related methods used to train the posterior hip muscles.

When considering knee pain in runners, clinicians must differentiate possible sources of the symptoms to determine symptom cause. Knee problems arise when runners increase the amount/frequency of loading through the lower limb. The way the loading is distributed through the knee determines which tissues are abnormally loaded, contributing to reported symptoms. Knee problems cannot be considered in isolation, requiring a thorough investigation of static and dynamic lower limb mechanics; footwear and running surfaces. This article examines potential sources of knee pain, exploring the role of the infrapatellar fat pad and plica in knee mechanics and their involvement in symptoms.

Exertional leg pain is a common condition seen in runners and the general population. Given the broad differential diagnosis of this complaint, this article focuses on the incidence, anatomy, pathophysiology, clinical presentation, diagnostic evaluation, and management of common causes that include medial tibial stress syndrome, tibial bone stress injury, chronic exertional compartment syndrome, arterial endofibrosis, popliteal artery entrapment syndrome, and entrapment of the common peroneal, superficial peroneal, and saphenous nerves. Successful diagnosis of these conditions hinges on performing a thorough history and physical examination followed by proper diagnostic testing and appropriate management.

Foot and ankle injuries account for nearly one-third of running injuries. Achilles tendinopathy, plantar fasciopathy, and ankle sprains are 3 of the most common types of injuries sustained in runners. Other common injuries include other tendinopathies of the foot and ankle, bone stress injuries, nerve conditions including neuromas, and joint disease including osteoarthritis. This review provides an evidence-based framework for the evaluation and optimal management of these conditions to ensure safe return to running participation and reduce risk for future injury.

Bone stress injuries (BSIs) are common running injuries and may occur at a rate of 20% annually. Both biological and biomechanical risk factors contribute to BSI. Evaluation of a runner with suspected BSI includes completing an appropriate history and physical examination. MRI grading classification for BSI has been proposed and may guide return to play. Management includes activity modification, optimizing nutrition, and addressing risk factors, including the female athlete triad. BSI prevention strategies include screening for risk factors during preparticipation physical examinations, optimizing nutrition (including adequate caloric intake, calcium, and vitamin D), and promoting ball sports during childhood and adolescence.

Female participation in running is at a historical high. Special consideration should be given to this population, in whom suboptimal nutritional intake, menstrual irregularity, and bone stress injury are common. Immature athletes should garner particular attention. Advances in the understanding of the Triad and Triad-related conditions have largely informed the approach to the health of this population. Clinicians should be well versed in the identification of Triad-related risk factors. A multidisciplinary team may be necessary for the optimal treatment of at-risk runners. Nonpharmacologic strategies to increase energy availability in athletes should be used as first-line treatment.

The validity of any research into the biomechanics of running should be questioned if the study has failed to look at whether pelvic malalignment was present and whether the altered, asymmetrical biomechanical changes attributable to the malalignment itself could have affected the results of the study.

Core muscles provide stability that allows generation of force and motion in the lower extremities, as well as distributing impact forces and allowing controlled and efficient body movements. Imbalances or deficiencies in the core muscles can result in increased fatigue, decreased endurance, and injury in runners. Core strengthening should incorporate the intrinsic needs of the core for flexibility, strength, balance, and endurance, and the function of the core in relation to its role in extremity function and dysfunction. Specific exercises are effective in strengthening the core muscles.

Musculoskeletal injuries in runners have been associated with faulty running mechanics. If left unaddressed, these injuries are likely to become chronic and/or repetitive. Increased hip adduction and vertical impact loading are two of the most common faulty mechanics associated with injury and have been the focus of retraining studies. While these programs have been successful, more work is needed in order to understand the optimal way to retrain gait patterns in runners. In summary, the human body has a considerable ability to adapt and leveraging this ability in order to reduce injury risk is very powerful.

PHYSICAL MEDICINE AND REHABILITATION CLINICS OF NORTH AMERICA

RELATED INTEREST

Radiologic Clinics of North America, July 2015 (Vol. 53, Issue 4)
Emergency and Trauma Radiology
Savvas Nicolaou, *Editor*

VISIT THE CLINICS ONLINE!
Access your subscription at:
www.theclinics.com

PHYSICAL MEDICINE AND REHABILITATION CLINICS OF NORTH AMERICA

Foreword

Supporting a Running Lifestyle

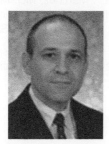

Santos F. Martinez, MD, MS
Consulting Editor

Running is a lifelong pursuit among many for which the destination may never be reached. Whether one is looking to complement fitness maintenance, to achieve endpoint goals, or to use running as a more introspective modality, it certainly plays a unique part of our contemporary fitness and sports culture. Much has evolved in our knowledge regarding complementary conditioning, injury prevention, mechanics of running injuries, and the unfortunate consequences of running-related injuries. It is with a sound knowledge of anatomy, biomechanics, nutrition, and rehabilitation strategies that we facilitate the patient's return to their pursuits, whether it is recreational, competitive, or just meeting the challenges of maintaining daily homeostasis in a hectic world. Sometimes, running serves as the only link for one's social camaraderie and at times a conduit for solitary contemplation. Others are driven by the clock, the distance, or maybe the terrain. They are fighting a personal challenge with a new battle to be gallantly pursued and conquered each day, overcoming perceived limitations. Optimal running tolerance and performance certainly are necessities for those involved with many sports, although it must be balanced with agility, strength training, and other requirements specific to the objective. There are other obvious benefits from running, such as improved cardiopulmonary fitness, leanness, bone mass, balance, and maintained functional independence. Reaction time improvement and maintenance are adjunctive benefits with many of these complementary activities. The numerous benefits from running need to be tempered by the potential for abuse and by observing signs of overtraining, which can take the individual down a deleterious avenue, which is not always perceived or accepted by one whose identity and balance are inherent and maintained through running.

Our subspecialty of Physiatry naturally approaches injuries, disability, and rehabilitation from a multidimensional viewpoint. Dr Fredericson and Dr Tenforde have met the challenge of putting together a great issue that will aid the Physiatrist in treating a wide spectrum of patients.

Phys Med Rehabil Clin N Am 27 (2016) xiii–xiv
http://dx.doi.org/10.1016/j.pmr.2015.11.001
1047-9651/16/$ – see front matter © 2016 Published by Elsevier Inc.

pmr.theclinics.com

Dr Fredericson has been an active mentor, speaker, researcher, and practitioner in this discipline for many years. We are certainly fortunate to have his gifted input and guidance for this project.

Santos F. Martinez, MD, MS
Campbell Clinic Orthopaedics
Memphis, TN, USA

E-mail address:
smartinez@campbellclinic.com

Preface

Running Injuries

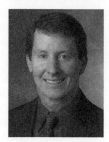 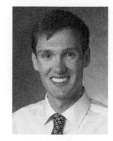

Michael Fredericson, MD, FACSM   Adam S. Tenforde, MD
Editors

We are honored with the opportunity to serve as guest editors for the issue, "Running Injuries" in *Physical Medicine and Rehabilitation Clinics of North America*. Running is of both professional and personal interest to us. We share the passion of the sport with our patients and desire to facilitate for each patient a successful return to running. Physiatrists have a unique perspective that can be very effective in evaluating and managing overuse injuries in runners, including an advanced understanding of the musculoskeletal system and influence of the kinetic chain in biomechanical stresses for injury.

Running injuries are very common and may recur, reflecting both the demands of the sport and the complexities of evaluating, treating, and preventing overuse injuries in this population. Review articles in this issue cover both the biomechanical and the biological risk factors for injury and advances in translational research for effective treatment strategies. This includes a discussion of common injuries by anatomical region; with added emphasis on specific knee conditions because knee injuries are a common class of injury in runners. Specific populations, including female runners, pediatric running injuries, and ultramarathoners, have unique health concerns, and each have dedicated reviews.

The review articles assembled reflect our advancement in knowledge for biomechanical risk factors for injury and the role of modifying running mechanics to address injuries. Discussion of gait evaluation, the concept of malalignment syndrome, core strengthening, and strategies for gait retraining to address running injuries are all included in this issue. We hope you enjoy reading this issue as much as we valued

Phys Med Rehabil Clin N Am 27 (2016) xv–xvi
http://dx.doi.org/10.1016/j.pmr.2015.10.001
1047-9651/16/$ – see front matter © 2016 Published by Elsevier Inc.

the opportunity to work with this talented and knowledgeable group of contributors. We thank the authors for their outstanding work in making this issue a success.

Michael Fredericson, MD, FACSM
Department of Orthopaedic Surgery
Division of Physical Medicine
and Rehabilitation
Stanford University
Redwood City, CA, USA

Adam S. Tenforde, MD
Department of Physical Medicine and Rehabilitation
Harvard Medical School
Spaulding Rehabilitation Hospital
Spaulding National Running Center
1575 Cambridge Street
Cambridge, MA 02138, USA

E-mail addresses:
mfred2@stanford.edu (M. Fredericson)
tenforde@stanford.edu (A.S. Tenforde)

Evaluation and Management of Hip and Pelvis Injuries

Bryan Heiderscheit, PT, PhD[a,b,c,*],
Shane McClinton, DPT, OCS, FAAOMPT, CSCS[d]

KEYWORDS

- Hamstring tendinopathy • Chronic groin pain • Greater trochanteric pain syndrome
- Piriformis syndrome • Iliopsoas tendinopathy • Femoroacetabular impingement
- Hip labral tear • Hip osteoarthritis

KEY POINTS

- Running-related injuries of the hip and pelvis can be particularly challenging to treat, often involving a prolonged period of recovery.
- Treatment decision-making is enhanced by corroboration of the history, symptoms, physical examination, and diagnostic imaging (when warranted), and decisions based on isolated tests or imaging are not recommended.
- Painful or aggravating activities such as running should be temporarily avoided or modified to reduce the mechanical load to the injured tissues.
- Treatment for hip-related tendinopathies should include an initial period to reduce tendon irritability, followed by a progressive loading program.
- Symptoms resulting from hip articular injuries, such as femoroacetabular impingement, labral tear, and osteoarthritis, can respond well to conservative management, including modification of running form to minimized loading to the hip joint.

INTRODUCTION

Injuries to the hip or pelvis comprise approximately 11% of running-related injuries[1,2] and can be among the most challenging to successfully treat, often involving a prolonged period of recovery. Unique risk factors that may predispose an individual to

Disclosure: Drs B. Heiderscheit and S. McClinton do not have any commercial or financial conflicts of interest to disclose.

[a] Department of Orthopedics & Rehabilitation, University of Wisconsin-Madison, 1300 University Avenue, Madison, WI 53706, USA; [b] UW Runners' Clinic, University of Wisconsin Health, 621 Science Dr, Madison, WI 53711, USA; [c] Badger Athletic Performance Research, University of Wisconsin-Madison, 1440 Monroe St, Madison, WI 53711, USA; [d] Doctor of Physical Therapy Program, Des Moines University, 3200 Grand Avenue, Des Moines, IA 50312, USA
* Corresponding author. Department of Orthopedics & Rehabilitation, UW Runners' Clinic, Badger Athletic Performance Research, University of Wisconsin-Madison, 1300 University Avenue, Madison, WI 53706.
E-mail address: heiderscheit@ortho.wisc.edu

hip or pelvis injury during running have not been clearly identified, although some evidence suggests women are at a greater risk.[3,4] The biomechanics of the hip and pelvis during running,[5,6] including the muscular demands,[7,8] have been characterized and provide useful insights into appropriate rehabilitation strategies to maximize recovery and return to full running. The purpose of this article is to review the more common running-related injuries to the hip and pelvis, with consideration of the cause, clinical presentation, and management.

INJURIES

Despite each injury having unique presentation and examination characteristics, certain aspects of the management strategy are common to all. For example, it is imperative that the irritability of the condition be controlled during the initial treatment stages using a variety of options including ice, non-steroidal anti-inflammatory drugs (NSAIDs), and activity modification. Running may need to be stopped temporarily or modified to reduce mechanical load to the injured area, such as decreased volume or intensity, avoiding hills, or using a higher step rate.[8-10] Body weight–supported running or deep water running may also be substituted.[11] Once symptoms are controlled and injured tissues are able to tolerate the demands of running, a progressive return is required to reacclimate to the mechanical loads of running. Retraining of running gait may be warranted to correct any pathomechanics in addition to a progressive return-to-running program to reduce the risk of reinjury. Also common to the management of all running-related hip and pelvis injuries is consideration of lumbopelvic dysfunction that can refer symptoms to, and affect function of, the primary area of injury. Lumbopelvic dysfunction, including myofascial trigger points (**Fig. 1**), joint and neurodynamic dysfunction, often occurs concurrently with hip and pelvis conditions and can affect the patient's presentation and rehabilitation. Hip mobility deficits are commonly observed in running-related hip and pelvis injuries and are amenable to mobilization procedures (**Fig. 2**).

Proximal Hamstring Tendinopathy

Proximal hamstring tendinopathy is a challenging injury owing to the prolonged course of treatment typically required to successfully return to full level of performance. Distinct from a hamstring strain injury, this condition often involves a progressive onset of symptoms localized near the ischial tuberosity, possibly involving the ischial bursa. Histologic evaluation frequently indicates a chronic tendinopathy with fibrosis, and occasional hyaline degeneration at the insertion site. In severe cases, MRI examination will reveal an associated stress reaction with marrow edema in the ischial tuberosity.[12]

Presentation

- Deep buttock pain is present near the ischial tuberosity and is aggravated when accelerating or running uphill, or with direct pressure on the injured area, including prolonged sitting. Pain is provoked near end-range hip flexion and with resisted hip extension in a hip flexed position.
- Pain provocation tests include the bent-knee stretch test,[13] modified bent-knee stretch test,[14] and Puranen-Orava test (**Table 1**).[15] All have been found to be reliable and valid, with the modified bent-knee stretch test having the highest values.[16]
- For cases that fail conservative management or are slow to progress, MRI may reveal a partial tendon tear.

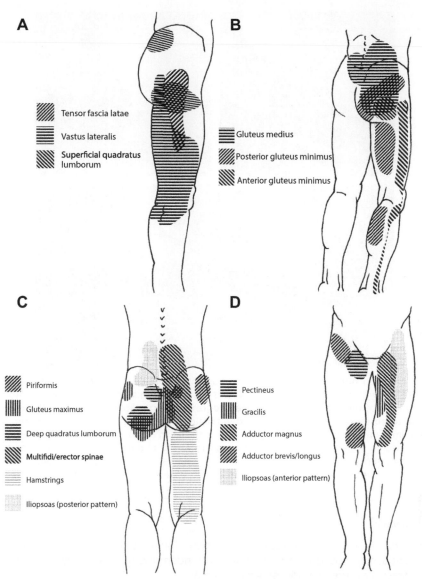

Fig. 1. Patterns of myofascial trigger points that refer symptoms to the hip and pelvis region as displayed from (*A*) lateral, (*B*) posterior lateral, (*C*) posterior, and (*D*) anterior perspectives. (*From* Travell JG, Simons DG. Myofascial pain and dysfunction: the trigger point manual: the lower extremities, vol. 2. Philadelphia: Lippincott Williams & Wilkins; 1983. p. 23–339.)

- If symptoms extend into the posterior thigh, contribution from the lumbar spine should also be ruled out and irritation of the sciatic or posterior femoral cutaneous nerves should be considered (slump test).[15,17]
- Differential diagnosis includes sacroiliac dysfunction, ischiogluteal bursitis, obturator internus bursitis, ischifemoral impingement, piriformis syndrome, lumbopelvic dysfunction, acetabular labral tear, and stress fracture of the pelvis and femoral head.

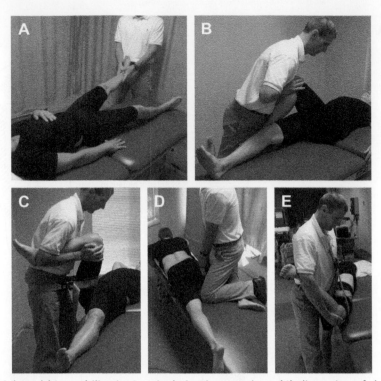

Fig. 2. Selected hip mobilization/manipulation interventions: (*A*) distraction of the hip is applied through manual contact at the lower leg and ankle starting in hip flexion, abduction, and external rotation and can be progressed into restricted ranges; (*B*) anterior-medial to posterior-lateral force applied with hip in adduction and internal rotation; (*C*) lateral/inferior distraction of the hip applied with hip in internal rotation; (*D*) posterior to anterior force applied in prone with the hip in flexion, abduction, and external rotation; and (*E*) posterior to anterior force applied in a unilateral prone position with the hip held in extension, slight adduction, and external rotation using the assistance of a belt.

Management

- Early treatment should include correction of lumbopelvic joint dysfunction and soft tissue mobilization to the involved tendon and adjacent muscles, avoiding direct pressure over the ischial tuberosity.
- Progressive loading guidelines (**Table 2**) should be followed with care to minimize tendon compression against the ischial tuberosity during the early stages of recovery.[18,19]
- Neuromuscular control exercises for the lumbopelvic region are recommended, with a particular focus on gluteal muscle activation.[13,20] Additional strengthening of the hamstrings with eccentric exercises may be considered once the tendon is less reactive; however, hip flexion angle may need to be initially constrained to prevent aggravation of the condition due to tendon wrapping around the ischial tuberosity.
- Corticosteroid injection under ultrasound guidance into the peritendinous soft tissues may be necessary in some more acute cases to enable performance of progressive loading program.[12]

Table 1
Clinical examination tests for hip and pelvis conditions

Test	Description of Positive Test	Reference Standard	Sensitivity (95% CI)	Specificity (95% CI)	+ Likelihood Ratio (95% CI)	− Likelihood Ratio (95% CI)
Proximal hamstring tendinopathy						
Bent-knee stretch test[16]	Pain with slow extension of the knee from a position of maximum hip flexion in supine	Pain in lower gluteal region, ischial tuberosity tenderness, and increased MRI signal intensity of proximal hamstring tendons	0.84 (0.71, 0.93)	0.87 (0.73, 0.95)	6.5 (3.1, 13.8)[a]	0.18 (0.09, 0.35)[a]
Modified bent-knee stretch test[16]	Pain with rapid extension of the knee from a position of maximum hip flexion in supine		0.89 (0.76, 0.96)	0.91 (0.79, 0.97)	10.3 (4, 26.3)[a]	0.12 (0.05, 0.27)[a]
Puranen-Orava test[16]	Pain with hamstring stretch in standing with foot supported so that hip is flexed 90° and knee is fully extended		0.76 (0.61, 0.87)	0.82 (0.68, 0.92)	4.4 (2.3, 8.4)[a]	0.29 (0.17, 0.49)[a]
GTPS						
Resisted external derotation test[29,108]	Pain when the patient internally rotates and extends the hip against examiner resistance from 90° hip flexion and full external rotation	MRI evidence of gluteus minimus or medius tendonitis, tendinosis, tear, or bursitis	0.88[b] (0.66, 0.97)[a]	0.97[b] (0.87, 1)[a]	33.5[a,b] (4.8, 233.7)	0.12[a,b] (0.03, 0.45)
Trendelenburg sign[108,109]	When standing unilaterally on the involved leg, patient unable to elevate and hold contralateral pelvis for 30 s		0.23 (0.05, 0.57)	0.94 (0.53, 1)	3.64 (0.2, 65.9)	0.82 (0.59, 1.15)
Resisted hip abduction[29,108,109]	1. Pain with resisted side-lying hip abduction up to 25° with the hip flexed 0°, 45°, and 90°		0.71[b] (0.47, 0.87)[a]	0.95[b] (0.83, 0.99)[a]	13.4[a,b] (3.4, 53.5)	0.31[a,b] (0.15, 0.65)
	2. Pain with resisted side-lying hip abduction with the hip 0° flexed and neutral rotation		0.47 (0.22, 0.73)	0.86 (0.42, 0.99)	3.27 (0.5, 21.7)	0.62 (0.4, 1)

(continued on next page)

Table 1
(continued)

Test	Description of Positive Test	Reference Standard	Sensitivity (95% CI)	Specificity (95% CI)	+ Likelihood Ratio (95% CI)	− Likelihood Ratio (95% CI)
FABER[31]	Lateral hip pain with the involved leg crossed (lateral malleolus just superior to the opposite patella) in supine and downward pressure applied to the medial knee and contralateral anterior superior iliac spine to externally rotate and abduct the leg toward the table.	Differentiation between GTPS and OA	0.83 (0.68, 0.93)	0.9 (0.68, 0.99)	8.3[a] (2.2, 31.1)	0.19[a] (0.1, 0.38)
Piriformis syndrome						
Test item cluster[39]	Two of the following 3: (1) pain at the intersection of the sciatic nerve and piriformis in side-lying FAIR position, (2) tenderness with palpation of the sciatic nerve and piriformis intersection, or (3) straight-leg raise <65° or 15° less than unaffected side	Delayed H-reflex between anatomic supine and side-lying FAIR position	0.92 (0.90, 0.94)[a]	0.85 (0.78, 0.90)[a]	6.1[a] (4.0, 9.3)	0.01[a] (0.07, 0.12)

Chronic groin pain

Test	Description	Reference standard				
Bilateral adductor test[108,110]	Groin pain with bilateral resisted hip adduction with both hips flexed 30°, slight hip internal rotation, and knees extended	MRI evidence of pubic bone marrow edema	0.54 (0.4, 0.68)	0.93 (0.81, 0.98)	7.8 (2.5, 23.9)	0.49 (0.35, 0.68)
Single adductor test[108,110]	Ipsilateral or contralateral groin pain with unilateral resisted hip adduction in supine with tested hip flexed 30° and knee extended; opposite hip is flat on the table in 0° hip flexion		0.30 (0.19, 0.45)	0.91 (0.78, 0.96)	3.3 (1.2, 9.2)	0.77 (0.62, 0.95)
Squeeze test[108,110]	Groin pain when patient maximally contracts adductors in supine with 45° hip flexion and 90° knee flexion and examiners fist between knees		0.43 (0.30, 0.58)	0.91 (0.78, 0.96)	4.7 (1.7, 12.6)	0.62 (0.48, 0.82)

FAI/labral tear

Test	Description	Reference standard				
FADIR[76]	Pain when hip is flexed 90° and then adducted and internally rotated with patient supine	Evidence of FAI or labral tear during surgery	0.99c (0.98, 1)	0.05c (0.01, 0.18)	1.04c (0.97, 1.12)	0.14c (0.02, 0.93)
FlexIR[76]	Pain when hip is flexed 90° and then internally rotated with patient supine		0.96c (0.81, 0.99)	0.25c (0.01, 0.81)	1.28c (0.72, 2.27)	0.15c (0.01, 1.99)
Squat test[111]	Pain when performing a maximum squat with feet shoulder width apart and arms held parallel to the floor	MRI evidence of cam-type FAI	0.75 (0.57, 0.89)	0.41 (0.27, 0.57)	1.3 (0.9, 1.7)	0.6 (0.3, 1.2)

(continued on next page)

Table 1
(continued)

Test	Description of Positive Test	Reference Standard	Sensitivity (95% CI)	Specificity (95% CI)	+ Likelihood Ratio (95% CI)	− Likelihood Ratio (95% CI)
Labral tear						
THIRD test[76]	Pain during hip compression and internal rotation that is absent or reduced with hip distraction and internal rotation with patient supine and hip flexed 90° and adducted 10°	Operative reports indicating labral tear	0.98 (0.93, 0.99)	0.75 (0.3, 0.95)	3.9 (0.7, 21.4)	0.03 (0, 0.12)
OA						
Sutlive et al,[112] test item cluster	1. Patient reports squatting aggravates symptoms 2. Pain in the groin or lateral hip during adduction of the scour test 3. Lateral hip pain with active hip flexion 4. Hip pain during active hip extension 5. Passive prone hip internal rotation ≤25°	Kellgren and Lawrence score of 2 or higher via radiographs	0.48 (0.26, 0.70) 0.71 (0.48, 0.88)	4/5 tests positive 0.98 (0.88, 1) 3/5 tests positive 0.86 (0.73, 0.94)	24.3 (4.4, 142.1) 5.2 (2.6, 10.9)	0.53 (0.35, 0.8) 0.33 (0.17, 0.66)
American College of Rheumatology test item cluster[113]	Positive in presence of either of the following test clusters: 1. Hip pain 2. Hip internal rotation ≤15° 3. Hip flexion ≤115° — 1. Hip internal rotation ≤25° with pain 2. Morning hip stiffness lasting ≤60 min 3. Age >50 y	Evidence of at least mild arthritis via radiographs	0.86 (0.78, 0.91)[a]	0.75 (0.65, 0.83)[a]	3.4[a] (2.4, 4.9)	0.19[a] (0.12, 0.3)

[a] Calculated by the authors of this article.
[b] Calculated from case control design. Sensitivity calculated from cases and MRI; Specificity calculated from control participants without use of MRI as the reference standard.
[c] Pooled diagnostic properties from meta-analysis.

Table 2
Tendinopathy management recommendations based on Kountouris and Cook[114]

Purpose	Treatment
Pain management and tendon load reduction	• Pain management ○ Ice and NSAIDs ○ Isometric exercises of the involved tendon: 30–60-s holds, 3–5 repetitions, 1–3 times; start with a lower frequency, repetition, and duration if tendon is highly reactive/irritable[18] ○ Corticosteroid injections may be considered for reactive tendons in early disrepair[115] • Reduce tendon load ○ Reduce running volume and load (increase step rate, avoid hills) to avoid exacerbation of symptoms ○ May need to temporarily avoid over-ground running and substitute other exercise options (cycling, deep water running, or body-weight–assisted treadmill) ○ Address local and adjacent impairments including trigger points, joint mobility, and posture
Tendon load adaptation	• Step 1: Improve muscle strength (higher load, 3 sets of 8–15 repetitions, 3–4 d/wk) and endurance (lower load, 3 sets of 20–30 repetitions, 5–7 d/wk) based on individual impairments and needs ○ Continue isometric exercises and ice for pain management ○ Consider non-weight-bearing exercise for lower load training and progress to weight-bearing exercises for higher load training that more closely reflect the demands of running ○ Emphasis on the eccentric phase initially but not exclusively ○ Consider neuromuscular control training of lumbopelvic region • Step 2: Improve muscle power ○ Increase speed of weight-bearing exercises ○ Progress to plyometric training, such as jump squats, skipping, jumping rope, double-leg progressing to single-leg hopping ○ 30–60-s repetitions, 4–6 sets with 60 s rest between sets, 2–3 d/wk

Progression should consider (1) pain behavior for 24 hours following the exercise to assess tendon irritability, and (2) similar performance between involved and uninvolved limbs with exercises and pain provocation tests.

Data from Kountouris A, Cook J. Rehabilitation of Achilles and patellar tendinopathies. Best Pract Res Clin Rheumatol 2007;21:295–316.

- Platelet-rich plasma injections may be useful in promoting symptom reduction and tissue recovery, although research is limited.[21,22] Limited evidence on shockwave therapy has shown promising benefits.[14]
- When pain persists despite multiple attempts of conservative management, surgery may be considered to relieve adhesions and facilitate normal sliding mechanics of the involved tissues. The proximal tendinous structures of the hamstrings are typically divided without releasing the muscle from the ischial tuberosity. Neurolysis may be performed if sciatic nerve compression is observed.[23,24]

Greater Trochanteric Pain Syndrome

Greater trochanteric pain syndrome (GTPS) is lateral hip pain that may occur due to a variety of disorders, including trochanteric and gluteus medius bursa irritation, external snapping hip (coxa saltans), and gluteus medius and minimus tendon tears and tendinopathy (**Fig. 3**). GTPS accounts for 5% of all running injuries, affecting

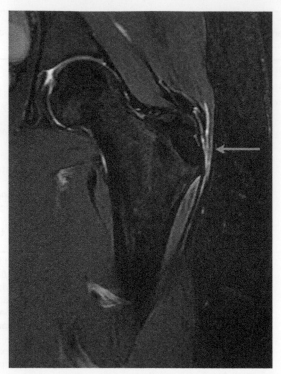

Fig. 3. Peritendinous edema involving the insertions of the left gluteus medius and minimus tendons (*arrow*) is present in a 29-year-old female runner with associated thickening in the gluteus medius tendon. Coronal image, T2 fat-saturation.

women up to 5 times more than men.[2,25–27] Consideration of peak muscle forces primarily of the gluteus medius and minimus during the loading response of running is important in the cause and rehabilitation of the runner with GTPS.[8]

Presentation

- Onset is often insidious but may be related to a change in running volume or intensity, running on a cambered surface,[28] and excessive peak hip adduction during stance phase.
- Pain is localized near the greater trochanter and may extend down the thigh in a nondermatomal pattern. Pain is exacerbated when lying on the affected side, sitting with legs crossed, unilateral standing, stair climbing, walking, or running, and can be reproduced with resisted hip abduction.
- Pain with resisted internal rotation from 90° of flexion and maximal hip external rotation implicates gluteal tendinopathy,[29] whereas a positive Trendelenburg test suggests a gluteal tear (see **Table 1**).[30]
- Hip internal or external rotation may be limited or painful; however, restricted motion in multiple directions is suggestive of an intra-articular disorder. In contrast to patients with hip osteoarthritis (OA), those with GTPS are able to localize lateral hip pain, have a FABER (flexion, abduction, external rotation) test provoking lateral hip pain (see **Table 1**), and do not have difficulty manipulating shoes and socks.[31]

- Prior or concurrent lumbar symptoms are common and warrant evaluation.[27] Trigger points of the spinal muscles, quadratus lumborum, gluteal muscles, piriformis, and tensor fascia latae may refer to the lateral hip (see **Fig. 1**).[32]
- With external snapping hip, the anterior gluteus maximus and iliotibial band snaps audibly when moved posterior to anterior over the greater trochanter during hip flexion from an extended position. Manual compression just proximal to the trochanter may alleviate the snapping.[33]
- MRI is typically reserved for recalcitrant cases to assess integrity of the gluteal tendons, bursa, and intra-articular structures.

Management

- Early treatment includes mobilization of adjacent soft tissues, hip (see **Fig. 2**), and lumbopelvic mobilization to include sacroiliac manipulation,[34] and the use of pillows to offload the hip when sleeping in side-lying.
- Progressive resistance training of the hip abductors and external rotators should be emphasized, starting with isometric activities and progressing to movements that maximize gluteus medius activity (**Figs. 4, 5**B**, 6, and 7, Table 3**).[35,36]
- Corticosteroid injection or extracorporeal shock-wave therapy may provide moderate improvement in symptoms and function in the short term that equals the response to exercise in the long term.[37]
- Surgical treatment may be considered if symptoms persist after 6 months of conservative management. Procedures include open or arthroscopic gluteal tendon repair or reconstruction, bursectomy, or iliotibial band release or lengthening.

Piriformis Syndrome

Piriformis syndrome is a neuromuscular disorder involving the sciatic nerve and piriformis muscle.[38] Lack of consensus on the definition of piriformis syndrome and valid diagnostic criteria make it difficult to determine the true incidence.[39] Piriformis

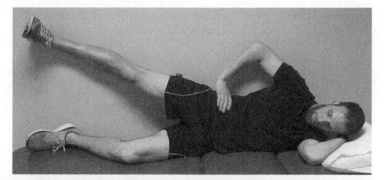

Fig. 4. Hip abduction exercise: In side-lying with the target hip on top and lower leg flexed at the hip and knee, the top hip is abducted with slight external rotation while the pelvis is stabilized perpendicular to the table. Additional internal or external rotation of the hip does not significantly change gluteus medius to tensor fascia latae ratio,[36] but stabilization of the pelvis perpendicular to the table is important to improve gluteus medius activation.[107] The back and heel can be placed at a wall to assure the pelvis remains perpendicular and to avoid compensatory hip flexion during abduction. An ankle weight can be used for additional resistance or a belt to achieve an isometric contraction. This can be progressed to a weight-bearing exercise by performing a side plank.

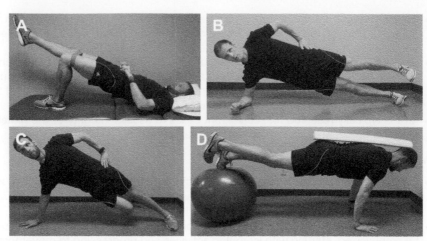

Fig. 5. Stabilization of lumbopelvic and hip regions through muscle performance training: (*A*) supine bridge to target gluteal muscles starting with bilateral bridge (not pictured) that can be progressed by adding a resistance band to emphasize hip abduction/external rotation and then a unilateral bridge; rotation of the pelvis is avoided via feedback from a dowel held on the front of the pelvis; (*B*) lateral side plank to target hip abductors that can be initiated from the knees (not pictured) and progressed to the feet, and then, by lifting the top leg, emphasis is placed on adequate abduction without rotation of the pelvis; (*C*) medial side plank to target hip adductors, emphasis is placed on adequate hip adduction without rotation of the pelvis; (*D*) prone plank that can be initiated with feet on the floor (not pictured) and progressed to both legs on a stability ball (placing ball closer to knees for less difficulty or closer to toes for greater difficulty), and by lifting one leg, emphasis is placed on a neutral spine (using a board or half foam roll for feedback) and avoidance of pelvic rotation.

syndrome is estimated to be the source of symptoms in 6% to 8% of individuals presenting with low back pain and sciatica.[40,41] During running, the piriformis has a similar activation pattern as the gluteal muscles, being most active during the loading response of stance, initially working eccentrically and then concentrically.[8]

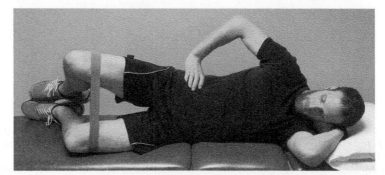

Fig. 6. Clam exercise: In side-lying position with the target hip on top in 30° of flexion, the hip is externally rotated and abducted. A resistance band can be added for greater difficulty or a belt used to perform an isometric contraction. This exercise targets the posterior fibers of the gluteus medius and minimus in addition to the piriformis, which are most active between 30° of hip flexion and 15° of hip extension during running.

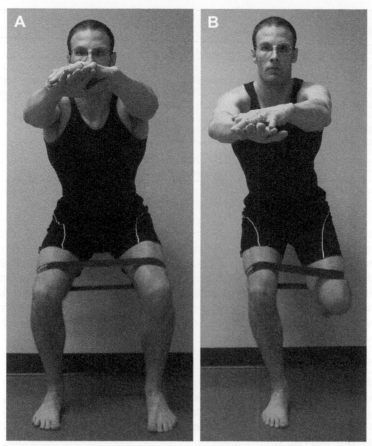

Fig. 7. Squat training: (*A*) bilateral squat or position to perform side-stepping and (*B*) unilateral squat. Emphasis is placed on avoidance of dynamic knee valgus (via hip internal rotation and adduction, and foot pronation). A band can be placed around the distal thigh to encourage the patient to react against the band using hip abductors and external rotators. A mirror is also encouraged initially for visual feedback of form.

Presentation

- Pain in the buttock is presented that may refer down the back of the leg in a sciatic distribution and is aggravated with sitting. Onset is typically insidious but may involve a traumatic impact, such as a fall. Tenderness is localized to the intersection of the sciatic nerve and piriformis in side-lying with hip flexed 60°, adducted, and internally rotated (FAIR), and supine straight leg raise is often limited (see **Table 1**).
- External rotation of the hip may be observed in standing or sitting. In supine with legs extended, increased external rotation of the involved leg may be present (Piriformis sign) and painful with forced internal rotation (Freiberg test).[42,43]
- During the loading response of walking or running, or during a single-leg step down test, excessive hip adduction and internal rotation may be observed, suggesting impaired eccentric piriformis function.[5,44]

Table 3
Exercises that target the gluteus medius

	Non-weight-bearing	Weight-bearing	Plyometric

Increased activation ↑	Side plank with top leg abducted
	Side-lying hip abduction
	Supine unilateral bridge with band
	Side-lying clam
	Supine bilateral bridge with band
		Single leg squat
		Unilateral hip hike/lower
		Lateral step up/down
		Side step with band
		  • Band around ankles
		  • Band around knees
		Forward or side lunge
		Bilateral squat with band
			Side hop onto involved leg, unilateral jump rope
			Forward hop onto involved leg
			Bilateral jump rope

————————————— Increased running specificity —————————————➤

Data from Refs.[35,36,116]

- In side-lying FAIR position, pain may be provoked with resisted abduction/ external rotation (Pace test), or simply abducting the hip with neutral rotation (Beatty test).[39,45,46] Diagnostic accuracy of these tests is unknown, and false positives are likely if symptom centralization occurs with lumbar movement testing.
- Differential diagnosis includes lumbar radiculopathy, sacoiliac joint dysfunction, intra-articular hip pathologic abnormality, proximal hamstring tendinopathy, greater trochanter pain syndrome, and referral from the gluteus medius or quadratus lumborum.

Management

- Mobilization of soft tissue restrictions and trigger points is useful for the piriformis, gluteals, and lumbosacral region. Aggressive piriformis stretching should be avoided when symptoms are irritable.
- Hip and lumbosacral mobilizations may also useful if restricted motion is observed (see **Fig. 2**).
- Neuromuscular training using rotational exercises may start with isometrics if symptom irritability is observed and progress to isotonics, with eventual progression into weight-bearing movements.
- Image-guided injections (corticosteroid, anesthetic, or botulinum toxin A) may be used in combination with the above for refractory cases to obtain short-term relief and determine potential surgical benefit.[47]
- A pelvic neurogram is recommended in refractory cases to better assess for anomalous sciatic nerve anatomy causing piriformis syndrome. There are 6 commonly described anatomic relationships, the most common being the sciatic nerve passing below the piriformis muscle.[48]

Iliopsoas Syndrome

The iliopsoas muscle functions eccentrically during the terminal stance phase of running to control hip extension and then acts concentrically during the initial swing to advance the thigh forward.[8] The iliopsoas tendon may be irritated by snapping over the anterior inferior iliac spine, the iliopectineal eminence, or the lesser trochanter (internal coxa saltans).[49] Iliopsoas impingement has also been described due to pressure, friction, or adhesions between the iliopsoas and the femoral head and anterior labrum.[50] Because iliopsoas tendinopathy, iliopsoas bursitis, and iliopsoas impingement may be hard to discriminate and can occur together, collectively, these conditions are called iliopsoas syndrome.

Presentation

- Onset is usually insidious but may involve increased uphill running. Pain is typically present in the anterior hip, and possibly the ipsilateral lower back (**Fig. 1C**).[51] Tenderness may be present over the anterior hip joint; however, this may also indicate femoroacetabular impingement (FAI) or labral pathologic abnormality.
- Pain is elicited with resistance of hip flexion, slight abduction, and external rotation in the supine position or when stabilizing with the involved leg in the prone plank position (**Fig. 5D**).
- Internal snapping can be reproduced with motion of the hip from flexion/abduction/external rotation to extension/adduction/internal rotation.
- Iliopsoas tightness may be present, contributing to impingement.[50] Iliopsoas impingement may be reproduced with supine hip flexion, adduction, and internal rotation (FADIR test) (see **Table 1**).[52]
- Imaging is typically reserved for cases that are unresponsive to conservative management. Radiographs may identify calcifications or femoroacetabular abnormalities associated with tendon or bursa irritation. MRI can provide further evidence of labral, tendon, and bursa pathologic abnormality.

Management

- General guidelines for tendon rehabilitation apply, including specific considerations for the iliopsoas muscle function and activities that load the tendon.
- Soft tissue mobilization, treatment of trigger points, and stretching of impairments identified in the iliopsoas should be emphasized with consideration of adjacent regions. Joint mobilization of the hip (see **Fig. 2**) and lumbosacral region may be considered.
- Once initial symptom irritability is managed, the tendon can be progressively loaded (see **Table 2**) complemented by hip strengthening (side-lying clam [see **Fig. 6**], seated hip internal and external rotation, and single-leg mini–wall squats [see **Fig. 7B**]) and lumbopelvic stabilization exercises (see **Fig. 5**).[49,53]
- Ultrasound-guided injections may be used in refractory cases to obtain short-term relief and coupled with conservative treatments indicated above. Endoscopic release or lengthening of iliopsoas may be considered if the patient continues to be unresponsive to conservative care.[54,55]

Chronic Groin Pain

Chronic groin pain has been attributed to a variety of sources, such as intra-abdominal, genitourinary, and musculoskeletal, with no clear consensus on definition or diagnostic criteria.[56,57] Involvement of the proximal adductor tendons is commonly recognized and often the focus of treatment programs. Rectus femoris and rectus abdominus have also been implicated,[58] and the presence of athletic pubalgia (sports hernia) should be considered.[59] Common in sports requiring high-speed cutting (ie, soccer, hockey, and American football),[57] chronic groin pain is less frequent among distance runners, although female runners during and after pregnancy may be at particular risk considering the structural and neuromuscular changes to the lumbopelvic region.[60] For the runner, intra-articular hip pathologic abnormality and femoral neck or lesser trochanteric bone stress injury needs to be ruled out.

Presentation

- Physical examination findings are often not specific enough to clearly differentiate between adductor tendinopathy, osteitis pubis (**Fig. 8**), and athletic

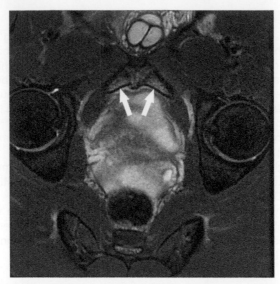

Fig. 8. Developing osteitis pubis in an 18-year-old male sprinter, as evidenced by mild T2 hyperintense edema (*arrows*). Oblique axial image, T2 fat-saturated.

pubalgia. Imaging techniques such as ultrasonography or MRI may prove useful during the diagnostic process.[61]

- Common symptoms include a dull aching pain involving the proximal adductor tendons and pubic symphysis region. Symptoms may radiate to the lower abdomen, perineum, and scrotum. Pain is typically aggravated with direct palpation, resisted hip adduction (see **Table 1**), and passive stretch of the hip adductors.
- Reduced force production during the adductor squeeze test is commonly observed[62] as well as reduced motion during hip internal rotation and bent knee fall-out test.[63]
- For athletic pubalgia, tenderness on the pubic tubercle and a potential palpable tear of the inguinal floor creating pain inside the external inguinal ring are considered the key physical examination findings.[64] Aggravating factors include athletic movements, coughing, sneezing, and a resisted situp.[64]

Management

- An 8- to 12-week neuromuscular training program was shown to effectively treat adductor-related chronic groin pain.[56] Examples of exercises include resisted isometric hip adduction, standing resisted hip adduction, trunk extensions, forward and oblique abdominal situps, single-leg balance, and side skating or lunging movements. In addition, a medial side plank can be used during later phases of rehabilitation to build load tolerance of the adductors (see **Fig. 5**C). Cross-friction massage, stretching, and electrophysical modalities (eg, electrical stimulation and laser) have been shown to be less effective for this condition.[56]
- If a pelvis bone stress injury is suspected, a common component of osteitis pubis, running should be avoided for a minimum of 6 weeks.[65] Dextrose injections have shown early modest success for osteitis pubis,[66] with corticosteroids being of limited benefit.[67]

- Chronic adductor tendinopathy that is resistant to conservative management may consider adductor longus tenotomy[68,69]; debridement and arthrodesis procedures have been described for recalcitrant osteitis pubis.[67] Athletic pubalgia is generally resistant to conservative management, with surgical repair or release often performed[59]; however, initial exercises should target hip adductors, gluteals, and deep abdominal muscles.

Femoroacetabular Impingement

FAI is increasingly recognized as a source of anterior hip pain, although the proportion of running-related hip injuries related to FAI is not known. Symptomatic FAI is pain due to the abutment of bony abnormalities between the proximal femur and acetabulum. Cam FAI involves a bump on the anterior or anterior-lateral femoral head or flattening of the usually concave femoral head-neck junction (**Fig. 9**). Pincer FAI is an overcoverage of the acetabulum due to focal anterior overgrowth, acetabular retroversion, or coxa profunda. Commonly, a combination of cam and pincer abnormalities is observed. Although hip morphology is an important aspect of FAI diagnosis, the distinction between normal morphologic variation and pathologic abnormality is challenging. In addition, FAI has been observed and associated with labral and chondral damage, but currently there is no conclusive evidence that FAI morphology leads to development of OA or early hip replacement.[70,71] There is moderate evidence that a greater cam deformity is associated with progression of FAI to labral tear, and when coupled with limited hip internal rotation, one study found increased risk of end-stage OA.[71,72] Because of the variability and uncertainty surrounding FAI diagnosis, the use of FAI syndrome has been recommended to define this condition.[70]

Presentation

- Pain is reported in the anterior and anterior-medial hip, although pain may also be reported in the lateral hip, anterior thigh, low back, and buttock.[73] Painful functions often involve flexion, adduction, and internal rotation, such sitting in a low

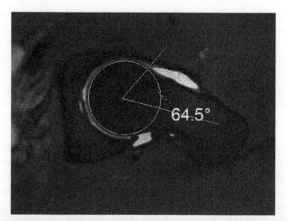

Fig. 9. Abnormal femoral head neck offset present in a 21-year-old man with hip pain, supporting a clinical diagnosis of cam-type FAI. An αangle of 65° is present as well as an abnormal bump at the anterior of the femoral head-neck junction. Oblique axial image of MR arthrogram, T1 fat-saturation sequence performed after intra-articular injection of contrast.

seat, squatting, and getting in and out of a car. During these functions, the patient may avoid impingement by leaning away from the affected side or bias position toward hip extension, external rotation, and abduction.

- Painful and reduced squat depth may present with less posterior pelvic tilt during squat (see **Table 1**).[74]
- Catching, clicking, or a giving-way sensation in the hip may be reported, which may implicate FAI and concurrent labral pathologic abnormality.
- Hip motion is limited in flexion and internal rotation in greater than 90° of hip flexion.[73,75] Hip adduction, internal rotation, and extension motion are reduced during walking and stair climbing.[75]
- Decreased strength of the hip adductors, abductors, flexors, and external rotators is common.[75]
- The FADIR and flexion/internal rotation (FlexIR) tests are the best clinical tests for FAI (see **Table 1**). Tests are more sensitive, and greater confidence is placed in using these tests to rule out FAI. The ability of these tests to discriminate between FAI and labral tears or other hip pathologic abnormality is limited.[76]
- Imaging can improve the certainty of FAI in cases unresponsive to initial conservative management and rule out alternate causes of pain. Plain radiographs are most commonly performed with anterior-posterior and modified Dunn views. Because of the high prevalence of FAI and labral pathologic abnormality in asymptomatic individuals, treatment decision should consider imaging results in light of the history and physical examination and differences from the uninvolved side.[77]
- MRI without intra-articular contrast may reveal labral tears, synovial pitting, or early acetabular chondromalacia. Evidence of labral injury has been found in 68% of asymptomatic individuals.[77]

Management

- Nonsurgical treatment is recommended initially for FAI and can reduce symptoms even though it will not alter structural deformities. Initial management includes avoidance of extreme ranges of hip flexion, internal rotation, and adduction.
- Mobilization and manipulation of the hip should be considered with an emphasis on lateral and inferior distraction (see **Fig. 2**A, C). Posterior capsule mobilization can also be performed below 90° of hip flexion in a manner that does not create impingement (see **Fig. 2**B). If hip mobilization is useful in reducing symptoms, the patient can perform self-mobilization at home using a belt or strap.[78–80]
- Stretching exercises should be performed outside of the impingement zone. Examples include hip internal rotation stretching in a half-kneeling position and piriformis stretch in supine, with thigh adducted and internally rotated below 90°.
- Neuromuscular training of the hip and lumbopelvic area is typically warranted. This training may include gluteus medius (see **Table 3**) and maximus exercises. Limitation of hip total range of motion or facilitation of posterior pelvic tilt and neutral lumbar spine at the peak of lunge and squat exercises can help to reduce impingement.
- Surgical treatment may be considered if nonsurgical management is ineffective. Indications for surgical management of FAI vary considerably, including a combination of clinical and imaging findings, symptom duration of at least 6 months, and a lack of response to exhaustive conservative management.[81] Consideration of surgery based solely on imaging is not recommended.[70,71,81] Arthroscopic

procedures are increasingly used, but open and mini-open procedures have similar outcomes.[81] Postoperative rehabilitation is guided by a physical therapist to restore mobility, neuromuscular performance, and overall function. Running may be initiated as early as 8 to 10 weeks after surgery, depending on the procedure performed.

Labral Tears

Running-related labral tears are postulated to arise from repetitive hip hyperextension and external rotation during terminal stance that results in subtle joint instability and stress at the chondrolabral junction,[82] typically at the 10 to 12 o'clock position (**Fig. 10**). Labral pathologic abnormality in runners may also be associated with iliopsoas impingement, which results in injury at the 3 o'clock position.[52] Runners may recall a traumatic event involving an audible pop or subluxation from a misstep on uneven ground, a hip-twisting event or fall, or a collision with a vehicle or bicycle. A runner with a labral injury often seeks treatment weeks to months after an acute tear, so often an acute event is unable to be identified. Although the prevalence of symptomatic running-related labral tears is not known, it is likely low. Of 162 arthroscopic hip surgeries performed over 3 years in 1 office, only 8 (3.7%) were identified as a competitive runner or a runner that participated in more than 5 marathons.[82] If a labral tear is identified via imaging, there is a chance it is asymptomatic, because 69% of the general population aged 18 to 66 had a labral tear, and those older than 30 years were 8 times more likely to have a tear than those younger than 30 years of age.[83]

Presentation

- A labral tear is difficult to distinguish from FAI and the 2 diagnoses commonly coexist. Contrary to FAI, pain from an isolated labral tear may be associated

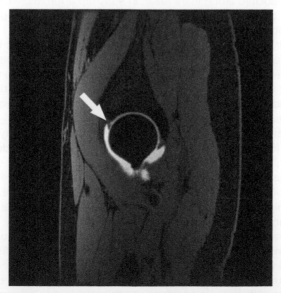

Fig. 10. Incomplete radial tear of the anterior superior labrum of the left hip (~1:30 position) (*arrow*) of a 21-year-old female cross-country runner. Sagittal image of MR arthrogram, 3D IDEAL sequence performed after intra-articular injection of contrast.

with hip extension or signs of instability/capsular laxity. In addition, iliopsoas tightness or pain with resisted testing may indicate iliopsoas impingement that has been associated with labral tearing but not FAI.[52]

- In addition to the FADIR and FlexIR tests (see **Table 1**), additional axial compression during the FADIR test and overpressure during the FlexIR test can be performed but does not improve sensitivity or specificity.[76] The internal rotation with distraction (THIRD) test demonstrates better diagnostic accuracy than the FADIR and FlexIR test (see **Table 1**), but has not been studied as rigorously.[76]

- Although there is no clinical examination test or test item cluster to confidently dissociate a labral tear from FAI, initial management does not seem to hinge on this dissociation. If the patient is not responsive to initial nonsurgical management, imaging can improve the diagnosis and identify labral pathologic abnormality, fracture, loose bodies, FAI, or hip dysplasia.

  ○ Anteroposterior pelvis and lateral hip radiographs may be normal in the presence of an isolated labral tear, but under chronic circumstances, labral calcifications may be seen. Radiographs may reveal cam or pincer FAI as already described. A radiographic feature unique to labral tears compared with pincer FAI is the acetabular dysplasia, defined by a lateral center-edge angle less than 20°.[84] Dysplasia may increase anterosuperior labral stress contributing to degeneration and tearing of the labrum.

  ○ MRI, MR angiography, and computed tomography are commonly used to assess labral integrity and have good to excellent sensitivity and specificity.[84] In addition, MRI is more sensitive than radiographs to detecting avascular necrosis, nondisplaced fracture (including stress fracture), and osseous lesions.[84]

Management

- Considering the prevalence of asymptomatic labral tears and lack of strong evidence that isolated labral tears result in early hip arthrosis,[85] nonsurgical management is a reasonable initial strategy with surgery reserved for cases that are not responsive to nonsurgical intervention.

- Initial nonsurgical management includes modification of weight-bearing rotation and extension activities. Neuromuscular training should be emphasized with a focus on the lumbopelvic and hip regions. This training includes trunk stabilizers (see **Fig. 5**); gluteus medius (see **Table 3**), minimus, and maximus; deep lateral rotators; and iliopsoas muscles while minimizing excessive contribution from the quadriceps femoris and hamstrings during exercises.[86,87]

- Runners with an isolated labral tear may not present with mobility impairments of the hip, but if FAI is also present, joint mobilization techniques described for FAI management are appropriate.

- Return to running is progressed gradually once symptoms are minimized and correction of running mechanics that can contribute to labral injury, such as excessive hip extension and external rotation during terminal stance, or hip adduction and internal rotation during initial to mid stance.

- For recalcitrant cases, a fluoroscopically or ultrasonography-guided intra-articular injection of anesthetic with corticosteroid can help to confirm the labrum's involvement and manage pain during rehabilitation.[85]

- If symptoms continue to persist beyond nonsurgical management, surgical debridement or repair of the labrum is performed arthroscopically. Concomitant surgery for FAI deformities may be performed if present, and if hip dysplasia is implicated in labral pathologic abnormality, periacetabular osteotomy may be performed.

Osteoarthritis

The articular cartilage of the femoral head and acetabulum can be prone to breakdown, causing arthrosis. However, no study has clearly defined an association between hip arthrosis and running.[88–90] In fact, a reduced incidence of osteoarthrosis and hip replacement has been found with long-term recreational running,[91] corresponding to a lower rate of disability progression among runners.[92,93] However, in those with OA, higher-impact exercise has been suggested to hasten disease progression and should be performed with caution.[94]

Presentation

- Progressive onset of pain and stiffness is presented with no specific traumatic event. Pain can vary in location (buttock, groin, and thigh) and character (dull or sharp) and often persists for hours following a pain-inducing activity.
- Reduced range of motion may be observed, most commonly internal rotation and abduction. Clinical examination test item clusters are able to assist with the diagnosis (see **Table 1**).
- Radiographs are routinely obtained to identify osteophytes, sclerosis, or a loss of joint space and are commonly used to confirm diagnosis and mark disease progression. Other diagnostic imaging, such as MRI with contrast, may be useful in better defining the extent of chondral involvement.

Management

- Neuromuscular training to the lumbopelvic and hip muscles should be emphasized and may prove beneficial in prolonged symptom reduction.[95]
- Hip joint mobilization and manipulation, such as lateral hip distraction (see **Fig. 2**C), can be of particular benefit in both reducing pain and increasing function.[78,96]
- If the patient intends to continue running despite the progressive pathologic abnormality, modification to the running form, such as reduced stride length, should be considered to minimize hip joint loading.[9,95]
- Injections (cortisone, platelet-rich plasma, hyaluronic acid) can improve pain and function.[97,98]
- Hip resurfacing arthroplasty and partial/total hip replacement may be considered for more advanced stages of arthrosis. Patients should be discouraged from running following a total hip replacement procedure due to component wear, subsidence, and implant fracture risks. Return to running following hip resurfacing may be possible; however, this should be done cautiously given the lack of long-term outcomes.[99]

Bone Stress Injuries

Although less common than other locations, bone stress injuries of the pelvis (**Fig. 11**) and femoral neck are considered medium and high risk, respectively.[100,101] Sacral stress injuries are more common in the long-distance runner compared with sprinters[102] and seem to increase in incidence during pregnancy and early postpartum and in those with osteopenia.[103] Sacral stress injuries can present similar to nonspecific low back pain and lumbar radiculopathy or sciatica, and therefore, the reported incidence may be greater due to underreporting.[104]

Femoral neck stress fractures account for approximately 11% of stress fractures in athletes.[105] They are more problematic than pelvic stress fractures, and a high index of

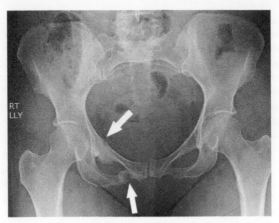

Fig. 11. Pelvis radiograph (anterior-posterior view) showing healing fractures of the right inferior and superior pubic rami (*arrows*) in a 45-year-old female distance runner. Injury occurrence was approximately 4.5 months earlier.

suspicion needs to be maintained in order to avoid serious complications, including fracture displacement, nonunion, and femoral head avascular necrosis.

Presentation

- Pain is usually insidious, often present throughout a run, and can linger for several days before dissipating with rest. Pain may also be reported in the buttock and can present similarly to lumbar radiculopathy.
- Most sacral stress injuries occur in the ala, and pain is typically localized to this region, although up to 25% of individuals with diagnosed sacral stress fractures present with pain on the contralateral side (**Fig. 12**).[106]
- Femoral neck stress injuries present with pain at the groin or anterior thigh, but may radiate to the knee. The pain intensifies with activity and is relatively relieved by rest. Pain with log rolling of the hip and tenderness to deep palpation at the hip joint and greater trochanter can be present.

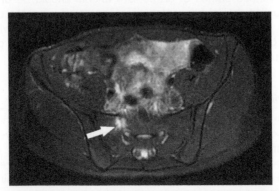

Fig. 12. Stress fracture of the right sacral ala at the level of S1 (*arrow*) in a 19-year-old female cross-country runner. Surrounding marrow edema is evident as well as a distinct fracture line without displacement. This fracture enters the right S1 neural foramen but there is no foraminal compromise. Axial image, T2 fat-suppression.

Management

- Management of sacrum and femoral neck stress injuries should comply with general recommendations for bone stress injuries, essentially involving a period of reduced loading followed by progressive reintroduction of load.
- Sacral stress injury: Initial management of sacral stress injuries includes rest from running and other impact-related activities. Daily weight-bearing activities such as walking should be promoted whenever possible; if painful, short-term use of crutches may be advised. Once pain and focal tenderness have resolved for at least 10 to 14 days, a gradual return to a running schedule can be initiated.
- Femoral neck stress injury: Compression-sided stress fractures are noted medially and are usually treated conservatively, including prolonged crutch weight-bearing and nonimpact aerobic exercise. Tension-sided stress fractures are found laterally and typically treated with urgent surgical fixation because they are more likely to displace. Rarely, conservative treatment such as for compression-side fractures is attempted for small, nondisplaced tension-sided stress fractures.

SUMMARY

Consistent with most running-related injuries, those injuries involving the hip and pelvis are largely regarded as overuse. The frequency of abnormal hip and pelvis diagnostic imaging in asymptomatic individuals and imperfect clinical diagnostic tests warrants correlation of diagnostic imaging with the history, symptoms, and physical examination when making treatment decisions. Conservative management that addresses the symptoms, underlying impairments, and faulty loading patterns often leads to successful recovery, including unrestricted running. When surgical management is warranted, current operative procedures may allow for a return to running.

REFERENCES

1. van Mechelen W. Running injuries. A review of the epidemiological literature. Sports Med 1992;14:320–35.
2. Taunton JE, Ryan MB, Clement DB, et al. A retrospective case-control analysis of 2002 running injuries. Br J Sports Med 2002;36:95–101.
3. Satterthwaite P, Norton R, Larmer P, et al. Risk factors for injuries and other health problems sustained in a marathon. Br J Sports Med 1999;33:22–6.
4. Taunton JE, Ryan MB, Clement DB, et al. A prospective study of running injuries: the Vancouver Sun Run "In Training" clinics. Br J Sports Med 2003;37: 239–44.
5. Schache AG, Bennell KL, Blanch PD, et al. The coordinated movement of the lumbo-pelvic-hip complex during running: a literature review. Gait Posture 1999;10:30–47.
6. Schache AG, Blanch P, Rath D, et al. Differences between the sexes in the three-dimensional angular rotations of the lumbo-pelvic-hip complex during treadmill running. J Sports Sci 2003;21:105–18.
7. Dorn TW, Schache AG, Pandy MG. Muscular strategy shift in human running: dependence of running speed on hip and ankle muscle performance. J Exp Biol 2012;215:1944–56.
8. Lenhart R, Thelen D, Heiderscheit B. Hip muscle loads during running at various step rates. J Orthop Sports Phys Ther 2014;44:766–74. A1–4.

9. Heiderscheit BC, Chumanov ES, Michalski MP, et al. Effects of step rate manipulation on joint mechanics during running. Med Sci Sports Exerc 2011;43: 296–302.

10. Chumanov ES, Wille CM, Michalski MP, et al. Changes in muscle activation patterns when running step rate is increased. Gait Posture 2012;36:231–5.

11. Moore MN, Vandenakker-Albanese C, Hoffman MD. Use of partial body-weight support for aggressive return to running after lumbar disk herniation: a case report. Arch Phys Med Rehabil 2010;91:803–5.

12. Zissen MH, Wallace G, Stevens KJ, et al. High hamstring tendinopathy: MRI and ultrasound imaging and therapeutic efficacy of percutaneous corticosteroid injection. AJR Am J Roentgenol 2010;195:993–8.

13. Fredericson M, Moore W, Guillet M, et al. High hamstring tendinopathy in runners: meeting the challenges of diagnosis, treatment, and rehabilitation. Phys Sportsmed 2005;33:32–43.

14. Cacchio A, Rompe JD, Furia JP, et al. Shockwave therapy for the treatment of chronic proximal hamstring tendinopathy in professional athletes. Am J Sports Med 2011;39:146–53.

15. Puranen J, Orava S. The hamstring syndrome. A new diagnosis of gluteal sciatic pain. Am J Sports Med 1988;16:517–21.

16. Cacchio A, Borra F, Severini G, et al. Reliability and validity of three pain provocation tests used for the diagnosis of chronic proximal hamstring tendinopathy. Br J Sports Med 2012;46:883–7.

17. Lew PC, Briggs CA. Relationship between the cervical component of the slump test and change in hamstring muscle tension. Man Ther 1997;2:98–105.

18. Cook JL, Purdam CR. The challenge of managing tendinopathy in competing athletes. Br J Sports Med 2014;48:506–9.

19. Rio E, Moseley L, Purdam C, et al. The pain of tendinopathy: physiological or pathophysiological? Sports Med 2014;44:9–23.

20. Jayaseelan DJ, Moats N, Ricardo CR. Rehabilitation of proximal hamstring tendinopathy utilizing eccentric training, lumbopelvic stabilization, and trigger point dry needling: 2 case reports. J Orthop Sports Phys Ther 2014;44:198–205.

21. Moraes VY, Lenza M, Tamaoki MJ, et al. Platelet-rich therapies for musculoskeletal soft tissue injuries. Cochrane Database Syst Rev 2014;(4):CD010071.

22. Fader RR, Mitchell JJ, Traub S, et al. Platelet-rich plasma treatment improves outcomes for chronic proximal hamstring injuries in an athletic population. Muscles Ligaments Tendons J 2014;4:461–6.

23. Young IJ, van Riet RP, Bell SN. Surgical release for proximal hamstring syndrome. Am J Sports Med 2008;36:2372–8.

24. Lempainen L, Sarimo J, Mattila K, et al. Proximal hamstring tendinopathy: results of surgical management and histopathologic findings. Am J Sports Med 2009; 37:727–34.

25. Strauss EJ, Nho SJ, Kelly BT. Greater trochanteric pain syndrome. Sports Med Arthrosc 2010;18:113–9.

26. Blank E, Owens BD, Burks R, et al. Incidence of greater trochanteric pain syndrome in active duty US military servicemembers. Orthopedics 2012;35: e1022–7.

27. Segal NA, Felson DT, Torner JC, et al. Greater trochanteric pain syndrome: epidemiology and associated factors. Arch Phys Med Rehabil 2007;88: 988–92.

28. Unfried B, Aguinaldo A, Cipriani D. What is the influence of cambered running surface on lower extremity muscle activity? J Appl Biomech 2013;29:421–7.

29. Lequesne M, Mathieu P, Vuillemin-Bodaghi V, et al. Gluteal tendinopathy in re-
    fractory greater trochanter pain syndrome: diagnostic value of two clinical tests.
    Arthritis Rheum 2008;59:241–6.
30. Bird PA, Oakley SP, Shnier R, et al. Prospective evaluation of magnetic reso-
    nance imaging and physical examination findings in patients with greater
    trochanteric pain syndrome. Arthritis Rheum 2001;44:2138–45.
31. Fearon AM, Scarvell JM, Neeman T, et al. Greater trochanteric pain syndrome:
    defining the clinical syndrome. Br J Sports Med 2013;47:649–53.
32. Travell JG, Simons DG. Myofascial pain and dysfunction: the trigger point
    manual: the lower extremities, vol. 2. Philadelphia: Lippincott Williams & Wilkins;
    1983. p. 23–339.
33. Mulligan EP, Middleton EF, Brunette M. Evaluation and management of greater
    trochanter pain syndrome. Phys Ther Sport 2015;16(3):205–14.
34. Cibulka MT, Delitto A. A comparison of two different methods to treat hip pain in
    runners. J Orthop Sports Phys Ther 1993;17:172–6.
35. Selkowitz DM, Beneck GJ, Powers CM. Which exercises target the gluteal mus-
    cles while minimizing activation of the tensor fascia lata? Electromyographic
    assessment using fine-wire electrodes. J Orthop Sports Phys Ther 2013;43:
    54–64.
36. Sidorkewicz N, Cambridge ED, McGill SM. Examining the effects of altering hip
    orientation on gluteus medius and tensor fascae latae interplay during common
    non-weight-bearing hip rehabilitation exercises. Clin Biomech (Bristol, Avon)
    2014;29:971–6.
37. Lustenberger DP, Ng VY, Best TM, et al. Efficacy of treatment of trochanteric
    bursitis: a systematic review. Clin J Sport Med 2011;21:447–53.
38. Miller TA, White KP, Ross DC. The diagnosis and management of Piriformis Syn-
    drome: myths and facts. Can J Neurol Sci 2012;39:577–83.
39. Fishman LM, Dombi GW, Michaelsen C, et al. Piriformis syndrome: diagnosis, treat-
    ment, and outcome–a 10-year study. Arch Phys Med Rehabil 2002;83:295–301.
40. Hallin RP. Sciatic pain and the piriformis muscle. Postgrad Med 1983;74:69–72.
41. Fishman SM, Caneris OA, Bandman TB, et al. Injection of the piriformis muscle
    by fluoroscopic and electromyographic guidance. Reg Anesth Pain Med 1998;
    23:554–9.
42. Freiberg A. Sciatic pain and its relief by operations on muscle and fascia. Arch
    Surg 1937;34:337–50.
43. Boyajian-O'Neill LA, McClain RL, Coleman MK, et al. Diagnosis and manage-
    ment of piriformis syndrome: an osteopathic approach. J Am Osteopath Assoc
    2008;108:657–64.
44. Tonley JC, Yun SM, Kochevar RJ, et al. Treatment of an individual with piriformis
    syndrome focusing on hip muscle strengthening and movement reeducation: a
    case report. J Orthop Sports Phys Ther 2010;40:103–11.
45. Pace JB, Nagle D. Piriform syndrome. West J Med 1976;124:435–9.
46. Beatty RA. The piriformis muscle syndrome: a simple diagnostic maneuver.
    Neurosurgery 1994;34:512–4 [discussion: 4].
47. Filler AG, Haynes J, Jordan SE, et al. Sciatica of nondisc origin and piriformis
    syndrome: diagnosis by magnetic resonance neurography and interventional
    magnetic resonance imaging with outcome study of resulting treatment.
    J Neurosurg Spine 2005;2:99–115.
48. Cassidy L, Walters A, Bubb K, et al. Piriformis syndrome: implications of
    anatomical variations, diagnostic techniques, and treatment options. Surg Ra-
    diol Anat 2012;34:479–86.

49. Johnston CA, Lindsay DM, Wiley JP. Treatment of iliopsoas syndrome with a hip rotation strengthening program: a retrospective case series. J Orthop Sports Phys Ther 1999;29:218–24.
50. Hammoud S, Bedi A, Voos JE, et al. The recognition and evaluation of patterns of compensatory injury in patients with mechanical hip pain. Sports Health 2014; 6:108–18.
51. Laible C, Swanson D, Garofolo G, et al. Iliopsoas syndrome in dancers. Orthop J Sports Med 2013;1:1–6.
52. Domb BG, Shindle MK, McArthur B, et al. Iliopsoas impingement: a newly identified cause of labral pathology in the hip. HSS J 2011;7:145–50.
53. Tyler TF, Fukunaga T, Gellert J. Rehabilitation of soft tissue injuries of the hip and pelvis. Int J Sports Phys Ther 2014;9:785–97.
54. Ilizaliturri VM, Buganza-Tepole M, Olivos-Meza A, et al. Central compartment release versus lesser trochanter release of the iliopsoas tendon for the treatment of internal snapping hip: a comparative study. Arthroscopy 2014;30:790–5.
55. El Bitar YF, Stake CE, Dunne KF, et al. Arthroscopic iliopsoas fractional lengthening for internal snapping of the hip: clinical outcomes with a minimum 2-year follow-up. Am J Sports Med 2014;42:1696–703.
56. Holmich P, Uhrskou P, Ulnits L, et al. Effectiveness of active physical training as treatment for long-standing adductor-related groin pain in athletes: randomised trial. Lancet 1999;353:439–43.
57. Macintyre J, Johson C, Schroeder EL. Groin pain in athletes. Curr Sports Med Rep 2006;5:293–9.
58. Karlsson J, Sward L, Kalebo P, et al. Chronic groin injuries in athletes. Recommendations for treatment and rehabilitation. Sports Med 1994;17:141–8.
59. Meyers WC, McKechnie A, Philippon MJ, et al. Experience with "sports hernia" spanning two decades. Ann Surg 2008;248:656–65.
60. Gutke A, Ostgaard HC, Oberg B. Pelvic girdle pain and lumbar pain in pregnancy: a cohort study of the consequences in terms of health and functioning. Spine (Phila Pa 1976) 2006;31:E149–55.
61. Santilli OL, Nardelli N, Santilli HA, et al. Sports hernias: experience in a sports medicine center. Hernia 2015. [Epub ahead of print].
62. Malliaras P, Hogan A, Nawrocki A, et al. Hip flexibility and strength measures: reliability and association with athletic groin pain. Br J Sports Med 2009;43:739–44.
63. Nevin F, Delahunt E. Adductor squeeze test values and hip joint range of motion in Gaelic football athletes with longstanding groin pain. J Sci Med Sport 2014; 17:155–9.
64. Caudill P, Nyland J, Smith C, et al. Sports hernias: a systematic literature review. Br J Sports Med 2008;42:954–64.
65. Verrall GM, Slavotinek JP, Fon GT, et al. Outcome of conservative management of athletic chronic groin injury diagnosed as pubic bone stress injury. Am J Sports Med 2007;35:467–74.
66. Topol GA, Reeves KD. Regenerative injection of elite athletes with career-altering chronic groin pain who fail conservative treatment: a consecutive case series. Am J Phys Med Rehabil 2008;87:890–902.
67. Hiti CJ, Stevens KJ, Jamati MK, et al. Athletic osteitis pubis. Sports Med 2011; 41:361–76.
68. Robertson IJ, Curran C, McCaffrey N, et al. Adductor tenotomy in the management of groin pain in athletes. Int J Sports Med 2011;32:45–8.
69. Gill TJ, Carroll KM, Makani A, et al. Surgical technique for treatment of recalcitrant adductor longus tendinopathy. Arthrosc Tech 2014;3:e293–7.

70. Reiman MP, Thorborg K. Femoroacetabular impingement surgery: are we moving too fast and too far beyond the evidence? Br J Sports Med 2015;49(12): 782–4.

71. Wright AA, Naze GS, Kavchak AE, et al. Radiological variables associated with progression of femoroacetabular impingement of the hip: a systematic review. J Sci Med Sport 2015;18:122–7.

72. Agricola R, Heijboer MP, Bierma-Zeinstra SM, et al. Cam impingement causes osteoarthritis of the hip: a nationwide prospective cohort study (CHECK). Ann Rheum Dis 2013;72:918–23.

73. Clohisy JC, Knaus ER, Hunt DM, et al. Clinical presentation of patients with symptomatic anterior hip impingement. Clin Orthop Relat Res 2009;467: 638–44.

74. Lamontagne M, Kennedy MJ, Beaulé PE. The effect of cam FAI on hip and pelvic motion during maximum squat. Clin Orthop Relat Res 2009;467:645–50.

75. Diamond LE, Dobson FL, Bennell KL, et al. Physical impairments and activity limitations in people with femoroacetabular impingement: a systematic review. Br J Sports Med 2015;49:230–42.

76. Reiman MP, Goode AP, Cook CE, et al. Diagnostic accuracy of clinical tests for the diagnosis of hip femoroacetabular impingement/labral tear: a systematic review with meta-analysis. Br J Sports Med 2015;49(12):811.

77. Frank JM, Harris JD, Erickson BJ, et al. Prevalence of femoroacetabular impingement imaging findings in asymptomatic volunteers: a systematic review. Arthroscopy 2015;31(6):1199–204.

78. Cook KM, Heiderscheit B. Conservative management of a young adult with hip arthrosis. J Orthop Sports Phys Ther 2009;39:858–66.

79. Wright AA, Hegedus EJ. Augmented home exercise program for a 37-year-old female with a clinical presentation of femoroacetabular impingement. Man Ther 2012;17:358–63.

80. Loudon JK, Reiman MP. Conservative management of femoroacetabular impingement (FAI) in the long distance runner. Phys Ther Sport 2014;15:82–90.

81. Ayeni OR, Wong I, Chien T, et al. Surgical indications for arthroscopic management of femoroacetabular impingement. Arthroscopy 2012;28:1170–9.

82. Guanche CA, Sikka RS. Acetabular labral tears with underlying chondromalacia: a possible association with high-level running. Arthroscopy 2005;21:580–5.

83. Register B, Pennock AT, Ho CP, et al. Prevalence of abnormal hip findings in asymptomatic participants: a prospective, blinded study. Am J Sports Med 2012;40:2720–4.

84. Reiman MP, Mather RC, Hash TW, et al. Examination of acetabular labral tear: a continued diagnostic challenge. Br J Sports Med 2014;48:311–9.

85. Hunt D, Prather H, Harris Hayes M, et al. Clinical outcomes analysis of conservative and surgical treatment of patients with clinical indications of prearthritic, intra-articular hip disorders. PM R 2012;4:479–87.

86. Lewis CL, Sahrmann SA. Acetabular labral tears. Phys Ther 2006;86:110–21.

87. Yazbek PM, Ovanessian V, Martin RL, et al. Nonsurgical treatment of acetabular labrum tears: a case series. J Orthop Sports Phys Ther 2011;41:346–53.

88. Konradsen L, Hansen EM, Sondergaard L. Long distance running and osteoarthrosis. Am J Sports Med 1990;18:379–81.

89. Chakravarty EF, Hubert HB, Lingala VB, et al. Long distance running and knee osteoarthritis. A prospective study. Am J Prev Med 2008;35:133–8.

90. Hansen P, English M, Willick SE. Does running cause osteoarthritis in the hip or knee? PM R 2012;4:S117–21.

91. Williams PT. Effects of running and walking on osteoarthritis and hip replacement risk. Med Sci Sports Exerc 2013;45:1292–7.
92. Bruce B, Fries JF, Lubeck DP. Aerobic exercise and its impact on musculoskeletal pain in older adults: a 14 year prospective, longitudinal study. Arthritis Res Ther 2005;7:R1263–70.
93. Chakravarty EF, Hubert HB, Lingala VB, et al. Reduced disability and mortality among aging runners: a 21-year longitudinal study. Arch Intern Med 2008;168: 1638–46.
94. Kettunen JA, Kujala UM. Exercise therapy for people with rheumatoid arthritis and osteoarthritis. Scand J Med Sci Sports 2004;14:138–42.
95. Siverling S, O'Sullivan E, Garofalo M, et al. Hip osteoarthritis and the active patient: will I run again? Curr Rev Musculoskelet Med 2012;5:24–31.
96. Hoeksma HL, Dekker J, Ronday HK, et al. Comparison of manual therapy and exercise therapy in osteoarthritis of the hip: a randomized clinical trial. Arthritis Rheum 2004;51:722–9.
97. Battaglia M, Guaraldi F, Vannini F, et al. Efficacy of ultrasound-guided intra-articular injections of platelet-rich plasma versus hyaluronic acid for hip osteoarthritis. Orthopedics 2013;36:e1501–8.
98. Lieberman JR, Engstrom SM, Solovyova O, et al. Is intra-articular hyaluronic acid effective in treating osteoarthritis of the hip joint? J Arthroplasty 2015;30: 507–11.
99. Fouilleron N, Wavreille G, Endjah N, et al. Running activity after hip resurfacing arthroplasty: a prospective study. Am J Sports Med 2012;40:889–94.
100. Fredericson M, Jennings F, Beaulieu C, et al. Stress fractures in athletes. Top Magn Reson Imaging 2006;17:309–25.
101. Nguyen JT, Peterson JS, Biswal S, et al. Stress-related injuries around the lesser trochanter in long-distance runners. AJR Am J Roentgenol 2008;190: 1616–20.
102. Bennell KL, Malcolm SA, Thomas SA, et al. The incidence and distribution of stress fractures in competitive track and field athletes. A twelve-month prospective study. Am J Sports Med 1996;24:211–7.
103. Longhino V, Bonora C, Sansone V. The management of sacral stress fractures: current concepts. Clin Cases Miner Bone Metab 2011;8:19–23.
104. Major NM, Helms CA. Sacral stress fractures in long-distance runners. AJR Am J Roentgenol 2000;174:727–9.
105. DeFranco MJ, Recht M, Schils J, et al. Stress fractures of the femur in athletes. Clin Sports Med 2006;25:89–103, ix.
106. Kiuru MJ, Pihlajamaki HK, Ahovuo JA. Fatigue stress injuries of the pelvic bones and proximal femur: evaluation with MR imaging. Eur Radiol 2003;13: 605–11.
107. Willcox EL, Burden AM. The influence of varying hip angle and pelvis position on muscle recruitment patterns of the hip abductor muscles during the clam exercise. J Orthop Sports Phys Ther 2013;43:325–31.
108. Reiman MP, Goode AP, Hegedus EJ, et al. Diagnostic accuracy of clinical tests of the hip: a systematic review with meta-analysis. Br J Sports Med 2013;47: 893–902.
109. Woodley SJ, Nicholson HD, Livingstone V, et al. Lateral hip pain: findings from magnetic resonance imaging and clinical examination. J Orthop Sports Phys Ther 2008;38:313–28.
110. Verrall GM, Slavotinek JP, Barnes PG, et al. Description of pain provocation tests used for the diagnosis of sports-related chronic groin pain: relationship of tests

to defined clinical (pain and tenderness) and MRI (pubic bone marrow oedema) criteria. Scand J Med Sci Sports 2005;15:36–42.

111. Ayeni O, Chu R, Hetaimish B, et al. A painful squat test provides limited diagnostic utility in CAM-type femoroacetabular impingement. Knee Surg Sports Traumatol Arthrosc 2014;22:806–11.

112. Sutlive TG, Lopez HP, Schnitker DE, et al. Development of a clinical prediction rule for diagnosing hip osteoarthritis in individuals with unilateral hip pain. J Orthop Sports Phys Ther 2008;38:542–50.

113. Altman R, Alarcon G, Appelrouth D, et al. The American College of Rheumatology criteria for the classification and reporting of osteoarthritis of the hip. Arthritis Rheum 1991;34:505–14.

114. Kountouris A, Cook J. Rehabilitation of Achilles and patellar tendinopathies. Best Pract Res Clin Rheumatol 2007;21:295–316.

115. Cook JL, Purdam CR. Is tendon pathology a continuum? A pathology model to explain the clinical presentation of load-induced tendinopathy. Br J Sports Med 2009;43:409–16.

116. Distefano LJ, Blackburn JT, Marshall SW, et al. Gluteal muscle activation during common therapeutic exercises. J Orthop Sports Phys Ther 2009;39:532–40.

Patellofemoral Pain

Rebecca A. Dutton, MD[a], Michael J. Khadavi, MD[b],
Michael Fredericson, MD[a],*

KEYWORDS

• Patellofemoral pain • Runner • Risk factors • Diagnosis • Management

KEY POINTS

• Patellofemoral pain (PFP) is a common condition, especially among runners.
• A variety of risk factors for PFP have been identified and may be loosely categorized by local joint abnormalities, aberrations in lower extremity biomechanics, and training errors.
• Proper diagnosis and management of PFP mandate close inspection and targeted intervention according to the individual's risk factor profile.
• Management strategies for PFP include quadriceps strengthening, stretching key muscle groups (quadriceps, hamstrings, and gastrocnemius), patellar taping, patellar bracing, hip strengthening, foot orthoses, gait re-education, and training modification.

INTRODUCTION

Patellofemoral pain (PFP) is characterized by anterior knee pain of insidious onset that is exacerbated under conditions of increased patellofemoral joint stress. It is commonly observed in runners and may arise in the setting of a variety of risk factors. PFP does not seem to be self-limited but rather can persist chronically if those factors contributing to its development are not properly recognized and addressed. Here, the epidemiology, risk factors, diagnosis, and management of PFP are reviewed.

DISCUSSION
Epidemiology

PFP accounts for up to 25% of knee injuries that present to sports medicine clinics.[1] PFP seems to be particularly common among runners, representing one of, if not the

Conflicts of Interest and Source of Funding: The authors have no conflicts of interest nor funding received for this work to declare.
[a] Division of Physical Medicine and Rehabilitation, Department of Orthopaedic Surgery, Stanford University, 450 Broadway Street, MC 6342, Redwood City, CA 94063-6342, USA; [b] Sports Medicine, Carondelet Orthopaedic Surgeons, 10777 Nall Avenue, Suite 300, Overland Park, KS 66211, USA
* Corresponding author.
E-mail address: mfred2@stanford.edu

most, common running-related musculoskeletal injury, particularly among longer-distance runners.[2-6]

PFP demonstrates a clear predilection for women with prevalence[5,7,8] and incidence[9] rates that are 2 to 3 times greater for women than men. This prevalence and incidence rate are thought to reflect specific anatomic and biomechanical variations in women that predispose to PFP. Women, for example, exhibit lower cartilage thickness and greater peak cartilage stress during stair-walking.[10-12] Disparities in lower extremity strength as well as both static and dynamic alignment have also been purported as contributing factors.[13] Comparative studies of lower extremity strength demonstrate greater hip abduction and external rotation strength in men when compared with women.[14] Meanwhile, increased Q-angle, as well as dynamic knee valgus angle and hip internal rotation angle, has also been reported in women compared with men.[15] Each of these variables has been independently implicated as risk factors for PFP and are discussed in greater detail in subsequent sections.

Traditionally, PFP has been considered an affliction of younger patients. Interestingly, a recent investigation of injury patterns in masters runners demonstrated similar rates of PFP between those older and younger than 40 years of age.[16] This trend may reflect greater involvement of older athletes in sport, and the increasingly recognized chronic nature of PFP. Certainly more current studies evaluating the incidence and prevalence of PFP across a wide age range are warranted.

Cause of Patellofemoral Pain

The precise pathogenesis of PFP remains poorly understood; however, the pain of PFP seems to represent the end result of increased stress at the patellofemoral joint.[12] The cause of exaggerated joint strain is a point of particular contention. Classically, aberrant patellar alignment and tracking were thought to signify the primary precipitant of patellofemoral stress and PFP. Nevertheless, it has become increasingly clear that patellofemoral malalignment, while representing one risk factor, cannot solely account for the development of PFP. Indeed, clinical and radiographic malalignment is observed in a mere subset of individuals presenting with PFP. Contrariwise, many with evidence of abnormalities in patellar position never develop symptoms of PFP.

Remedying this incongruity, Dye[17] proposed his "theory of tissue homeostasis." He suggested that alterations in tissue homeostasis may occur under any circumstance that supersedes the so-called envelope of function or load acceptance capacity of the joint. According to his model, gross structural abnormalities and repetitive overload alike may challenge the envelope of function, exceeding the force across the joint that can be safely tolerated and ultimately result in disruption to the osseous and periosseous tissues. Among the tissues thought to cause pain in PFP are the subchondral bone (by way of disrupted articular cartilage), medial and lateral retinacula, and infrapatellar fat pad.[18]

Risk Factors

PFP is thought to be multifactorial, with a variety of risk factors that may contribute to its inception. Although the significance of these risk factors in isolation is debatable, it is more likely the culmination of multiple predisposing conditions that challenges the load-bearing tolerance of the joint and results in symptoms. In order to develop a framework for the diagnosis of PFP, then, it is critical to first understand these underlying risk factors, which may be categorized broadly as local joint impairments, deficits in lower extremity biomechanics, and training errors (Table 1). Moreover, recognition of these factors allows for a more targeted approach to treatment and may help prevent recurrence.

Table 1		
Risk factors for patellofemoral pain		
Local Joint Factors	**Lower Extremity Biomechanics**	**Training Considerations**
Patellar maltracking or hypermobility	Hip muscle dysfunction	Female gender
Quadriceps weakness	• Hip abductor/ER weakness	Novice runners
Delayed VMO activation	• Impaired hip muscle endurance	Abrupt escalation in exercise
Soft tissue inflexibility	• Neuromuscular incoordination	• Increased intensity
• Quadriceps	Foot overpronation	• Increased frequency
• Gastrocnemius	Gait deviations	Excessive hill work (especially downhill)
• Iliotibial band	• Excessive hip adduction/femoral IR	Inadequate recovery time
• Hamstring	• Increased peak GRF	High weekly mileage
	• Heel foot-strike pattern	

Risk factors for the development of PFP may be broadly categorized as local joint factors, lower extremity biomechanics, and training considerations.

Abbreviations: ER, external rotator; GRF, ground reaction force; IR, internal rotation.

Local joint impairments

To begin, it is important to consider the stabilizing structures of the knee joint itself, because these local structures have a direct effect on patellofemoral function, including patellar position and tracking.

Quadriceps muscle weakness The quadriceps muscle complex represents one such structure that influences the patellofemoral joint. Quadriceps muscle weakness has long been implicated in PFP. Observational studies have reported an association between reduced quadriceps torque[19–21] and volume[20,22] in patients with PFP. A recent meta-analysis further established a significant correlation between quadriceps atrophy and PFP, both when compared with the asymptomatic limb and when compared with a distinct control group.[23] More directed attention has been given to vastus medialis oblique (VMO) strength in particular, as VMO fibers insert more distally and horizontally on the patella and are thought to impart dynamic medial patellar stability.[24,25] Accordingly, studies have also found an association between reduced VMO volume and PFP.[26,27]

However, such studies fail to define the presence of quadriceps weakness in PFP as causal or secondary. Two prospective studies have attempted to clarify the relationship between quadriceps strength and PFP with varying results.[15,28] When normalized for body weight, Milgrom and colleagues[28] reported no relationship between knee extension strength and the development of PFP, whereas Boling and colleagues[15] found that individuals with reduced quadriceps strength had an apparent predisposition to PFP. Pooled analysis of the 2 studies demonstrated a significant ($P<.01$) association between decreased knee extension strength and the development of PFP,[29] suggesting that quadriceps weakness may play a causal role in PFP, although more prospective studies are needed to confirm this notion.

Delayed vastus medialis activation In addition to quadriceps strength, vastus medialis (VM) and vastus lateralis (VL) activation seems closely entwined with PFP. Delayed VM activation relative to that of VL has been implicated in multiple studies of PFP.[30–33] It has been postulated that the role of vasti muscle activation is especially relevant among a subset of individuals with PFP who demonstrate evidence of lateral patellar maltracking. Pal and colleagues[34,35] identified patellar maltrackers based on the presence of patellar tilt and bisect offset as measured from weight-bearing MRI and found that, within this group specifically, the degree of maltracking was closely correlated with delay in VM activation. As with quadriceps strength, additional prospective evidence is necessary to more clearly define the cause-and-effect relationship between vasti muscle activation and PFP.

Soft tissue inflexibility Inflexibility of the soft tissues surrounding the knee joint seems to represent another risk factor for PFP. Excessive tension involving the lateral restraints of the knee, and especially the lateral retinaculum, has been heavily implicated for its role in patellar maltracking. The midportion of the lateral retinaculum represents the strongest and most substantial layer and derives its fibers from the iliotibial band. The transverse orientation of these fibers resists medial displacement of the patella and when excessively taught may result in disproportionate lateral translation. It follows that dysfunction of the iliotibial band could result in aberrant patellar tracking and increased contact forces across the patellofemoral joint, and in turn contribute to the development of PFP. In support of this, several cross-sectional studies have observed a relationship between iliotibial band tightness and the presence of PFP.[36,37] It has been reported that among runners with PFP specifically, a high proportion (67%) have tightness of the iliotibial band.[38]

Inflexibility of the quadriceps, gastrocnemius, and hamstring muscles likewise seems to correlate with PFP. Tightness of the quadriceps femoris seems to represent a risk factor for the development of PFP.[39,40] Mechanistically, quadriceps tightness is theorized to increase the posterior force of the patella against the femoral trochlea, in turn elevating patellofemoral joint stress, especially with activity.[40] Hamstring inflexibility has also been linked to PFP. Several case-controlled studies have reported a significant difference in hamstring flexibility between PFP and control groups.[41] It has been theorized that tightness of the hamstring exerts a constant flexion moment to the patella, thereby requiring greater quadriceps power to extend the knee, and increasing patellofemoral joint reaction forces[41,42]; however, such a causal relationship has yet to be confirmed. Finally, inflexibility of the gastrocnemius has been prospectively associated with the development of PFP.[40] The precise role of gastrocnemius tightness in the pathophysiology of PFP remains unclear, although alterations in foot position and excessive subtalar joint pronation have been proposed.[39]

Deficits in lower extremity biomechanics

By way of a closed kinetic chain, function of the entire lower extremity can alter movement and stress patterns at the patellofemoral joint. Thus, lower extremity biomechanics, including those involving the hip, trunk, foot, and ankle, are important to consider in the pathogenesis and treatment of PFP. Excessive internal rotation of the femur, in particular, can increase patellofemoral stress and in turn predispose to PFP. Internal rotation of the femur under a fairly fixed patella generates a relative lateral displacement of the patella with respect to the femur. Dynamic MRI studies have helped define the influence of femoral internal rotation in PFP, demonstrating increased femoral rotation and consequent lateral patellar displacement and tilt across degrees of knee flexion during weight-bearing in women with PFP.[43,44]

Hip weakness Weakness involving the external rotators and abductors of the hip can contribute to excessive internal rotation of the femur and, in turn, has been implicated in the development of PFP. A correlation between isometric hip abductor and external rotator weakness to PFP is supported by several studies.[39,45,46] Further corroborating the role of hip strength in PFP are numerous randomized controlled trials, which upheld hip abductor strengthening in the treatment of PFP to improve both symptoms and function.[47–51] However, such studies fail to define hip weakness as causative of PFP. It is worth noting that more recent prospective investigations found no association between hip abductor or external rotator strength to the eventual development of

PFP.[15,52] Separately, a meta-analysis likewise failed to identify a causal relationship of hip weakness to PFP.[53] It may be that hip weakness is consequential rather than contributory to PFP. In support of this, Finnoff and colleagues[54] discovered a significant decrement over time in hip abductor and external rotator strength among individuals who developed PFP. These findings may reflect a greater role for hip muscle performance rather than static strength in the dynamic control of femoral internal rotation. Indeed, as is later discussed, hip muscle performance during dynamic tasks seems to represent a distinct risk factor for PFP, independent of hip strength.[55,56]

Foot pronation Foot pronation is important for force absorption during walking and running. However, excessive pronation is thought to predispose to increased patellofemoral stress and PFP. The precise mechanism by which this occurs is unproven, although compensatory internal rotation of the femur has been conjectured.[57] In normal gait, the foot pronates and the tibia internally rotates during early contact. Once the foot reaches midstance and the foot is in full contact with the ground, the subtalar joint supinates and the tibia follows, externally rotating, in order to move the knee into extension. In situations of excessive pronation, the subtalar joint remains in a pronated position at midstance, preventing the tibia from externally rotating. Tiberio[57] has theorized that to compensate and promote knee extension, the femur internally rotates on the tibia. As was previously discussed, increased internal rotation of the femur beneath the patella yields lateral displacement of the patella and increased patellofemoral joint strain. Most prospective studies to date have suggested a predisposition to PFP under conditions of overpronation.[15,58] Furthermore, a recent meta-analysis for the role of foot posture in overuse injuries concluded that evidence, albeit limited, maintains overpronation of the foot as a risk factor for PFP.[59] It seems, however, that the changes in foot position necessary to increase one's risk of PFP are quite subtle with differences in navicular drop or hindfoot motion of 1 mm and 1° to 2°, respectively.[15,60]

Gait aberrations By definition, running-related injuries are the consequence of circumstances related to the act of running, including dynamic biomechanics and training habits. Thus, such factors must be considered potential contributors, especially in runners presenting with PFP. Excessive hip adduction and internal rotation during dynamic activities, for example, have been strongly implicated in PFP. Studies have shown greater hip internal rotation during single leg squat,[61] jump landing tasks,[15] and running[62] in women with PFP. It is interesting that targeted hip-strengthening regimens, while improving strength, may not affect these associated gait impairments.[55,56] It seems that muscle performance including endurance and neuromuscular coordination likely also play a role in the dynamic control of femoral internal rotation. Souza and Powers[62] reported an association between greater hip internal rotation during running and diminished hip extension endurance. As well, altered neuromuscular activity of the gluteus medius and maximus muscles has been associated with PFP.[61,62]

Other gait deviations that have been implicated in PFP include accelerated foot pronation,[63,64] increased peak ground reaction force, reduced step rate,[65,66] and decreased knee flexion angle at initial contact.[67] However, such findings to date are observational, and further research is needed to confirm their association and any causal relationship to PFP.

Training errors
A proportion of running-related injuries, inclusive of PFP, are undoubtedly related to errors in training. Training errors, including improper or overly worn footwear, hard or irregular training surfaces, abrupt escalation in exercise including rapid increases

in duration, frequency, speed, intensity, or hill work, and inadequate time for recovery, represent mechanisms by which the athlete may exceed Dye's proposed envelope of function or load acceptance capacity of the joint.[68] Although not enough to produce an immediate structural damage, these repetitive stresses result in loss of tissue homeostasis over time and consequent injury.[17] Athletes who are new to running may be at particularly high risk.[69,70] A recent analysis of 874 novice runners demonstrated that those who increased their weekly distances by more than 30% over a 2-week period were more likely to develop running-related injuries, including PFP.[71] In addition, high weekly mileage has been associated with a greater risk of running-related injuries, with 20 to 40 miles per week representing a critical threshold beyond which injury becomes significantly more likely.[69,70,72]

Other considerations: generalized laxity

Generalized ligamentous laxity has been implicated in PFP. It is rational to assume that diffuse laxity would not spare the knee, but rather predispose to increased patellar mobility and patellar maltracking. Although logical, few studies have investigated the relationship between generalized ligamentous laxity and PFP. al-Rawi and Nessan[73] observed greater joint laxity in patients with chondromalacia patellae, noting a higher proportion of patients with hypermobile joints when compared with controls, as well as greater total mobility scores within the patient group. Witvrouw and colleagues[40] prospectively evaluated the role of generalized ligamentous laxity in PFP and found that, among various measures of joint laxity, only thumb-to-forearm mobility correlated with development of PFP.

Diagnosis

History

An important first step in the diagnosis of PFP is a thorough history. The history should emphasize symptom onset, location, and aggravating factors, as well as an investigation to underlying risk factors for the development of PFP.

The pain of PFP is typically described as spontaneous and insidious, without any clear precipitating event. Patients tend to describe a vague ache localized diffusely to the anterior knee.[18] Pain will typically be exacerbated by activities that increase stress to the patellofemoral joint, including prolonged knee flexion (the so-called positive theater sign), as well as walking down stairs, running, jumping, or squatting.[74] Patients may relate associated symptoms of knee catching or buckling while walking. They may also endorse subjective sensations of stiffness or swelling; however, significant swelling of the knee joint is not a prominent feature of PFP in isolation and should evoke consideration for alternative pathologic abnormalities.[18]

In addition to a complete symptom inventory, it is critical to elicit a history of risk factors for PFP. In particular, the practitioner should evaluate for training habits resulting in repetitive overload to the patellofemoral joint (see **Table 1**, column 3, Training Considerations).[75] The provider should inquire regarding the initiation of any new activities. In the running population specifically, it is important to consider any abrupt escalation in training, including sudden increases in duration, frequency, or intensity of workouts. In addition, it is important to consider the presence of excessive hill training, and in particular, running steep descents, because this may increase stress about the knee joint by up to 6 times body weight.[76]

Physical examination

PFP is a clinical diagnosis and should be based on the amalgamation of historical features and examination findings (**Table 2**). The physical examination serves to more precisely localize the patient's pain, exclude alternative diagnoses (**Box 1**), and also

Table 2
Physical examination of patellofemoral pain

Position	Physical Examination Technique or Maneuver Suggesting PFP	
Standing	Static inspection	*Genu valgum* or *genu varum*
		Squinting patella
		Excessive foot pronation
		Generalized joint laxity
	Dynamic tests	*Poor single-leg squat*: exaggerated knee valgum or femoral internal rotation
		Impaired landing task: exaggerated knee valgum or femoral internal rotation
		Altered gait mechanics: excessive hip adduction, accelerated foot pronation, decreased step rate, increased peak ground reaction force
Sitting	Tests	*Positive J-sign*: patella shifts laterally with knee extension, creating an inverted "J" shape
Lying	Inspection	*Absence of marked swelling, erythema, warmth*
		Atrophy of VMO and/or quadriceps complex
		Delayed VM oblique activation relative to VL
	Palpation	Tenderness over the *lateral retinaculum*
	Tests	*Excessive lateral glide*: lateral displacement of patella by >0.5 cm
		Positive lateral patellar tilt: increased height of the medial patella border relative to the lateral patellar border
		Altered patellar mobility: limited medial or excessive mediolateral mobility
		Muscle inflexibility (popliteal angle, Obers test, Ely test, GN stretch)

A comprehensive physical examination should evaluate alignment and biomechanical factors that may contribute to PFP in standing, sitting, and lying positions.
Abbreviation: GN, gastrocnemius.

identify any underlying factors predisposing to the development of PFP. The recognition of risk factors not only further supports the diagnosis but also represents a critical first step in designing an appropriate and targeted rehabilitation protocol.

Beginning with the patient standing, lower extremity alignment should first be observed statically. The examiner may assess the presence of either genu valgum or genu varum deformities of the knee. In addition to genu valgum, it is important to make note of any excessive internal rotation of the femur, which is indicated by an inward-pointing patella (or so-called squinting patella), external rotation of the tibia, and hindfoot valgus.[77] The finding of a femoral internal rotation is common in PFP and is often associated with a tight iliotibial band or weak hip abductors and external rotators.[18] Moving distally, one may also ascertain foot position, and in particular, the presence of excessive foot pronation.[78]

An assessment for generalized ligamentous laxity should also be undertaken. Joint laxity may be ascertained based on the criteria defined by Beighton and Horan.[79] This criteria include the presence of hyperextension of the elbows and knees beyond 10°, passive dorsiflexion of the fifth digit metacarpophalangeal joints beyond 90°, passive thumb-to-forearm apposition, and forward flexion of the trunk with the knees held straight such that the hands rest on the floor with palms flat. Three of 5 positive

---

Box 1
Differential diagnosis of anterior knee pain

Patellar tendinopathy

Prepatellar or infrapatellar bursitis

Infrapatellar fat pad syndrome

Plica syndrome

Chondromalacia patellae

Patellofemoral osteoarthritis

Osteochondritis dissecans

Patellar stress fracture

Patellar instability

Osgood-Schlatter disease[a]

Sinding-Larsen-Johansson disease[a]

A variety of conditions may cause anterior knee pain. These should be considered and excluded when evaluating a patient with suspected PFP.
  [a] Indicates pediatric-specific conditions.
  Data from Hiemstra LA, Karslake S, Irving C. Anterior knee pain in the athlete. Clin Sports Med 2014;33:437–59.

---

tests indicate generalized laxity. In instances of suspected generalized laxity, it is important to look for other phenotypic features that may suggest an underlying syndrome, such as Ehler-Danlos or Marfan, that would warrant further evaluation for systemic manifestations and consultation to appropriate specialists for management.

With the patient still standing, an evaluation of dynamic lower extremity biomechanics is critical, particularly for the athlete presenting with suspected PFP. A single leg squat is useful to identify hip abductor weakness. The patient is asked to stand with full weight on the affected limb and slowly squat with the knee flexed to 45° to 60°. The examiner should observe for exaggerated knee valgus or femoral internal rotation as the patient descends.[80] The squat should also be evaluated for proper form, ensuring that the knee does not extend beyond the toes. Alternatively, a unilateral or bilateral landing task may be similarly used to assess for the presence of dynamic knee valgus.[80,81]

For runners in particular, a running gait analysis may provide additional information. It is important to scrutinize the position of the hip, knee, and foot, taking note of excessive hip internal rotation or adduction, increased dynamic knee valgus, and excessive foot pronation. Other factors that are worth considering, although their precise clinical significance requires further investigation, include ground reaction force, step rate, running speed, and body orientation at initial contact.

Moving next to a seated position, it is possible to evaluate dynamic patellar tracking. The J-sign is used to describe pathologic tracking and may be observed by having the patient actively extend the knee from 90° of flexion to full extension. Normal patellar motion is characterized by nearly straight movement of the patella proximally with only slight lateral shift near terminal extension. Improper patellar tracking is demonstrated when the patella frankly deviates laterally with extension, creating an inverted "J" shape and thus representing a positive J-sign.[82]

With the patient supine, gross static inspection of the knee joint is typically relatively unremarkable. Findings of marked swelling, erythema, or warmth should prompt investigation to alternative causes for pain. Astute inspection may reveal atrophy of the VM or the quadriceps complex more generally. This finding may be accentuated when the patient is asked to contract the muscle.[83] With this, the examiner might also make note of the timing of VM, and in particular, VMO contraction relative to VL, looking for any delay in onset between VMO and VL.[83,84]

The quadriceps angle, or Q-angle, is designed to quantify risk for lateral patellar displacement and patellar maltracking. It is measured as the angle formed by the intersection of 2 lines: the line formed between the anterosuperior iliac spine to the center of the patella, and the line generated from the center of the patella to the middle of the anterior tibial tuberosity. The significance of the Q-angle in the diagnosis of PFP has been widely debated. The variable association of Q-angle with PFP is likely in part related to inconsistency in measurement technique and poor interobserver as well as interrater reliability.[77] Indeed, a properly gauged clinical Q-angle has demonstrated moderate correlation with MRI-derived Q-angles.[85] Accurate measurement mandates a neutral position of the leg. Any outward rotation of the foot will superficially increase the Q-angle, while internal rotation of the thigh will spuriously reduce the Q-angle.[82] In addition, a modified, long-arm goniometer may enhance the reliability of Q-angle assessment.[85] Q-angles exceeding 15° to 20° denote increased lateral pull about the patella and greater propensity for patellar malalignment.[85]

Next, gentle palpation over the anterior knee while passively flexing the joint may yield crepitus, although this finding is poorly specific for PFP and has limited diagnostic bearing.[82] More directed palpation should include, in particular, the medial and lateral retinacula. With the knee extended, the examiner may begin with palpation over portions of the retinacula. If tolerated, the patella may be gently displaced both medially and laterally, which not only further stresses each retinacula but also permits more direct palpation of the retinacular fibers.[86]

From this position, the examiner may also evaluate patellar position and mobility by way of the mediolateral glide, patellar tilt, and patellar mobility tests, which when positive suggest deficits or tightness of the medial or lateral soft tissue restraints. Mediolateral glide represents the position of the patella relative to the trochlea in the coronal plane. It is assessed with the knee flexed to 20°, and by comparing the distance from the mid-patella to the lateral femoral condyle and to the medial femoral condyle. Under normal conditions, the patella should rest equidistant from each epicondyle.[18] Instances whereby the distance to the medial femoral epicondyle exceeds the distance to the lateral femoral epicondyle (ie, lateral displacement) by greater than 0.5 cm indicate a positive test and suggest excessive tightness of the lateral restraints and reduced VMO tension.[87] Patellar tilt describes the inclination of the patella in the transverse plane. With the knee extended, the examiner palpates the height of the medial and lateral patellar borders. The 2 heights should be equal. Increased height of the medial patellar border implies that the patella is tilted laterally, while reciprocally, increased height of the lateral patellar border indicates medial patellar tilt.[82,87] Use of a pluri-cal caliber applied to the medial and lateral aspects of the patella to measure the respective tilt angles has also been described and may enhance intrarater and interrater reliability of the test.[88] Finally, the patellar mobility test quantifies the mediolateral range of motion of the patella. The knee is placed in 20° of flexion, and the patella is divided into 4 longitudinal quadrants. With the quadriceps fully relaxed, the examiner translates the patella medially and laterally. Medial glide to a distance less than that of one quadrant is consistent with tightness of the lateral restraints. Conversely, motion in the medial or lateral direction exceeding the distance of 3 quadrants suggests hypermobility of the patella.[77]

Another important risk factor for PFP that should be assessed in the course of examination is soft tissue flexibility. With the patient remaining supine, hamstring and gastroc soleus flexibility may be approximated by measurement of the popliteal angle, and passive ankle dorsiflexion with the knee in extension, respectively.[83] Next, with the patient side-lying, iliotibial band tightness may be assessed via Ober test. Last, quadriceps flexibility is ascertained with the patient prone via Ely test. The examiner should stabilize the pelvis while flexing the knee and bringing the heel toward the buttock until reaching a point of firm resistance. The distance between the heel and buttock is measured, most conveniently by way of finger breadths and compared side to side.[83]

Imaging

Because PFP is a clinical diagnosis, there is limited utility for imaging in the diagnosis of PFP. Imaging plays the greatest role in excluding alternative diagnoses. Nevertheless, plain radiographs of the knee are often a reasonable first-line study in the evaluation of knee pain, and specific risk factors for PFP (especially patellar position) can be inferred from such images. An axial radiograph taken at 30° to 45° of knee flexion, or Merchant view, is ideal for interpreting the position of the patella within the trochlear groove and thus establishing the presence of lateral displacement or tilt. Measures that may be obtained from the axial view include the sulcus angle, congruence angle, lateral displacement, and lateral patellofemoral angle (**Fig. 1**A–D).[89,90] The lateral view may be useful to assess the superior-inferior relation of the patella. Pal and colleagues[91] found that a high-riding patella (patella alta) predisposed to PFP, possibly due to reduced osseous contact and subsequent instability of a patella that articulates superior to the trochlea.[92] Measures of vertical patellar position include the Insall-Salvati and Blackburne-Peel indices (see **Fig. 1**E–F).[90]

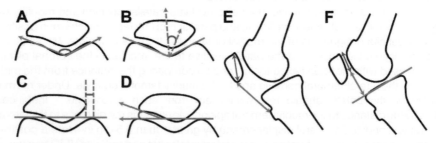

Fig. 1. Radiographic measures associated with PFP. (*A*) The sulcus angle is the angle formed at the trough of the femoral sulcus. A shallower trochlear groove (ie, greater sulcus angle) may predispose to PFP. (*B*) The congruence angle is measured by first bisecting the sulcus angle to produce a reference line and then creating a second line between the apex of the sulcus and the lowest point of the patellar articular surface. Angles lateral to the reference line are designated positive, with greater positive angles suggesting greater lateral shift. (*C*) Lateral displacement may also be quantified by the distance between the medial patellar facet and the apex of the medial femoral condyle. (*D*) The lateral patellofemoral angle is a measure of patellar tilt and is calculated as the angle between a horizontal line across the peaks of the 2 femoral condyles and a line along the lateral patellar facet. An angle opening medially indicates lateral tilt. (*E*) The Insall-Salvati index is calculated in the sagittal plane as the ratio of patella length to patellar tendon length. Ratios greater than 1.2 are suggestive of patella alta. (*F*) The Blackburne-Peel index similarly quantifies patellar height and is the ratio of the distance of the articular surface of the patella to the distance measured between the inferior patellar articular surface and the tibial plateau.

Investigations relating each of these measures to PFP have shown variable and conflicting results. These conflicting results are consistent with patterns observed for risk factors and clinical examination findings and underscores the importance of a holistic approach to diagnosis that considers the entirety of an individual's risk factor profile, rather than discrete elements, when making a diagnosis of PFP.

Management

Management of PFP can be challenging, with persistent symptoms reported in as many as 91% of patients with PFP after extended follow-up.[93] Initial management should include activity modification, analgesics such as a short course of nonsteroidal anti-inflammatory drugs, and modalities to acutely control pain. In addition, it is critical that the clinician generate a tailored and comprehensive rehabilitation program, unique to the individual and based on those risk factors and examination findings previously discussed (**Table 3**).[94–96]

Quadriceps strengthening

Quadriceps strengthening has and continues to represent a mainstay in the treatment of PFP. There is strong evidence that isolated quadriceps strengthening is superior to

Table 3
Treatment strategies in patellofemoral pain

Risk Factor	Examination Correlate	Treatment Considerations
Quadriceps weakness	Muscle atrophy Knee extensor weakness	Quadriceps strengthening
Delayed VMO activation	Delayed VMO contraction	Biofeedback
Patellar maltracking	Patella alta Lateral patellar tilt Lateral patellar glide	Patellar taping/bracing
Patellar hypermobility	Excessive patellar mobility Generalized ligamentous laxity	Patellar taping/bracing
Soft tissue inflexibility	Quadriceps tightness Gastrocnemius tightness Positive Obers test Hamstring tightness	Stretching
Hip muscle weakness	Hip abductor weakness Dynamic knee valgum with SLS Excessive hip adduction with SLS Excessive contralateral pelvic drop with SLS	Hip strengthening
Foot malposition	Foot overpronation	Foot orthosis
Gait deviations	Excessive ipsilateral hip adduction Excessive contralateral pelvic drop Forceful heel strike	Gait retraining • Visual feedback • Forefoot strike
Training errors	Self-report of an abrupt increase in training intensity or insufficient recovery time	Relative rest Correct training errors Patient education

Management of PFP mandates careful consideration of the underlying risk factors for its development, with targeted treatment strategies applied accordingly.
Abbreviation: SLS, single leg squat.
Adapted from Dutton RA, Khadavi MJ, Fredericson M. Update on rehabilitation of patellofemoral pain. Curr Sports Med Rep 2014;13(3):173; with permission.

education alone in the management of PFP.[97] The ideal approach to quadriceps strengthening should incorporate both open and closed kinetic chain exercises to promote strengthening throughout the arc of motion.[98,99] In general, open kinetic chain exercises (especially in the range of 90°–45°) are better tolerated under circumstances of acute pain or weakness. However, closed kinetic chain exercises with an emphasis on cocontractions seem more beneficial to improve function.[100–102] Thus, quadriceps strengthening for PFP should begin with open kinetic chain exercises and progress to closed kinetic chain strengthening as early as the patient is able to tolerate.[103,104]

Given the perceived importance of the VMO in PFP, several studies have compared overall quadriceps strengthening to selective VMO training programs. Efforts aimed at selective VMO strengthening have included the incorporation of hip adduction strengthening[105] and electromyography (EMG) biofeedback.[106–108] Neither of these strategies have demonstrated benefit in the management of PFP. Thus, specific exercises to isolate the VMO are not indicated, but rather, a well-rounded quadriceps strengthening program is recommended and should correct any imbalance in strength between the quadriceps muscles.

Electromyography biofeedback
EMG biofeedback measures neuromuscular contractions and provides auditory or visual feedback signals designed to increase awareness and voluntary control of muscle activation. As was previously discussed, EMG biofeedback has no proven role for targeted VMO strengthening in the management of PFP.[106–108] However, there is limited evidence to suggest its utility in promoting VMO activation patterns. When combined with therapeutic exercise, EMG biofeedback aimed at increasing VMO activation while maintaining constant VL activity and has been shown to improve VMO:VL activation ratios.[109] Given the correlation between patellar maltracking and delayed VMO activation,[34,35] it may be reasonably inferred that EMG biofeedback could improve VMO activation and in turn PFP, especially among identified patellar maltrackers. Controlled trials in this regard are lacking, and certainly further research is necessary to confirm this notion.

Taping
Patellar taping represents a common adjuvant in the management of PFP, with a variety of taping methods reported in the literature. The tailored McConnell taping technique perhaps offers the greatest merit, aimed at controlling patellar tilt, glide, or spin based on physical examination findings.[110] This method has been shown to increase VMO activity and augment temporal activation of the VMO.[111,112] In addition, McConnell taping seems to enhance patellar position within the trochlear groove and increase patellofemoral contact area under dynamic MRI.[113] It has been suggested that improved contact area produces a wider distribution of forces across the patella and may relieve contact in sensitive areas, thereby reducing PFP.[114] The explicit impact of McConnell taping to promote pain reduction and function has been demonstrated in several studies.[115,116] Whittingham and colleagues[116] found that pain and function scores were significantly better among patients managed with a combination of McConnell taping and exercise when compared with patients managed with placebo taping and exercise or exercise alone. Mason and colleagues[115] evaluated the effect of quadriceps strengthening, quadriceps stretching, and McConnell taping in isolation and in combination. Although improvements in pain and strength were demonstrated across all intervention groups in isolation, more significant and pervasive improvements were observed when the 3 modalities were combined. Current consensus guidelines purport level 1 evidence for the role of medially directed patellar

taping in immediate pain reduction for PFP. It is suggested that this has value to gain patient trust, facilitate active engagement, and optimize outcomes.[103]

Bracing

Patellar braces have likewise been proposed to modify patellofemoral kinematics and in turn improve PFP.[114,117] Medially directed patellofemoral stabilization braces, in particular, demonstrate reduced lateral translation and tilt of the patella, although it is worth noting that alignment is not fully restored to normal with bracing alone.[114,117] Furthermore, such braces, akin to taping, seem to increase patellofemoral contact area, which is suggested to be a driving factor in pain reduction.[114] Immediate pain reduction following application of a brace has been reported.[114] In fact, current guidelines suggest strong evidence in support of patellar braces for immediate pain reduction in PFP.[103] However, the longer-term impact of patellar bracing is debated.[103,118,119] This debate may reflect inconsistencies in patient selection or the type of brace used. A recent investigation demonstrated minimal accord among specialists regarding the criteria to prescribe a patellofemoral brace.[120] Although further studies are needed to clarify the most appropriate subpopulations for brace utilization, a properly fitted patellar stabilization brace is considered good practice, especially in those patients with documented patellar maltracking or for whom taping may be inappropriate (for example, due to skin irritation).[103]

Stretching/flexibility

Based on the apparent association between muscle inflexibility and PFP, it is logical to incorporate stretching procedures as a part of the rehabilitation prescription, especially for those individuals who reveal muscle tightness on physical examination. Evidence to support lower limb stretching in isolation is lacking; however, generalized stretching protocols comprising the quadriceps, hamstring, gastrocnemius, and iliotibial band, when combined with an exercise program, have established benefit. In a randomized, controlled single-blind trial, Moyano and colleagues[121] demonstrated significant reductions in pain among individuals managed with a stretching routine combined with strengthening or aerobic exercise. Proprioceptive neuromuscular facilitation stretching in particular, a technique combining passive and isometric stretching, may yield enhanced pain control and function. Halabchi and colleagues[95] also demonstrated that an individualized rehabilitation regimen incorporating targeted stretching for individuals who demonstrated inflexibility on examination resulted in significantly greater improvements in pain and function. Further investigation is necessary to identify whether specific muscles or stretches are more significant in PFP. Nevertheless, available evidence indicates that, particularly in instances of demonstrable inflexibility, it is prudent to include stretching of the quadriceps, gastrocnemius, hamstring, or iliotibial band in the treatment of PFP. Given the role of the iliotibial tract on lateral patellar tilt and compression, an emphasis on relieving iliotibial band tightness may prove particularly high yield, especially in individuals with concurrent tightness of the lateral retinaculum and paterllar tilt on examination.[94]

Hip strengthening

Although controversy exists regarding the cause-and-effect relationship of hip weakness and PFP, it is clear that weakness of the hip abductors and external rotators exists commonly in patients with PFP.[39,45,46,54] Therefore, irrespective of cause or consequence, it stands to reason that hip strengthening would play an important role in PFP rehabilitation; this is supported by an increasing body of evidence, especially among women with PFP. Nakagawa and colleagues[51] published the first randomized controlled trial investigating the utility of a hip strengthening protocol. This study demonstrated that the addition of hip abductor and external rotator strength exercises to a traditional rehabilitation program resulted in less pain and improved gluteus medius neuromuscular activation.[51] Since that time, 4 additional randomized controlled trials have supported hip strengthening in reducing PFP and optimizing function in women with PFP.[47–50] Importantly, when compared with knee stretching and strengthening alone, the addition of targeted hip exercise seems to provide more lasting benefits at 1 year and minimizes the risk of pain relapse.[49] This finding is further supported by a recent *Cochrane Review*, which upholds the combination of hip and knee exercises when compared with knee exercise alone in the treatment of PFP.[122] Thus, targeted hip muscle strengthening is encouraged for PFP rehabilitation, particularly in women who demonstrate static or dynamic evidence of hip weakness and medial femoral collapse on physical examination.

Foot orthoses

The precise role of foot orthoses in the management of PFP remains somewhat ambiguous. As was previously discussed, excessive pronation seems to represent one possible risk factor for the development of PFP. However, results of foot orthoses to correct overpronation in the management of PFP have been mixed. Some studies have indicated positive effects in both pain reduction and functional performance immediately following use[123] and over a period of time up to 3 months.[124,125] On the other hand, in a randomized controlled trial comparing the efficacy of prefabricated foot orthoses, flat inserts, and physical therapy, Collins and colleagues[126] failed to distinguish any cumulative benefit from the addition of a prefabricated orthosis to a standard physical therapy program when treating PFP. Moreover, evidence supporting the use of foot orthoses in PFP according to several systematic reviews is at best limited.[127,128] A recent *Cochrane Review* concluded that "while foot orthoses may help relieve knee pain over the short term, the benefit may be marginal."[129]

Several issues may explain the discrepancies and minimal effects of foot orthoses reported in the literature, including underpowered sample sizes[130] and a failure to screen for lower-extremity mechanics that may influence response to an orthosis. Predictors for response to foot orthoses include lower baseline pain levels, increased midfoot mobility (change in midfoot width between non-weight-bearing and weight-bearing), reduced ankle dorsiflexion, and use of less supportive shoes.[131,132] In addition, it has been suggested that those who report immediate pain reduction with an orthosis when performing a single-leg squat are more likely to benefit from one.[123,131] Although there are no specific criteria to identify those individuals who warrant a trial of an orthosis in the management of PFP, it is reasonable to trial an orthosis in conjunction with, or following, an appropriate course of physical therapy in individuals with excessive pronation on dynamic examination.[103] If an over-the-counter orthosis is not sufficient, a custom, full-contact orthosis with a stiffer medial heel wedge may be indicated.[133,134]

Gait retraining

Despite a lack of objective evidence, expert opinions endorse movement pattern and gait retraining in the management of PFP.[103] Several case series have aimed to reduce dynamic hip adduction and internal rotation through a variety of mechanisms, including visual feedback from an instrumented treadmill,[135] real-time hip adduction measurements,[63] adoption of a forefoot strike pattern[136] and direct mirror feedback.[137] All of these have promise in the treatment of PFP-associated gait aberrations, reporting both biomechanical and clinical success.

Additional efforts to reduce ground reaction forces and transmitted patellofemoral stress through gait modification have been investigated. Higher step-rate has been associated with a decreased foot inclination angle, step length, center of mass vertical excursion, and horizontal distance from center of mass and heel at initial contact.[65,66] As well, barefoot running has been shown to reduce patellofemoral joint reaction forces and, in turn, patellofemoral stress.[67]

Although each of these interventions imply potential benefits, additional trials are necessary to establish the safest and most effective clinical approach to gait retraining in PFP.

Correcting training errors

Initial management of the runner with PFP must emphasize activity modification to a pain-free level.[17] Activity modification is important in both controlling pain and stimulating recovery. During this period, it is also critical to analyze the runner's training program for any overt errors, including increasing exercise intensity too quickly, inadequate time for recovery, and excessive hill work.[133] The athlete must be educated regarding safe training to promote recovery and, more notably, to prevent recurrence. As a general rule, most experts conservatively recommend increases in volume or intensity of no more than 10% per week, although a recent study proposed that increases of up to 30% over 2 weeks may be equally safe.[71] Activity should not be reintroduced or advanced beyond a rate that can be reasonably tolerated without reproduction of pain or associated symptoms. A mild hill incline is usually well tolerated, although downhill running is typically problematic.

SUMMARY

In summary, PFP is a common and potentially debilitating ailment among runners. Its origin seems to be multifactorial and successful treatment mandates a comprehensive yet customized approach, targeting those risk factors unique to the individual. In addition to biomechanical corrections, activity modification to a pain-free level is critical for the runner especially. As well, any errors in training must be acknowledged and corrected before return to sport. Gait retraining is an emerging area in PFP research that shows great promise and is likely to prove particularly relevant for the runner in the management of this condition. Further research is yet needed to clarify the safest and most effective methods of gait retraining in the management of PFP.

REFERENCES

1. Devereaux MD, Lachmann SM. Patello-femoral arthralgia in athletes attending a sports injury clinic. Br J Sports Med 1984;18(1):18–21.
2. Fallon KE. Musculoskeletal injuries in the ultramarathon: the 1990 Westfield Sydney to Melbourne run. Br J Sports Med 1996;30(4):319–23.
3. Fields KB. Running injuries - changing trends and demographics. Curr Sports Med Rep 2011;10(5):299–303.
4. Fredericson M, Misra AK. Epidemiology and aetiology of marathon running injuries. Sports Med 2007;37(4–5):437–9.
5. Taunton JE, Ryan MB, Clement DB, et al. A retrospective case-control analysis of 2002 running injuries. Br J Sports Med 2002;36(2):95–101.
6. Scheer BV, Murray A. Al Andalus Ultra Trail: an observation of medical interventions during a 219-km, 5-day ultramarathon stage race. Clin J Sport Med 2011; 21(5):444–6.

7. DeHaven KE, Lintner DM. Athletic injuries: comparison by age, sport, and gender. Am J Sports Med 1986;14(3):218–24.
8. Stracciolini A, Casciano R, Levey Friedman H, et al. Pediatric sports injuries: a comparison of males versus females. Am J Sports Med 2014; 42(4):965–72.
9. Boling M, Padua D, Marshall S, et al. Gender differences in the incidence and prevalence of patellofemoral pain syndrome. Scand J Med Sci Sports 2010; 20(5):725–30.
10. Besier TF, Pal S, Draper CE, et al. The role of cartilage stress in patellofemoral pain. Med Sci Sports Exerc 2015;1. http://dx.doi.org/10.1249/MSS.0000000000000685.
11. Draper CE, Besier TF, Gold GE, et al. Is cartilage thickness different in young subjects with and without patellofemoral pain? Osteoarthritis Cartilage 2006; 14(9):931–7.
12. Farrokhi S, Keyak JH, Powers CM. Individuals with patellofemoral pain exhibit greater patellofemoral joint stress: a finite element analysis study. Osteoarthritis Cartilage 2011;19(3):287–94.
13. Boles CA, Ferguson C. The female athlete. Radiol Clin North Am 2010;48(6): 1249–66.
14. Leetun DT, Ireland ML, Willson JD, et al. Core stability measures as risk factors for lower extremity injury in athletes. Med Sci Sports Exerc 2004;36(6): 926–34.
15. Boling MC, Padua DA, Marshall SW, et al. A prospective investigation of biomechanical risk factors for patellofemoral pain syndrome: the Joint Undertaking to Monitor and Prevent ACL Injury (JUMP-ACL) cohort. Am J Sports Med 2009; 37(11):2108–16.
16. McKean KA, Manson NA, Stanish WD. Musculoskeletal injury in the masters runners. Clin J Sport Med 2006;16(2):149–54.
17. Dye SF. The pathophysiology of patellofemoral pain: a tissue homeostasis perspective. Clin Orthop 2005;436:100–10.
18. McConnell J. The physical therapist's approach to patellofemoral disorders. Clin Sports Med 2002;21(3):363–87.
19. Dvir Z, Shklar A, Halperin N, et al. Concentric and eccentric torque variations of the quadriceps femoris in patellofemoral pain syndrome. Clin Biomech (Bristol, Avon) 1990;5(2):68–72.
20. Kaya D, Citaker S, Kerimoglu U, et al. Women with patellofemoral pain syndrome have quadriceps femoris volume and strength deficiency. Knee Surg Sports Traumatol Arthrosc 2011;19(2):242–7.
21. Werner S. An evaluation of knee extensor and knee flexor torques and EMGs in patients with patellofemoral pain syndrome in comparison with matched controls. Knee Surg Sports Traumatol Arthrosc 1995;3(2):89–94.
22. Callaghan MJ. Quadriceps atrophy: to what extent does it exist in patellofemoral pain syndrome? Br J Sports Med 2004;38(3):295–9.
23. Giles LS, Webster KE, McClelland JA, et al. Does quadriceps atrophy exist in individuals with patellofemoral pain? A systematic literature review with meta-analysis. J Orthop Sports Phys Ther 2013;43(11):766–76.
24. Farahmand F, Senavongse W, Amis AA. Quantitative study of the quadriceps muscles and trochlear groove geometry related to instability of the patellofemoral joint. J Orthop Res 1998;16(1):136–43.
25. Lin F, Wang G, Koh JL, et al. In vivo and noninvasive three-dimensional patellar tracking induced by individual heads of quadriceps. Med Sci Sports Exerc 2004;36(1):93–101.

26. Jan M-H, Lin D-H, Lin J-J, et al. Differences in sonographic characteristics of the vastus medialis obliquus between patients with patellofemoral pain syndrome and healthy adults. Am J Sports Med 2009;37(9):1743–9.
27. Pattyn E, Verdonk P, Steyaert A, et al. Vastus medialis obliquus atrophy: does it exist in patellofemoral pain syndrome? Am J Sports Med 2011;39(7):1450–5.
28. Milgrom C, Finestone A, Eldad A, et al. Patellofemoral pain caused by overactivity. A prospective study of risk factors in infantry recruits. J Bone Joint Surg Am 1991;73(7):1041–3.
29. Pappas E, Wong-Tom WM. Prospective predictors of patellofemoral pain syndrome: a systematic review with meta-analysis. Sports Health 2012;4(2): 115–20.
30. Chester R, Smith TO, Sweeting D, et al. The relative timing of VMO and VL in the aetiology of anterior knee pain: a systematic review and meta-analysis. BMC Musculoskelet Disord 2008;9:64.
31. Cowan SM, Hodges PW, Bennell KL, et al. Altered vastii recruitment when people with patellofemoral pain syndrome complete a postural task. Arch Phys Med Rehabil 2002;83(7):989–95.
32. Voight ML, Wieder DL. Comparative reflex response times of vastus medialis obliquus and vastus lateralis in normal subjects and subjects with extensor mechanism dysfunction. An electromyographic study. Am J Sports Med 1991;19(2): 131–7.
33. Witvrouw E, Sneyers C, Lysens R, et al. Reflex response times of vastus medialis oblique and vastus lateralis in normal subjects and in subjects with patellofemoral pain syndrome. J Orthop Sports Phys Ther 1996;24(3):160–5.
34. Pal S, Besier TF, Draper CE, et al. Patellar tilt correlates with vastus lateralis: vastus medialis activation ratio in maltracking patellofemoral pain patients. J Orthop Res 2012;30(6):927–33.
35. Pal S, Draper CE, Fredericson M, et al. Patellar maltracking correlates with vastus medialis activation delay in patellofemoral pain patients. Am J Sports Med 2011;39(3):590–8.
36. Hudson Z, Darthuy E. Iliotibial band tightness and patellofemoral pain syndrome: a case-control study. Man Ther 2009;14(2):147–51.
37. Puniello MS. Iliotibial band tightness and medial patellar glide in patients with patellofemoral dysfunction. J Orthop Sports Phys Ther 1993;17(3):144–8.
38. Waryasz GR, McDermott AY. Patellofemoral pain syndrome (PFPS): a systematic review of anatomy and potential risk factors. Dyn Med 2008;7:9.
39. Piva SR, Goodnite EA, Childs JD. Strength around the hip and flexibility of soft tissues in individuals with and without patellofemoral pain syndrome. J Orthop Sports Phys Ther 2005;35(12):793–801.
40. Witvrouw E, Lysens R, Bellemans J, et al. Intrinsic risk factors for the development of anterior knee pain in an athletic population. A two-year prospective study. Am J Sports Med 2000;28(4):480–9.
41. White LC, Dolphin P, Dixon J. Hamstring length in patellofemoral pain syndrome. Physiotherapy 2009;95(1):24–8.
42. Kwon O, Yun M, Lee W. Correlation between intrinsic patellofemoral pain syndrome in young adults and lower extremity biomechanics. J Phys Ther Sci 2014;26(7):961–4.
43. Powers CM, Ward SR, Fredericson M, et al. Patellofemoral kinematics during weight-bearing and non-weight-bearing knee extension in persons with lateral subluxation of the patella: a preliminary study. J Orthop Sports Phys Ther 2003;33(11):677–85.

44. Souza RB, Draper CE, Fredericson M, et al. Femur rotation and patellofemoral joint kinematics: a weight-bearing magnetic resonance imaging analysis. J Orthop Sports Phys Ther 2010;40(5):277–85.
45. Bolgla LA, Malone TR, Umberger BR, et al. Hip strength and hip and knee kinematics during stair descent in females with and without patellofemoral pain syndrome. J Orthop Sports Phys Ther 2008;38(1):12–8.
46. Ireland ML, Willson JD, Ballantyne BT, et al. Hip strength in females with and without patellofemoral pain. J Orthop Sports Phys Ther 2003;33(11):671–6.
47. Dolak KL, Silkman C, Medina McKeon J, et al. Hip strengthening prior to functional exercises reduces pain sooner than quadriceps strengthening in females with patellofemoral pain syndrome: a randomized clinical trial. J Orthop Sports Phys Ther 2011;41(8):560–70.
48. Fukuda TY, Rossetto FM, Magalhães E, et al. Short-term effects of hip abductors and lateral rotators strengthening in females with patellofemoral pain syndrome: a randomized controlled clinical trial. J Orthop Sports Phys Ther 2010;40(11): 736–42.
49. Fukuda TY, Melo WP, Zaffalon BM, et al. Hip posterolateral musculature strengthening in sedentary women with patellofemoral pain syndrome: a randomized controlled clinical trial with 1-year follow-up. J Orthop Sports Phys Ther 2012;42(10):823–30.
50. Khayambashi K, Mohammadkhani Z, Ghaznavi K, et al. The effects of isolated hip abductor and external rotator muscle strengthening on pain, health status, and hip strength in females with patellofemoral pain: a randomized controlled trial. J Orthop Sports Phys Ther 2012;42(1):22–9.
51. Nakagawa TH, Muniz TB, Baldon Rde M, et al. The effect of additional strengthening of hip abductor and lateral rotator muscles in patellofemoral pain syndrome: a randomized controlled pilot study. Clin Rehabil 2008;22(12):1051–60.
52. Thijs Y, Pattyn E, Van Tiggelen D, et al. Is hip muscle weakness a predisposing factor for patellofemoral pain in female novice runners? A prospective study. Am J Sports Med 2011;39(9):1877–82.
53. Rathleff MS, Rathleff CR, Crossley KM, et al. Is hip strength a risk factor for patellofemoral pain? A systematic review and meta-analysis. Br J Sports Med 2014;48(14):1088.
54. Finnoff JT, Hall MM, Kyle K, et al. Hip strength and knee pain in high school runners: a prospective study. PM R 2011;3(9):792–801.
55. Earl JE, Hoch AZ. A proximal strengthening program improves pain, function, and biomechanics in women with patellofemoral pain syndrome. Am J Sports Med 2011;39(1):154–63.
56. Willy RW, Davis IS. The effect of a hip-strengthening program on mechanics during running and during a single-leg squat. J Orthop Sports Phys Ther 2011; 41(9):625–32.
57. Tiberio D. The effect of excessive subtalar joint pronation on patellofemoral mechanics: a theoretical model. J Orthop Sports Phys Ther 1987;9(4):160–5.
58. Hetsroni I, Finestone A, Milgrom C, et al. A prospective biomechanical study of the association between foot pronation and the incidence of anterior knee pain among military recruits. J Bone Joint Surg Br 2006;88(7):905–8.
59. Neal BS, Griffiths IB, Dowling GJ, et al. Foot posture as a risk factor for lower limb overuse injury: a systematic review and meta-analysis. J Foot Ankle Res 2014;7(1):55.
60. Thijs Y, De Clercq D, Roosen P, et al. Gait-related intrinsic risk factors for patellofemoral pain in novice recreational runners. Br J Sports Med 2008;42(6):466–71.

61. Nakagawa TH, Moriya ÉTU, Maciel CD, et al. Trunk, pelvis, hip, and knee kinematics, hip strength, and gluteal muscle activation during a single-leg squat in males and females with and without patellofemoral pain syndrome. J Orthop Sports Phys Ther 2012;42(6):491–501.
62. Souza RB, Powers CM. Differences in hip kinematics, muscle strength, and muscle activation between subjects with and without patellofemoral pain. J Orthop Sports Phys Ther 2009;39(1):12–9.
63. Noehren B, Scholz J, Davis I. The effect of real-time gait retraining on hip kinematics, pain and function in subjects with patellofemoral pain syndrome. Br J Sports Med 2011;45(9):691–6.
64. Rodrigues P, TenBroek T, Van Emmerik R, et al. Evaluating runners with and without anterior knee pain using the time to contact the ankle joint complexes' range of motion boundary. Gait Posture 2014;39(1):48–53.
65. Heiderscheit BC, Chumanov ES, Michalski MP, et al. Effects of step rate manipulation on joint mechanics during running. Med Sci Sports Exerc 2011;43(2):296–302.
66. Lenhart RL, Thelen DG, Wille CM, et al. Increasing running step rate reduces patellofemoral joint forces. Med Sci Sports Exerc 2014;46(3):557–64.
67. Bonacci J, Vicenzino B, Spratford W, et al. Take your shoes off to reduce patellofemoral joint stress during running. Br J Sports Med 2014;48(6):425–8.
68. Fredericson M. Common injuries in runners. Diagnosis, rehabilitation and prevention. Sports Med 1996;21(1):49–72.
69. Macera CA, Pate RR, Powell KE, et al. Predicting lower-extremity injuries among habitual runners. Arch Intern Med 1989;149(11):2565–8.
70. Marti B, Vader JP, Minder CE, et al. On the epidemiology of running injuries. The 1984 Bern Grand-Prix study. Am J Sports Med 1988;16(3):285–94.
71. Nielsen RØ, Parner ET, Nohr EA, et al. Excessive progression in weekly running distance and risk of running-related injuries: an association which varies according to type of injury. J Orthop Sports Phys Ther 2014;44(10):739–47.
72. Walter SD, Hart LE, McIntosh JM, et al. The Ontario cohort study of running-related injuries. Arch Intern Med 1989;149(11):2561–4.
73. al-Rawi Z, Nessan AH. Joint hypermobility in patients with chondromalacia patellae. Br J Rheumatol 1997;36(12):1324–7.
74. Green S. Patellofemoral syndrome. J Bodyw Mov Ther 2005;9:16–26.
75. Fairbank JC, Pynsent PB, van Poortvliet JA, et al. Mechanical factors in the incidence of knee pain in adolescents and young adults. J Bone Joint Surg Br 1984;66(5):685–93.
76. Andriacchi TP, Andersson GB, Fermier RW, et al. A study of lower-limb mechanics during stair-climbing. J Bone Joint Surg Am 1980;62(5):749–57.
77. Lester JD, Watson JN, Hutchinson MR. Physical examination of the patellofemoral joint. Clin Sports Med 2014;33(3):403–12.
78. Barton CJ, Bonanno D, Levinger P, et al. Foot and ankle characteristics in patellofemoral pain syndrome: a case control and reliability study. J Orthop Sports Phys Ther 2010;40(5):286–96.
79. Boyle KL, Witt P, Riegger-Krugh C. Intrarater and interrater reliability of the Beighton and Horan joint mobility index. J Athl Train 2003;38(4):281–5.
80. Herrington L. Knee valgus angle during single leg squat and landing in patellofemoral pain patients and controls. Knee 2014;21(2):514–7.
81. Myer GD, Ford KR, Barber Foss KD, et al. The incidence and potential pathomechanics of patellofemoral pain in female athletes. Clin Biomech 2010;25(7):700–7.

82. Fredericson M, Yoon K. Physical examination and patellofemoral pain syndrome. Am J Phys Med Rehabil 2006;85(3):234–43.
83. Post WR. Clinical evaluation of patients with patellofemoral disorders. Arthroscopy 1999;15(8):841–51.
84. Halabchi F, Mazaheri R, Seif-Barghi T. Patellofemoral pain syndrome and modifiable intrinsic risk factors; how to assess and address? Asian J Sports Med 2013; 4(2):85–100.
85. Draper CE, Chew KTL, Wang R, et al. Comparison of quadriceps angle measurements using short-arm and long-arm goniometers: correlation with MRI. PM R 2011;3(2):111–6.
86. Fulkerson JP. Awareness of the retinaculum in evaluating patellofemoral pain. Am J Sports Med 1982;10(3):147–9.
87. Watson CJ, Propps M, Galt W, et al. Reliability of McConnell's classification of patellar orientation in symptomatic and asymptomatic subjects. J Orthop Sports Phys Ther 1999;29(7):378–85 [discussion: 386–93].
88. Tomsich DA, Nitz AJ, Threlkeld AJ, et al. Patellofemoral alignment: reliability. J Orthop Sports Phys Ther 1996;23(3):200–8.
89. Elias D, White L. Imaging of patellofemoral disorders. Clin Radiol 2004;59(7): 543–57.
90. Schulz B, Brown M, Ahmad CS. Evaluation and imaging of patellofemoral joint disorders. Oper Tech Sports Med 2010;18(2):68–78.
91. Pal S, Besier TF, Beaupre GS, et al. Patellar maltracking is prevalent among patellofemoral pain subjects with patella alta: an upright, weightbearing MRI study. J Orthop Res 2013;31(3):448–57.
92. Stefanik JJ, Zumwalt AC, Segal NA, et al. Association between measures of patella height, morphologic features of the trochlea, and patellofemoral joint alignment: the MOST study. Clin Orthop Relat Res 2013;471(8):2641–8.
93. Stathopulu E, Baildam E. Anterior knee pain: a long-term follow-up. Rheumatology (Oxford) 2003;42(2):380–2.
94. Dutton RA, Khadavi MJ, Fredericson M. Update on rehabilitation of patellofemoral pain. Curr Sports Med Rep 2014;13(3):172–8.
95. Halabchi F, Mazaheri R, Mansournia MA, et al. Additional effects of an individualized risk factor-based approach on pain and the function of patients with patellofemoral pain syndrome: a randomized controlled trial. Clin J Sport Med 2015. http://dx.doi.org/10.1097/JSM.0000000000000177.
96. Selhorst M, Rice W, Degenhart T, et al. Evaluation of a treatment algorithm for patients with patellofemoral pain syndrome: a pilot study. Int J Sports Phys Ther 2015;10(2):178–88.
97. Kooiker L, Van De Port IGL, Weir A, et al. Effects of physical therapist-guided quadriceps-strengthening exercises for the treatment of patellofemoral pain syndrome: a systematic review. J Orthop Sports Phys Ther 2014;44(6). 391–B1.
98. Escamilla RF, Fleisig GS, Zheng N, et al. Biomechanics of the knee during closed kinetic chain and open kinetic chain exercises. Med Sci Sports Exerc 1998;30(4):556–69.
99. Steinkamp LA, Dillingham MF, Markel MD, et al. Biomechanical considerations in patellofemoral joint rehabilitation. Am J Sports Med 1993;21(3):438–44.
100. Bakhtiary AH, Fatemi E. Open versus closed kinetic chain exercises for patellar chondromalacia. Br J Sports Med 2008;42(2):99–102 [discussion: 102].
101. Stiene HA, Brosky T, Reinking MF, et al. A comparison of closed kinetic chain and isokinetic joint isolation exercise in patients with patellofemoral dysfunction. J Orthop Sports Phys Ther 1996;24(3):136–41.

102. Witvrouw E, Lysens R, Bellemans J, et al. Open versus closed kinetic chain exercises for patellofemoral pain. A prospective, randomized study. Am J Sports Med 2000;28(5):687–94.
103. Barton CJ, Lack S, Hemmings S, et al. The "best practice guide to conservative management of patellofemoral pain": incorporating level 1 evidence with expert clinical reasoning. Br J Sports Med 2015;49(14):923–34.
104. Collado H, Fredericson M. Patellofemoral pain syndrome. Clin Sports Med 2010; 29(3):379–98.
105. Song C-Y, Lin Y-F, Wei T-C, et al. Surplus value of hip adduction in leg-press exercise in patients with patellofemoral pain syndrome: a randomized controlled trial. Phys Ther 2009;89(5):409–18.
106. Dursun N, Dursun E, Kiliç Z. Electromyographic biofeedback-controlled exercise versus conservative care for patellofemoral pain syndrome. Arch Phys Med Rehabil 2001;82(12):1692–5.
107. Syme G, Rowe P, Martin D, et al. Disability in patients with chronic patellofemoral pain syndrome: a randomised controlled trial of VMO selective training versus general quadriceps strengthening. Man Ther 2009;14(3):252–63.
108. Yip SLM, Ng GYF. Biofeedback supplementation to physiotherapy exercise programme for rehabilitation of patellofemoral pain syndrome: a randomized controlled pilot study. Clin Rehabil 2006;20(12):1050–7.
109. Ng GYF, Zhang AQ, Li CK. Biofeedback exercise improved the EMG activity ratio of the medial and lateral vasti muscles in subjects with patellofemoral pain syndrome. J Electromyogr Kinesiol 2008;18(1):128–33.
110. Crossley K, Cowan SM, Bennell KL, et al. Patellar taping: is clinical success supported by scientific evidence? Man Ther 2000;5(3):142–50.
111. Christou EA. Patellar taping increases vastus medialis oblique activity in the presence of patellofemoral pain. J Electromyogr Kinesiol 2004;14(4):495–504.
112. Cowan SM, Bennell KL, Hodges PW. Therapeutic patellar taping changes the timing of vasti muscle activation in people with patellofemoral pain syndrome. Clin J Sport Med 2002;12(6):339–47.
113. Derasari A, Brindle TJ, Alter KE, et al. McConnell taping shifts the patella inferiorly in patients with patellofemoral pain: a dynamic magnetic resonance imaging study. Phys Ther 2010;90(3):411–9.
114. Powers CM, Ward SR, Chan L-D, et al. The effect of bracing on patella alignment and patellofemoral joint contact area. Med Sci Sports Exerc 2004;36(7): 1226–32.
115. Mason M, Keays SL, Newcombe PA. The effect of taping, quadriceps strengthening and stretching prescribed separately or combined on patellofemoral pain. Physiother Res Int 2011;16(2):109–19.
116. Whittingham M, Palmer S, Macmillan F. Effects of taping on pain and function in patellofemoral pain syndrome: a randomized controlled trial. J Orthop Sports Phys Ther 2004;34(9):504–10.
117. Draper CE, Besier TF, Santos JM, et al. Using real-time MRI to quantify altered joint kinematics in subjects with patellofemoral pain and to evaluate the effects of a patellar brace or sleeve on joint motion. J Orthop Res 2009;27(5):571–7.
118. Arazpour M, Notarki TT, Salimi A, et al. The effect of patellofemoral bracing on walking in individuals with patellofemoral pain syndrome. Prosthet Orthot Int 2013;37(6):465–70.
119. Miller MD, Hinkin DT, Wisnowski JW. The efficacy of orthotics for anterior knee pain in military trainees. A preliminary report. Am J Knee Surg 1997; 10(1):10–3.

120. Solinsky R, Beaupre GS, Fredericson M. Variable criteria for patellofemoral bracing among sports medicine professionals. PM R 2014;6(6):498–505.
121. Moyano FR, Valenza MC, Martin LM, et al. Effectiveness of different exercises and stretching physiotherapy on pain and movement in patellofemoral pain syndrome: a randomized controlled trial. Clin Rehabil 2013;27(5):409–17.
122. Van der Heijden RA, Lankhorst NE, van Linschoten R, et al. Exercise for treating patellofemoral pain syndrome. Cochrane Database Syst Rev 2015;(1):CD010387.
123. Barton CJ, Menz HB, Crossley KM. The immediate effects of foot orthoses on functional performance in individuals with patellofemoral pain syndrome. Br J Sports Med 2011;45(3):193–7.
124. Barton CJ, Menz HB, Crossley KM. Effects of prefabricated foot orthoses on pain and function in individuals with patellofemoral pain syndrome: a cohort study. Phys Ther Sport 2011;12(2):70–5.
125. Johnston LB, Gross MT. Effects of foot orthoses on quality of life for individuals with patellofemoral pain syndrome. J Orthop Sports Phys Ther 2004;34(8): 440–8.
126. Collins N, Crossley K, Beller E, et al. Foot orthoses and physiotherapy in the treatment of patellofemoral pain syndrome: randomised clinical trial. Br J Sports Med 2009;43(3):169–71.
127. Barton CJ, Munteanu SE, Menz HB, et al. The efficacy of foot orthoses in the treatment of individuals with patellofemoral pain syndrome: a systematic review. Sports Med 2010;40(5):377–95.
128. Swart NM, van Linschoten R, Bierma-Zeinstra SMA, et al. The additional effect of orthotic devices on exercise therapy for patients with patellofemoral pain syndrome: a systematic review. Br J Sports Med 2012;46(8):570–7.
129. Hossain M, Alexander P, Burls A, et al. Foot orthoses for patellofemoral pain in adults. Cochrane Database of Systematic Reviews 2011;1. Art. No.:CD008402. http://dx.doi.org/10.1002/14651858.CD008402.pub2.
130. Collins NJ, Bisset LM, Crossley KM, et al. Efficacy of nonsurgical interventions for anterior knee pain: systematic review and meta-analysis of randomized trials. Sports Med 2012;42(1):31–49.
131. Barton CJ, Menz HB, Crossley KM. Clinical predictors of foot orthoses efficacy in individuals with patellofemoral pain. Med Sci Sports Exerc 2011;43(9): 1603–10.
132. Vicenzino B, Collins N, Cleland J, et al. A clinical prediction rule for identifying patients with patellofemoral pain who are likely to benefit from foot orthoses: a preliminary determination. Br J Sports Med 2010;44(12):862–6.
133. Fredericson M, Powers CM. Practical management of patellofemoral pain. Clin J Sport Med 2002;12(1):36–8.
134. Powers CM, Berke GM, Clary MD, et al. Patellofemoral pain: is there a role for orthoses? PM R 2010;2(8):771–6.
135. Crowell HP, Milner CE, Hamill J, et al. Reducing impact loading during running with the use of real-time visual feedback. J Orthop Sports Phys Ther 2010;40(4): 206–13.
136. Cheung RTH, Davis IS. Landing pattern modification to improve patellofemoral pain in runners: a case series. J Orthop Sports Phys Ther 2011;41(12):914–9.
137. Willy RW, Scholz JP, Davis IS. Mirror gait retraining for the treatment of patellofemoral pain in female runners. Clin Biomech (Bristol, Avon) 2012;27(10): 1045–51.

Iliotibial Band Syndrome in Runners

Biomechanical Implications and Exercise Interventions

Robert L. Baker, BS, MBA[a],*, Michael Fredericson, MD[b]

KEYWORDS

- Iliotibial band syndrome • Biomechanics • Running • Exercises • Strength

KEY POINTS

- Iliotibial band syndrome is the most common cause of lateral knee pain in runners, but needs further epidemiologic study to better understand differences among various types of runners.
- Contributing factors include strain and strain rate, kinematic deviations in the frontal and transverse plane, and weakness in the lateral and posterior hip musculature.
- The pathophysiology has 2 models, enthesopathy and compression versus impingement and friction.
- Neuromuscular coordination is a developing area of interest as a contributing factor and training method.
- Exercises are debated regarding the effect on changing running mechanics with attention to dosing and postures.

INTRODUCTION

Iliotibial band syndrome (ITBS) has been reported as the second most common running injury and most common reason for lateral knee pain in runners[1] (Fig. 1). In a prospective study of 400 female runners over 4 years in the University of Delaware community, the reported incidence of ITBS was 16%.[2] Gender comparison has no definitive study, although Taunton and colleagues[1] analyzed 2002 consecutive running injuries in a Vancouver running clinic, finding 63 cases of ITBS in 926 males

---

Disclosure: No financial interests exist in the materials presented in this article. One illustration requires specific wording to credit JOSPT and Chris Powers as written under **Fig. 9**.
a Emeryville Sports Physical Therapy, 2322 Powell Street, Emeryville, CA 94608, USA;
b Orthopedic Medicine, Stanford University, Stanford, CA, USA
* Corresponding author.
E-mail address: Rb415@comcast.net

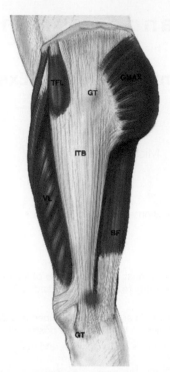

Fig. 1. Iliotibial band syndrome. Red mark indicates site of injury: insertion of the iliotibial band into and just proximal to the lateral femoral epicondyle. BF, biceps femoris; GMAX, gluteus maximus; GT, greater trochanter; ITB, iliotibial band; TFL, tensor fasciae latae; VL, vastus lateralis.

and 105 cases of ITBS in 1076 females, indicating 6.8% male prevalence and 9.8% female prevalence. Interestingly no contributing factors were identified among the following: varus and valgus knee, pes planus, pes cavus, Q angle, and leg length. Tenforde and colleagues[3] analyzed surveys for 442 female and 306 male runners aged 13 to 18 years old, finding lifetime self-reported prevalence of 7% female and 5% male. During an ultramarathon running event, Fallon[4] reported 3 cases of ITBS in 29 runners, translating to an incidence of 10.3%. Epidemiologic understanding is limited by a lack of prospective studies measuring the incidence of ITBS. In addition, information is limited regarding incidence and prevalence of ITBS in various running populations: elite versus casual; and triathlon, 5 to 10 km, marathon, and ultramarathon. It is possible that these varying populations have different contributing factors.

Runners inflicted with ITBS are challenged by lateral knee pain. The first well-documented cases were performed by Lieutenant Commander James Renne, a medical corps officer who documented on 16 ITBS cases out of 1000 military recruits.[5] The onset occurred most frequently at the lateral knee after 2 miles of running, or hiking over 10 miles. Walking with the knee extended relieved the symptoms. All of the patients had focal tenderness over the lateral femoral epicondyle at 30° of flexion, and 5 patients had an unusual palpation described as "rubbing of a finger over a wet balloon."

These descriptions were further clarified 5 years later in 1980 by Clive Noble.[6,7] In his South African clinic 100 consecutive cases of ITBS were evaluated. Ninety-eight percent of these injuries were in males of age range 19 to 48 years old. Six patients exhibited bilateral symptoms. In 21 cases, soft-tissue swelling was described over the lateral epicondyle of the femur. The pain was often reproduced by standing on the involved leg with knee flexed to 30°. Varus stress to the knee did not reproduce the symptoms, and intra-articular knee tests were negative for joint disorder. However, the confirmation test present in all cases was pain to pressure over the lateral femoral epicondyle region at 30° of knee flexion when moving from 90° of knee flexion, the Noble compression test.

ANATOMY

The iliotibial band has been a long-standing fascination of evolutionary biologists and functional anatomists. Emanuel Kaplan described the iliotibial band as an "independent structure," suggesting the description "anterolateral ligament of support."[8] The ligament was described as firmly attached to the lateral edge of the linea aspera of the femur and lateral femoral epicondyle, with distal course to the Gerdy tubercle. Fascial relationships were described among the iliotibial band, fascia lata, vastus lateralis, biceps femoris, and lateral surface of the tibia. With the tensor fascia lata and gluteus maximus as a focus, Kaplan determined through concentric muscle contraction by electrical stimulation that the role of the muscle was at the hip, and therefore that the function of the iliotibial band at the knee was ligamentous. However, this analysis lacked the current technology and research demonstrating isometric and eccentric control of femur rotation at the knee through muscle function at the hip.[9,10] Absent from Kaplan's explanation is the current understanding of torque-producing and postural muscles, where isometric stabilization at the lumbar spine and hip may be related to torque-producing muscle action for the knee.[11–13] Histologic and dissection study of the iliotibial band at the lateral femoral epicondyle and gluteus maximus and fascia lata suggest a mechanosensory role acting proximally on the anterolateral knee.[14,15] The mechanosensory role of the iliotibial band may affect the interpretation of the ligament versus tendon function of the iliotibial band from hip to lateral femoral epicondyle.[15]

The iliotibial band is a dynamic and multidimensional structure with relationships that span the lumbar spine to the anterolateral knee[15,16] (**Fig. 2**). Anatomic understanding of the iliotibial band was furthered functional anatomy descriptions of the gluteus maximus by Jack Stern.[17] Specifically, the upper gluteus maximus accounted for the vast changes in man in comparison with other primates. In particular, the human gluteus maximus is much heavier than that of other primates, with more cranial attachment to the ilium, sacrum, and multifidus fascia. This description is consistent with functional anatomy in other studies that have reported the upper gluteus maximus functioning in the frontal plane in synergy with the gluteus medius.[18] By contrast, the lower gluteus maximus has more control in the transverse plane, with deceleration along with the quadriceps and during acceleration at toe-off.[18,19] Stern and Kaplan perspectives offer a viewpoint that the upper regions of the iliotibial band have fascial connections from the lower back, sacrum, and ilium that connect by way of the gluteus maximus to the femur, fascia lata, and iliotibial band. These structural interrelationships are potentially relevant to understanding the strain on the iliotibial band, and treatment strategy.

Two theories compete for the anatomic explanation of iliotibial syndrome: compression and enthesopathy versus friction and impingement[14,20,21] (**Figs. 3** and **4**). Fairclough and colleagues[14] described a tendinous insertion into the region just proximal and over the lateral femoral epicondyle. This region was marked by a fan-shaped insertion into the periosteum with compression of fat, blood vessels, nerves,

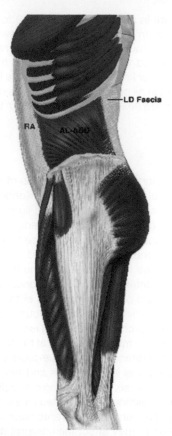

Fig. 2. Relationships of the iliotibial band lumbar spine to knee. The iliotibial band connects superiorly through the gluteus maximus to the lumbodorsal fascial; and inferiorly to the femur, vastus lateralis, lateral retinaculum knee, biceps femoris, and anterolateral tibia. The interactions of the iliotibial band suggest a coordinated effort among the structures of the lumbar spine, hip, femur, and knee, including the lumbodorsal fascia, gluteal fascia, fascia lata, and anterolateral knee. AL-ABD, anterolateral abdominals; LD Fascia, lumbodorsal fascia; RF, rectus abdominis.

and Pacinian corpuscles. The role of fat and Pacinian corpuscle needs further clarification in regard to monitoring velocity, pressure, and vibration, and effects on proximal musculature.[22–24] Abnormal tensioning and mechanosensory disturbance have biometric and training considerations. Orchard and colleagues[21] described a friction model in which the posterior fibers attach tightly to the femur and then glide over the lateral femoral epicondyle. This process occurs in an anterior to posterior direction during knee flexion.[25] This mechanism of anterior to posterior motion is related to normal tibia internal rotation, bowing of the vastus lateralis and biceps femoris, and tensioning of the fascia lata and iliotibial band.[14,21] The abnormal and excessive tensioning of the iliotibial band may be related to hypertonicity of the gluteus maximus,[15] increased activation of the tensor fascia lata and gluteus maximus,[15] and rapid rate of loading of the iliotibial band.[26,27]

The compression and friction models overlap. Jelsing and colleagues[25] demonstrated using sonographic evaluation that the iliotibial band at the lateral femoral

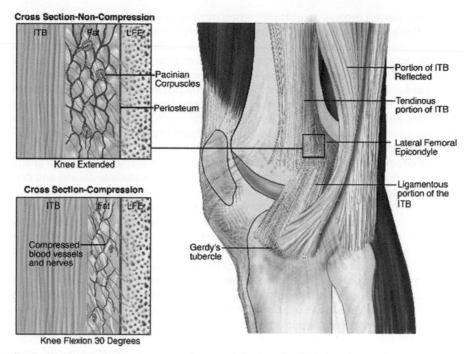

Fig. 3. Enthesopathy and compression model. ITB, iliotibial band; LFE, lateral femoral epicondyle.

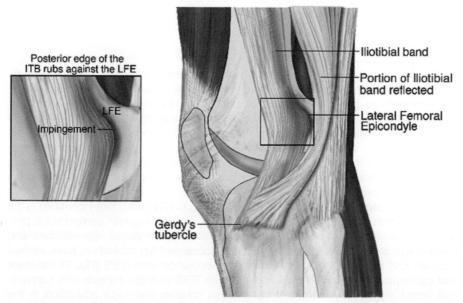

Fig. 4. Friction and impingement model. ITB, iliotibial band; LFE, lateral femoral epicondyle.

epicondyle moved anterior to posterior when moving from 0° to 30° and 45° of knee flexion. Participants included 20 subjects, including 5 men and 15 women. Iliotibial band borders were measured anteriorly (n = 20) and posteriorly (n = 4) in both supine and standing subjects. Posterior fibers were noted as more difficult to capture because of stronger blending into the fascia. These findings are consistent with those of Orchard and colleagues,[21] who reported that the posterior borders of the iliotibial band in 6 of 11 cadaver knees had anterior to lateral femoral epicondyle in full knee extension, with a high degree of variation in width. Both of these studies[21,25] draw attention to anatomic factors that support friction and impingement, and the unique posterior fiber attributes in ITBS.

The anatomic factors in ITBS at the knee have further evolved through ongoing dissection, histologic, sonography, and magnetic resonance studies. Jelsing and colleagues[28] used sonography in 12 unembalmed cadaver knees after injecting saline solution to create an effusion, then monitored below the iliotibial band at the lateral femoral epicondyle. All knees demonstrated fluid deep and anterior to the iliotibial band insertion whether or not the knee was extended or flexed. This finding leads to the consideration of a lateral synovial recess extending deep to the iliotibial band insertion as a source of pain. Ekman and colleagues[29] used MRI in 7 cases of ITBS, reporting thickening of the iliotibial band insertion in comparison with a control group. Ekman and colleagues performed a 1-year follow up MRI of 1 ITBS patient who returned to full activity but exhibited mild tenderness at the lateral femoral epicondyle, demonstrating a significant reduction in the fluid collection deep to the iliotibial band. Nemeth and Sanders[30] observed for the synovial recess and iliotibial band a relationship in 8 cadaver knees, in surgeries including 35 total knee arthroplasties, 350 knee arthroscopies, and 21 surgical approaches for ITBS, and 3 MRI studies for ITBS. These findings support the theory that there is no bursa under the iliotibial band insertion at the lateral femoral epicondyle. However, a consistent finding was a synovial fold of the lateral synovial recess. Histologic examination of ITBS biopsies versus controls demonstrated signs of inflammation, hyperplasia, fibrosis, and mucoid degeneration. The presence of fluid, synovial recess, and soft-tissue thickening implicate abnormal inflammation and soft-tissue remodeling at the iliotibial band insertion.

KINEMATIC AND MUSCLE PERFORMANCE FACTORS

ITBS occurs in the deceleration phase of stance-phase running[19,21,31] (**Figs. 5** and **6**). The preceding swing phase and muscle preactivation may have a role in the quality and performance of the deceleration phase.[19,32,33] The sagittal plane has not been firmly established as a risk factor for injury except for the impingement zone at around 30° of flexion.[21] Miller and colleagues[34] analyzed kinematics in 8 runners during an exhaustive run (ie, self-selected pace at 20 minutes) and compared kinematic measures with those in age-matched controls. The investigators reported that fatigue measurements were different, including greater knee-flexion angles at heel strike near voluntary exhaustion.

More consistently, kinematic factors contributing to ITBS have been identified in the frontal and transverse planes.[2,26,35,36] Noehren and colleagues[2] completed a prospective study of 18 female runners with ITBS and compared age-matched and mileage-matched controls. Findings included increased hip adduction, knee internal rotation, and femur external rotation in the population with ITBS (**Fig. 7**). Noehren and colleagues[36] studied 17 male runners with ITBS in a comparison with controls, and found significantly increased hip internal rotation and knee adduction in the injured group (**Fig. 8**).

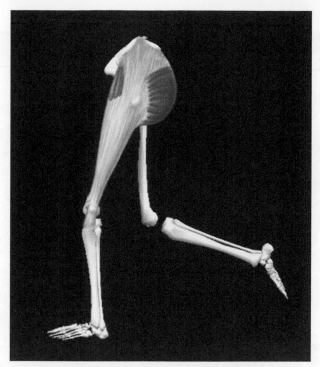

Fig. 5. Heel-strike runner.

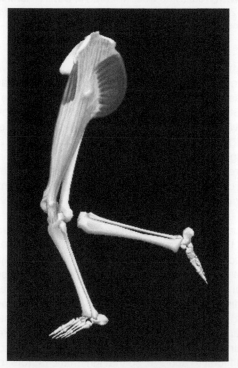

Fig. 6. Peak knee flexion at mid-stance. The deceleration phase of running is heel strike to peak knee flexion and is associated with ITBS.

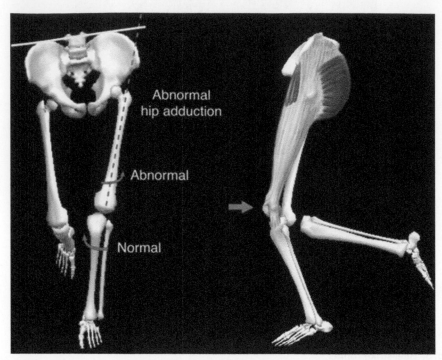

Fig. 7. Female runner with ITBS. (*Data from* Noehren B, Davis I, Hamill J. ASB clinical biome-chanics award winner 2006 prospective study of the biomechanical factors associated with iliotibial band syndrome. Clin Biomech (Bristol, Avon) 2007;22(9):951–6.)

Hamill and colleagues[26] analyzed 17 female runners who developed ITBS from a sample size of 400 in a prospective study that was part of a larger ongoing study. Strain was defined as the change in iliotibial band length while running divided by the original length. Strain rate was defined as the change in strain divided by the change in time. Software for interactive musculoskeletal modeling was used to model each subject, defining the iliotibial band as an elastic structure arising from the iliac crest and terminating on the Gerdy tubercle. The strain was not different for the involved limb compared with the contralateral limb, although the effect size suggested a clinically significant difference at touchdown but not at maximum knee flexion. Strain rate was significantly greater in the involved leg than in the uninvolved leg and either matched control leg.

Foch and colleagues[37] reported compensatory trunk ipsilateral flexion in female runners with current ITBS compared with runners with previous ITBS and controls. The sample size included 9 runners per group, and 8 of 9 currently injured participants had received treatment before testing. The gap between the onset of injury and data collection was 21 months. Given the gap between injury and data collection and prior treatment, these findings may be influenced by patient treatments such as gluteus medius strengthening and iliotibial band stretching. The Internet has made readily available front-line approaches to treating ITBS, such as stretching the iliotibial band and strengthening the gluteus medius. It is possible that motor control changes in running are more difficult to achieve, so that kinematic factors may sustain influence by early self-directed and clinically managed treatment. However, the finding by Foch

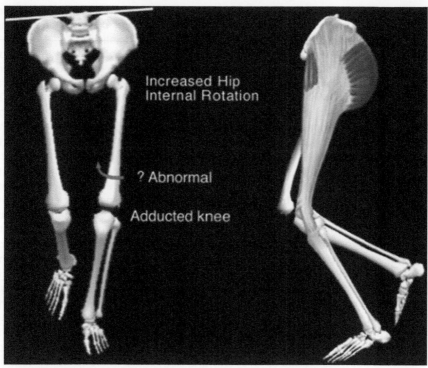

Fig. 8. Male runner with ITBS. The femur may or may not exhibit increased internal rotation. The investigators did not report on the mechanism of increased hip internal rotation. (*Data from* Noehren B, Schmitz A, Hempel R, et al. Assessment of strength, flexibility, and running mechanics in men with iliotibial band syndrome. J Orthop Sports Phys Ther 2014;3:217–22.)

and colleagues[37] of ipsilateral trunk flexion in stance-phase running may be one compensation of slackening the iliotibial band and reducing strain.

Kinematics in ITBS have been investigated from a variety of aspects. Tateuchi and colleagues[38] measured iliotibial band hardness in 16 healthy participants, both male and female. The method used Shear-wave elastography from the superior border of the patella to the posterior border of the iliotibial band. Subjects performed no pelvic drop, 10° pelvic drop, pelvic drop and trunk lean away, pelvic rise, and pelvic rise and trunk lean toward. Results indicated that the pelvic drop and trunk lean away increased iliotibial band hardness. Conversely, iliotibial band hardness reduced with pelvic rise and trunk lean toward. The investigators noted trends in electromyography data of increased gluteus maximus, gluteus medius, and tensor fasciae latae activation in the pelvic rise condition, and decreased activation in the pelvic drop. Meardon and Derrick[39] studied the iliotibial band strain and strain rate in 8 male and 7 female runners without injury. The research design evaluated a narrow, preferred, and wide-foot placement in stance-phase running. The narrow foot placement exhibited higher iliotibial strain, strain rate, and hip adduction. The investigators suggested that this was a possible source of passive strain on the iliotibial tract caused by excessive lengthening of the iliotibial band. Miller and colleagues[40] evaluated 8 runners with ITBS and 8 runners without ITBS to compare kinematics during an exhaustive run. Participants had been pain free for 4 months before data collection. The ITBS group showed low variability in coupling involving thigh adduction/abduction to foot inversion/eversion, a coordination factor. The investigators suggested that low variability in kinematic positions may be related to fewer choices of coordination patterns, which was described as a factor involving segmental coordination.

The classic study of muscle-related factors in ITBS was by Fredericson and colleagues,[41] who identified and treated hip abductor weakness in male and female runners with ITBS. Weakness was identified at baseline compared with the noninjured limb and with control noninjured runners. Unique to the design was recruitment of 24 consecutive cases with recent-onset injury (within 2 months) and excluding participants who had undergone prior treatment by a physical therapist. Strength testing controlled for hip flexion and hip internal rotation with neutral trunk alignment of limb to trunk. The break test was used starting with an isometric contraction that was overcome by an eccentric force, a good representation of the forces that challenge the gluteus medius and upper gluteus maximus muscles in deceleration-phase running. Over a 6-week multimodal training program, strength changes were identified in 34.9% of female and 51.4% of male runners. At 6 weeks, 22 of 24 runners were pain free and returned to running. Treatment was multimodal, including nonsteroidal anti-inflammatory medication and ultrasound, with corticosteroid medication at the lateral femoral epicondyle region over 1 to 2 sessions. Stretching included the iliotibial band and biceps femoris/iliotibial band. Strengthening emphasized the gluteus medius in both side lying and standing. The strength training repetitions were performed slowly downward with emphasis on isometric holds and eccentric training. Repetitions and sets started at 1 set of 15 repetitions with progression to 3 sets of 30 repetitions.

Noehren and colleagues[36] assessed strength and flexibility in male runners with and without ITBS. The external rotators of the hip were significantly weaker using handheld dynamometry normalized to lever arm and body mass at 7.8 ± 1.2 for controls and 6.6 ± 2.2 for ITBS cases ($P = .03$). The investigators suggested that excessive hip internal rotation may be due to weakness of the hip, tight iliotibial band, or altered neuromuscular control. Participant selection criteria were strict but lacked screening for prior treatment by a physical therapist.

TREATMENT STRATEGY AND PRACTICE
Phases of Recovery in Iliotibial Band Syndrome

Orientation to gait and kinematics in iliotibial band syndrome in comparison with patellofemoral pain syndrome
The interaction of the pelvis and trunk on knee moments is illustrated by Powers[13] (**Fig. 9**). Using biomechanical theory, Powers suggested that varus torque on the knee through poor pelvic control may be a factor in ITBS; this might present as in **Fig. 9**B, illustrating the shift of center of mass away from the stance knee and the stance knee outside the foot, whereas the kinematics for patellofemoral pain may be as shown in **Fig. 9**C with a valgus knee position and shift in center of mass over the stance limb. The similarities between these 2 running injuries include ability to control the trunk, pelvis, and knee when lowering the body weight. In the case of ITBS, one key biomechanical goal is to reduce strain related to excessive lengthening of the iliotibial band and stress related to the insertion at the lateral femoral epicondyle. In patellofemoral syndrome the kinematics of the valgus knee may relate to an internally rotated femur and contact pressure at the patellofemoral joint.[10,13,42–44] These improved kinematics might present as illustrated in **Fig. 9**A.

Acute phase of iliotibial band syndrome
The acute phase of ITBS[45] is described well by Noble[7] in reviewing 100 consecutive cases of ITBS (**Table 1**) in South African runners. Seventy-three cases continued

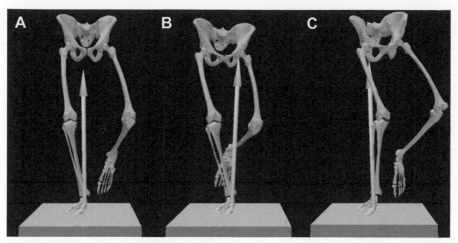

Fig. 9. Frontal plane motions of the trunk and pelvis and moments at the knees. (*A*) Normal alignment. (*B*) Trendelenburg sign. (*C*) Compensated Trendelenburg sign. (*From* Powers CM. The influence of abnormal hip mechanics on knee injury: a biomechanical perspective. J Orthop Sports Phys Ther. 2010;40:44; with permission.)

with follow-up, and the pain was "remarkably resistant" to treatment. The approach consisted of corticosteroid injections, repeated several times in some cases. The most notable contributory factor was a rapid increase in mileage in 64% of runners.

Given pain and inflammation at the insertion and passive and active tension factors of the iliotibial band,[15,26,38,46] the acute phase is ideal for myofascial treatment addressing trigger points in the biceps femoris, vastus lateralis, gluteus maximus, and tensor fasciae latae muscles.[47–49] Fredericson and colleagues[47] initiated myofascial mapping for trigger points in the anterior gluteus minimus, central belly of the vastus lateralis, and fascial attachment among the iliotibial band, vastus lateralis, and biceps femoris. **Fig. 10** demonstrates one method used to separate fascia and release trigger points using a manual therapy technique. Roach and colleagues[48] demonstrated a method to identify and treat trigger points in the gluteus medius using applied pressure through the thumbs. Iontophoresis with dexamethasone may be useful as an anti-inflammatory modality.[50]

The acute phase may also be useful to instruct runners on how to walk to control for pelvic drop, pelvic rise, and trunk deviation if present. The evaluation process may include a 6-inch step-down test to represent lowering the body weight on one leg with mirror feedback or video to better appreciate control of the trunk, pelvis, and knee[51] (**Fig. 11**). Because runners are walking, motor control can be initiated with simple walking strategies such as slightly forward trunk posture to promote a hip strategy[52,53] (**Fig. 12**). Barrios and colleagues[54] were able to reduce knee external adduction movement in a sample of 8 varus-aligned knees in otherwise healthy participants using faded feedback on knee adduction. The motor cues were 3 similar phrases including "walk with your knees closer together." Participants were treated with 8 sessions using treadmill walking and visual feedback through a video monitor. Although Barrios and colleagues[54] emphasized control of excess knee adduction in healthy subjects, this technique may be useful for ITBS patients in the acute and subacute phase during which motor control can start with a walking technique. Male runners who exhibit increased knee varus in stance may benefit from this type of cue to bring the knees inward in stance running.

Table 1
Phases of recovery in ITBS

Phase	Functional Problem	Medication	Hands on	Modalities	Exercise
Acute: 3 d–1 wk	Running causes pain	Anti-inflammatory medication	Myofascial: hands-on ITB. TPs in vastus lateralis, biceps femoris, and GMAX	Ice, iontophoresis with dexamethasone	Walking technique: activate core and gluteal muscles, soft landing
Subacute: 3 d–2 wk	Running causes pain	If still focal pain, consider ultrasound-guided corticosteroid injection	Manual Stretching ITB, VL, and BF	Wean ice	Stretch ITB and lateral hamstrings; activate posterolateral hip muscles
Recovery strength: 1–6 wk	Running causes pain	—	Facilitate anterolateral abdominals and posterolateral hip muscles	Observe, palpate, and cue for posterolateral hip muscles	Standing exercises and progressive resistance posterolateral hip. Stretch ITB, VL, and BF
Return to running: 6 wk	Every other day and avoid downhill	—	Motor control cues to core and posterolateral gluteal	Observe for pelvic control. Consider 2D point-and-shoot motion capture	6-inch step-down with control of pelvis. Hip strategy
Notes	Consider easy sprints in first week	—	Run softly with feel under the body	Emphasize control for varus knee, pelvis, and trunk; avoid overstride	Technique emphasizes posterolateral hip muscles

Abbreviations: 2D, 2-dimensional; BF, biceps femoris; GMAX, gluteus maximus muscle; ITB, iliotibial band; TPs, trigger points; VL, vastus lateralis.

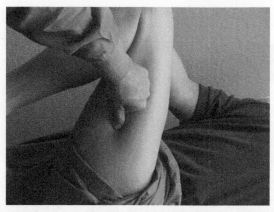

Fig. 10. Soft-tissue mobilization for the iliotibial band. The soft-tissue approach emphasizes fascial connections between the vastus lateralis, iliotibial band, and biceps femoris. Trigger-point methods may be used, including deep pressure holds at 60 seconds per painful trigger point. (*Data from* Fredericson M, Guillet M, Debenedictis L. Innovative solutions for iliotibial band syndrome. Phys Sportsmed 2000;2:53–68; and Roach S, Sorenson E, Headley B, et al. Prevalence of myofascial trigger points in the hip in patellofemoral pain. Arch Phys Med Rehabil 2013;3:522–6.)

The subacute phase

The subacute phase is marked by a reduction in acute pain and inflammation.[45] If focal pain persists at the lateral femoral epicondyle, ultrasound-guided corticosteroid injection should be considered.[55] Fredericson and colleagues[56] compared 3 types of

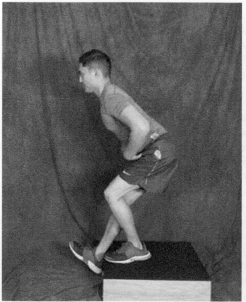
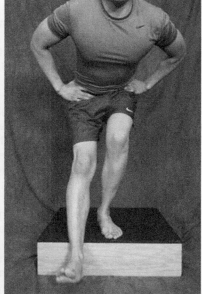

Fig. 11. Single-leg step-down test and exercise. If tolerated, several repetitions can be performed with assessment of trunk lean, pelvic drop or rise, and knee valgus or varus. This information may provide a benchmark for the patient. The single-leg step-down promotes awareness of movement issues but should not be used for treatment until pain is gone.

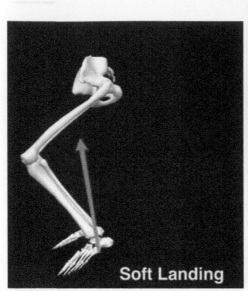
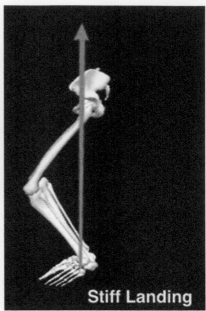

Soft Landing   Stiff Landing

Fig. 12. Soft and stiff landing and hip strategy. This simulation image is based on a drop jump measured from touch down to peak knee flexion. The intention is to illustrate how the forward trunk position may assist a hip strategy and reduce stress at the knees-soft landing. The drop jump is not intended for training patients with ITBS. The illustration is intended for early strategy about hip strategy in walking and, eventually, running.

iliotibial band stretches, showing a significant improvement in range of motion in all 3 (**Fig. 13**). Given the fascial relationship among the iliotibial band, vastus lateralis, and biceps femoris, foam roller and manual therapy type stretches may be useful to reduce passive tension in the iliotibial band (**Fig. 14**).

The recovery strengthening phase

The recovery strengthening phase begins as fascial restrictions and range of motion have progressed and symptoms have eased.[45] The muscles that interact with the iliotibial band and related kinematic factors are extensive[57] (**Figs. 15** and **16**). Initial emphasis should be isometric and eccentric training for the gluteus medius with focus on the posterior gluteus medius, given the findings of Fredericson and colleagues.[41] Training the gluteus medius has been studied with emphasis on leg to trunk alignment, isometric and eccentric emphasis, and avoiding muscle substitution[41,58,59] (**Figs. 17–20**). Training the gluteus maximus and hip external rotators has a more general research foundation given the increased hip internal rotation in male runners, weakness in the external rotators of the hip in male runners, and the increased strain rate in the iliotibial band in female runners.[60] The single-leg step down (see **Fig. 11**), single-leg wall squat (**Fig. 21**), and single-leg dead lift (**Fig. 22**) are recommended, given the relationship of lowering body weight on one leg and neuromuscular control.[61] Training is emphasized to reduce abnormal lengthening of the iliotibial band (ie, excess strain) and abnormal compression or friction at the lateral femoral epicondyle (ie, excess stress). Specifically, as appropriate to clinical evaluation, male runners may train for reduced varus knees (ie, bring knees inward and align with the foot and

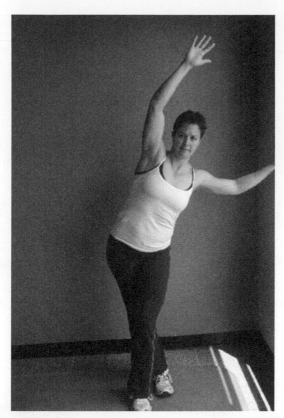

Fig. 13. Iliotibial band stretch. This iliotibial band stretch outperformed 2 other stretches using 30-second holds at 3 stretches. (*Data from* Fredericson M, White JJ, Macmahon JM, et al. Quantitative analysis of the relative effectiveness of 3 iliotibial band stretches. Arch Phys Med Rehabil 2002;5:589–92.)

ankle) and females may train to control for excessive hip adduction (ie, level hips, trunk forward, and hip strategy in lowering body weight).[2,26,36,52,53]

Debate exists in the literature about the ability of exercise to modify kinematic changes in runners. Willy and Davis[62] treated 20 healthy runners with excessive hip adduction over 6 weeks using exercises specific to single-leg squat. The participants used mirror feedback and verbal guidance on knee alignment. Progression was to weight-bearing single-leg squat in weeks 4 to 6. The dosing was generally 10 repetitions at 2 sets, and some exercises used isometric holds at 5 or 10 seconds. Strength improvement was noted in the hip abductors and external rotators, and alignment improved in the single-leg squat. However, during running no change was reported for hip adduction compared with preintervention. The investigators suggested that neuromuscular training specific to running may be needed to transfer strength to skill. Snyder and colleagues[60] trained 15 female participants using closed-chain hip abduction and rotation exercises. The exercises involved standing with a pulley for resistance to the hips, including hip-hike and hip-drop exercises. Training lasted 6 weeks at 3 times per week. Four standing exercises were performed for the entire 6 weeks. Resistance was based on achieving 60% of the maximal contraction and repetitions to fatigue with emphasis on trunk posture. Strength changes were

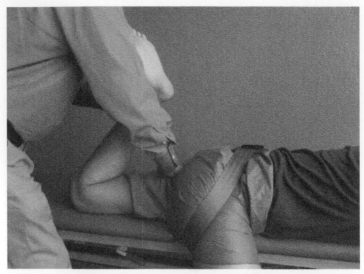

Fig. 14. Manual therapy stretch of rectus femoris and vastus lateralis. Controlling the pelvis in the frontal plane and posterior hip stabilization assists in isolating the anterolateral thigh.

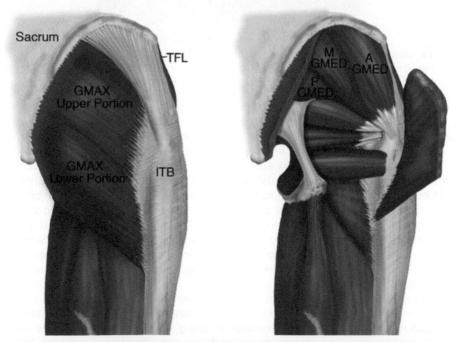

Fig. 15. Hip muscles interacting with iliotibial band. The illustrated muscles function to stabilize the hip and pelvis in stance running. The training may focus on isometric and eccentric function, endurance, timing, and coordination. A, anterior; GMAX, gluteus maximus; GMED, gluteus medius; ITB, iliotibial band; M, middle; P, posterior; TFL, tensor fasciae latae.

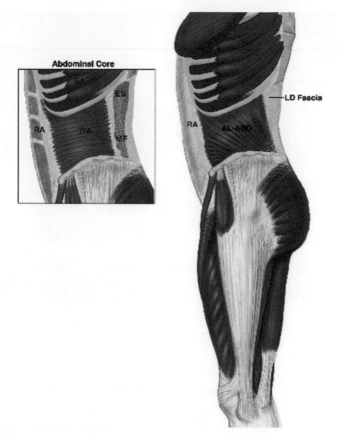

Fig. 16. Abdominal and lumbar muscles interacting with the iliotibial band. The trunk muscles have not been fully analyzed in iliotibial band syndrome. However, the close interaction between the trunk, pelvis, and hip suggests a training relationship between the lumbar muscles and hip muscles. AL-ABD, anterolateral abdominal muscles; ES, erector spinae; LD Fascia, lumbodorsal fascia; MF, multifidus; RA, rectus abdominis; SA, serratus anterior; TrA, transversus abdominis.

significant in the hip abductors and hip external rotators. The findings also included a reduction in rear foot inversion and knee abduction moment, and a trend toward reduced hip internal rotation in running. The investigators mentioned that kinematic data of the trunk was not captured, although trunk compensation and improvement may be a reason for kinetic improvement. If so, kinematic changes in the trunk might explain the kinetic improvement. More research is needed to better understand the interaction of positioning and trunk, dosing and exercise, and training and kinematics.

The return to running phase
The return to running phase is marked by pain-free exercise and good form in all exercises.[45] While 6 weeks is a benchmark, the range is variable based on successful completion of earlier phase recovery. Graded progression is achieved by running every other day with emphasis on good running form. The initial week of running may include easy sprints on level ground, based on the assumption that deeper knee positions may reduce the iliotibial band impingement. Downhill running is not

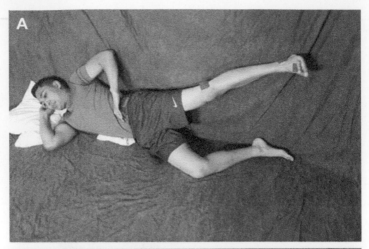

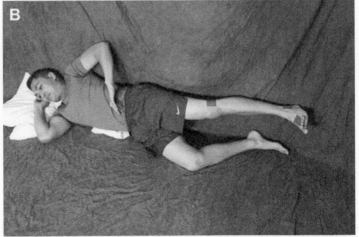

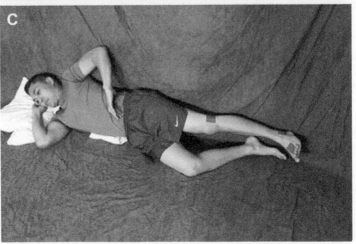

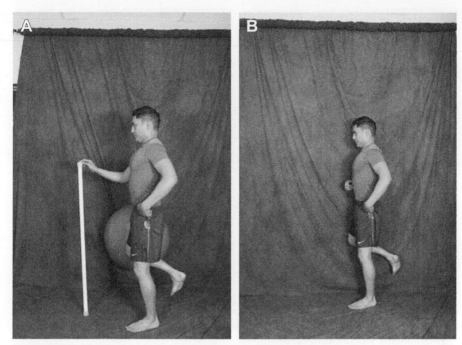

Fig. 18. (*A, B*) Gluteus medius in standing leg facilitated with abduction into the wall. Isometric gluteus medius wall with and without the ball facilitates the stance-leg gluteus medius, with emphasis on posterior gluteus medius. A stick can be used for balance. Isometric holds of 5 to 15 seconds are recommended to simulate postural function. (*Data from* Refs.[11,41,59])

recommended in the first 2 weeks given the risk of higher ground-reaction force. Motor control emphasis is recommended to focus on pelvic control, forward trunk, and softer landing.

CASE EXAMPLE USING RUNNING TECHNIQUE RETRAINING

Physical therapist Darrell J. Allen[63] reported an ITBS case study whereby he instructed the runner to increase the step rate by 5%. The patient had no prior treatment. Video analysis was performed with a single camera and analyzed in slow motion at 60 frames per second. Stride rate was calculated at 168 steps per minute. The heel strike

Fig. 17. (*A–C*) Side-lying hip abduction. Gowda and colleagues used the wall for guidance to assist extended hip posture to target the posterior gluteus medius. Dosing started at 6 to 8 repetitions at 2 sets and progressed to 15 repetitions at 3 sets. Weights were then added as tolerance improved using 6 to 8 repetition sets. Fredericson emphasized slow eccentric sets of from 15 to 30 repetitions and 3 sets, avoiding hip internal rotation and flexion (tensor fasciae latae substitution), and avoiding hip hiking (quadratus lumborum substitution). (*Data from* Fredericson M, Cookingham CL, Chaudhari AM, et al. Hip abductor weakness in distance runners with iliotibial band syndrome. Clin J Sport Med 2000;3:169–75; and Gowda AL, Mease SJ, Donatelli R, et al. Gluteus medius strengthening and the use of the Donatelli drop leg test in the athlete. Phys Ther Sport 2014;1:15–9.)

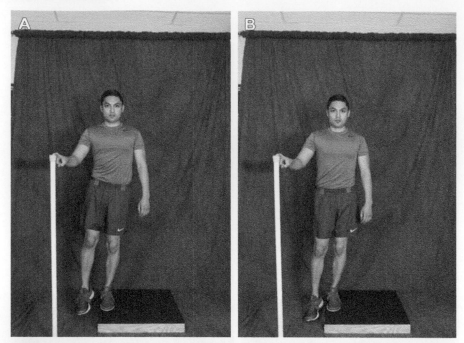

Fig. 19. (*A, B*) Gluteus medius and upper gluteus maximus using the pelvic drop in standing leg with minimal support as needed.

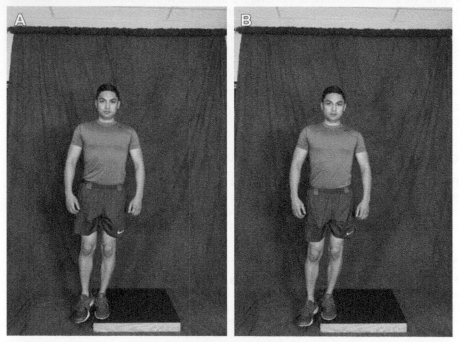

Fig. 20. (*A, B*) Gluteus medius and upper gluteus maximus in standing leg using the pelvic drop without support. Slow eccentric pelvic drops were used by Fredericson and colleagues in sets of 15 to 30 repetitions, progressing from 1 to 3 sets. (*Data from* Fredericson M, Cookingham CL, Chaudhari AM, et al. Hip abductor weakness in distance runners with ilio-tibial band syndrome. Clin J Sport Med 2000;3:169–75.)

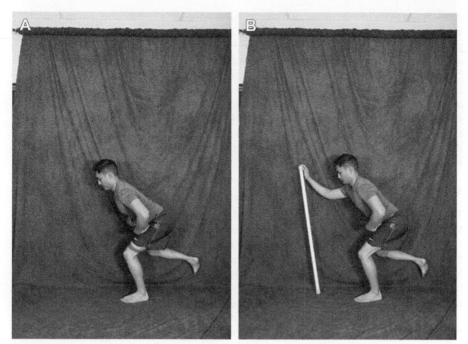

Fig. 21. (*A*, *B*) Single-leg wall squat with and without support. Trunk forward will challenge the gluteus maximus. Abduction Into the wall further activates the stance posterolateral hip musculature.

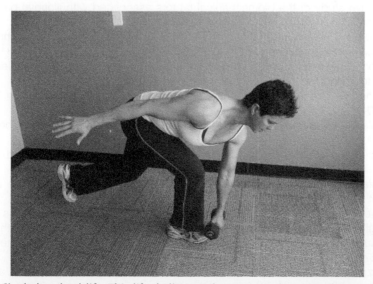

Fig. 22. Single-leg dead lift. This lift challenges the posterior hip musculature, including gluteus maximus, to control internal rotation of the hip and balance in the frontal plane.

occurred in front of the center of mass with the knee in 10° of flexion. No forward lean was observed during stance phase. Based on recommendations by Heiderscheit and colleagues,[64] the step rate was increased by 5% to 176 steps per minute using a metronome to increase pace. The running instructions also included the phrases "run quietly" and "let your feet strike under your body as you fall forward." Weight-bearing and hip-oriented exercises were performed. At 4 weeks the patient was able to run at a cadence of 176 steps per minute, with tolerance of 3.5 miles of running. At 6 weeks the patient could run 7 miles. At 4 months' follow-up the patient was able to run 13.1 miles without pain. Neuromuscular training specific to running has potential in the treatment of ITBS as part of a multimodal program that includes hip and pelvis exercise.

SUMMARY

The biomechanical approach to ITBS includes improved force distribution into the iliotibial band insertion at the knee. Iliotibial band strain and strain rate are competing risk factors for ITBS. Researchers suggest further exploration of neuromuscular control at the hip. The hip control mechanism may be influenced by mechanoreceptors at the knee and coordination of the trunk and pelvis. Passive and active tension in the iliotibial band is a possible contributing factor. Researchers propose 3 recurring factors that influence the iliotibial band: reduced length, altered neuromuscular control, and weakness of the posterior and lateral hip musculature. Muscle performance factors focus on isometric and eccentric function in the deceleration phase of running. Research is needed to better understand the influences of the trunk on pelvis and motor control strategies.

REFERENCES

1. Taunton JE, Ryan MB, Clement DB, et al. A retrospective case-control analysis of 2002 running injuries. Br J Sports Med 2002;2:95–101.
2. Noehren B, Davis I, Hamill J. ASB clinical biomechanics award winner 2006 prospective study of the biomechanical factors associated with iliotibial band syndrome. Clin Biomech (Bristol, Avon) 2007;9:951–6.
3. Tenforde AS, Sayres LC, McCurdy ML, et al. Overuse injuries in high school runners: lifetime prevalence and prevention strategies. PM R 2011;2:125–31.
4. Fallon KE. Musculoskeletal injuries in the ultramarathon: the 1990 Westfield Sydney to Melbourne run. Br J Sports Med 1996;4:319–23.
5. Renne JW. The iliotibial band friction syndrome. J Bone Joint Surg Am 1975;8:1110–1.
6. Noble CA. The treatment of iliotibial band friction syndrome. Br J Sports Med 1979;2:51–4.
7. Noble CA. Iliotibial band friction syndrome in runners. Am J Sports Med 1980;4:232–4.
8. Kaplan EB. The iliotibial tract; clinical and morphological significance. J Bone Joint Surg Am 1958;4:817–32.
9. Powers CM, Ward SR, Fredericson M, et al. Patellofemoral kinematics during weight-bearing and non-weight-bearing knee extension in persons with lateral subluxation of the patella: a preliminary study. J Orthop Sports Phys Ther 2003;11:677–85.
10. Souza RB, Powers CM. Predictors of hip internal rotation during running: an evaluation of hip strength and femoral structure in women with and without patellofemoral pain. Am J Sports Med 2009;3:579–87.

11. Hodges PW. Core stability exercise in chronic low back pain. Orthop Clin North Am 2003;2:245–54.
12. Macconaill MA. The function of intra-articular fibrocartilages, with special reference to the knee and inferior radio-ulnar joints. J Anat 1932;66(Pt 2):210–27.
13. Powers CM. The influence of abnormal hip mechanics on knee injury: a biomechanical perspective. J Orthop Sports Phys Ther 2010;2:42–51.
14. Fairclough J, Hayashi K, Toumi H, et al. The functional anatomy of the iliotibial band during flexion and extension of the knee: implications for understanding iliotibial band syndrome. J Anat 2006;3:309–16.
15. Stecco A, Gilliar W, Hill R, et al. The anatomical and functional relation between gluteus maximus and fascia lata. J Bodyw Mov Ther 2013;4:512–7.
16. Vieira EL, Vieira EA, da Silva RT, et al. An anatomic study of the iliotibial tract. Arthroscopy 2007;3:269–74.
17. Stern JT Jr. Anatomical and functional specializations of the human gluteus maximus. Am J Phys Anthropol 1972;3:315–39.
18. Lyons K, Perry J, Gronley JK, et al. Timing and relative intensity of hip extensor and abductor muscle action during level and stair ambulation. An EMG study. Phys Ther 1983;10:1597–605.
19. Novacheck TF. The biomechanics of running. Gait Posture 1998;1:77–95.
20. Fairclough J, Hayashi K, Toumi H, et al. Is iliotibial band syndrome really a friction syndrome? J Sci Med Sport 2007;2:74–6 [discussion: 77–8].
21. Orchard JW, Fricker PA, Abud AT, et al. Biomechanics of iliotibial band friction syndrome in runners. Am J Sports Med 1996;3:375–9.
22. Benjamin M, Redman S, Milz S, et al. Adipose tissue at entheses: the rheumatological implications of its distribution. A potential site of pain and stress dissipation? Ann Rheum Dis 2004;12:1549–55.
23. Jozsa L, Balint J, Kannus P, et al. Mechanoreceptors in human myotendinous junction. Muscle Nerve 1993;5:453–7.
24. Zimny ML, Wink CS. Neuroreceptors in the tissues of the knee joint. J Electromyogr Kinesiol 1991;3:148–57.
25. Jelsing EJ, Finnoff JT, Cheville AL, et al. Sonographic evaluation of the iliotibial band at the lateral femoral epicondyle: does the iliotibial band move? J Ultrasound Med 2013;7:1199–206.
26. Hamill J, Miller R, Noehren B, et al. A prospective study of iliotibial band strain in runners. Clin Biomech (Bristol, Avon) 2008;8:1018–25.
27. Meardon SA, Campbell S, Derrick TR. Step width alters iliotibial band strain during running. Sports Biomech 2012;4:464–72.
28. Jelsing EJ, Maida E, Finnoff JT, et al. The source of fluid deep to the iliotibial band: documentation of a potential intra-articular source. PM R 2014;2: 134–8.
29. Ekman EF, Pope T, Martin DF, et al. Magnetic resonance imaging of iliotibial band syndrome. Am J Sports Med 1994;6:851–4.
30. Nemeth WC, Sanders BL. The lateral synovial recess of the knee: anatomy and role in chronic iliotibial band friction syndrome. Arthroscopy 1996;5:574–80.
31. Dugan SA, Bhat KP. Biomechanics and analysis of running gait. Phys Med Rehabil Clin N Am 2005;3:603–21.
32. Phinyomark A, Osis S, Hettinga BA, et al. Gender differences in gait kinematics in runners with iliotibial band syndrome. Scand J Med Sci Sports 2015;10:12394.
33. Potthast W, Bruggemann GP, Lundberg A, et al. The influences of impact interface, muscle activity, and knee angle on impact forces and tibial and femoral accelerations occurring after external impacts. J Appl Biomech 2010;1:1–9.

34. Miller RH, Lowry JL, Meardon SA, et al. Lower extremity mechanics of iliotibial band syndrome during an exhaustive run. Gait Posture 2007;3:407–13.
35. Ferber R, Noehren B, Hamill J, et al. Competitive female runners with a history of iliotibial band syndrome demonstrate atypical hip and knee kinematics. J Orthop Sports Phys Ther 2010;2:52–8.
36. Noehren B, Schmitz A, Hempel R, et al. Assessment of strength, flexibility, and running mechanics in men with iliotibial band syndrome. J Orthop Sports Phys Ther 2014;3:217–22.
37. Foch E, Reinbolt JA, Zhang S, et al. Associations between iliotibial band injury status and running biomechanics in women. Gait Posture 2015;2:706–10.
38. Tateuchi H, Shiratori S, Ichihashi N. The effect of angle and moment of the hip and knee joint on iliotibial band hardness. Gait Posture 2015;41:522–8.
39. Meardon SA, Derrick TR. Effect of step width manipulation on tibial stress during running. J Biomech 2014;11:2738–44.
40. Miller RH, Meardon SA, Derrick TR, et al. Continuous relative phase variability during an exhaustive run in runners with a history of iliotibial band syndrome. J Appl Biomech 2008;3:262–70.
41. Fredericson M, Cookingham CL, Chaudhari AM, et al. Hip abductor weakness in distance runners with iliotibial band syndrome. Clin J Sport Med 2000;3: 169–75.
42. Powers CM. The influence of altered lower-extremity kinematics on patellofemoral joint dysfunction: a theoretical perspective. J Orthop Sports Phys Ther 2003;11: 639–46.
43. Souza RB, Draper CE, Fredericson M, et al. Femur rotation and patellofemoral joint kinematics: a weight-bearing magnetic resonance imaging analysis. J Orthop Sports Phys Ther 2010;5:277–85.
44. Souza RB, Powers CM. Differences in hip kinematics, muscle strength, and muscle activation between subjects with and without patellofemoral pain. J Orthop Sports Phys Ther 2009;1:12–9.
45. Fredericson M, Wolf C. Iliotibial band syndrome in runners: innovations in treatment. Sports Med 2005;5:451–9.
46. Stecco C, Gagey O, Belloni A, et al. Anatomy of the deep fascia of the upper limb. Second part: study of innervation. Morphologie 2007;292:38–43.
47. Fredericson M, Guillet M, Debenedictis L. Innovative solutions for iliotibial band syndrome. Phys Sportsmed 2000;2:53–68.
48. Roach S, Sorenson E, Headley B, et al. Prevalence of myofascial trigger points in the hip in patellofemoral pain. Arch Phys Med Rehabil 2013;3:522–6.
49. Simons DG, Mense S. Understanding and measurement of muscle tone as related to clinical muscle pain. Pain 1998;1:1–17.
50. Gurney AB, Wascher DC. Absorption of dexamethasone sodium phosphate in human connective tissue using iontophoresis. Am J Sports Med 2008;4: 753–9.
51. Earl JE, Monteiro SK, Snyder KR. Differences in lower extremity kinematics between a bilateral drop-vertical jump and a single-leg step-down. J Orthop Sports Phys Ther 2007;5:245–52.
52. Farrokhi S, Pollard CD, Souza RB, et al. Trunk position influences the kinematics, kinetics, and muscle activity of the lead lower extremity during the forward lunge exercise. J Orthop Sports Phys Ther 2008;7:403–9.
53. Pollard CD, Sigward SM, Powers CM. Limited hip and knee flexion during landing is associated with increased frontal plane knee motion and moments. Clin Biomech (Bristol, Avon) 2010;2:142–6.

54. Barrios JA, Crossley KM, Davis IS. Gait retraining to reduce the knee adduction moment through real-time visual feedback of dynamic knee alignment. J Biomech 2010;11:2208–13.
55. Gunter P, Schwellnus MP. Local corticosteroid injection in iliotibial band friction syndrome in runners: a randomised controlled trial. Br J Sports Med 2004;3: 269–72 [discussion: 72].
56. Fredericson M, White JJ, Macmahon JM, et al. Quantitative analysis of the relative effectiveness of 3 iliotibial band stretches. Arch Phys Med Rehabil 2002;5: 589–92.
57. Baker RL, Souza RB, Fredericson M. Iliotibial band syndrome: soft tissue and biomechanical factors in evaluation and treatment. PM R 2011;6:550–61.
58. Gowda AL, Mease SJ, Donatelli R, et al. Gluteus medius strengthening and the use of the Donatelli drop leg test in the athlete. Phys Ther Sport 2014;1:15–9.
59. O'Sullivan K, Smith SM, Sainsbury D. Electromyographic analysis of the three subdivisions of gluteus medius during weight-bearing exercises. Sports Med Arthrosc Rehabil Ther Technol 2010;2:17.
60. Snyder KR, Earl JE, O'Connor KM, et al. Resistance training is accompanied by increases in hip strength and changes in lower extremity biomechanics during running. Clin Biomech (Bristol, Avon) 2009;1:26–34.
61. Distefano LJ, Blackburn JT, Marshall SW, et al. Gluteal muscle activation during common therapeutic exercises. J Orthop Sports Phys Ther 2009;7:532–40.
62. Willy RW, Davis IS. The effect of a hip-strengthening program on mechanics during running and during a single-leg squat. J Orthop Sports Phys Ther 2011;9: 625–32.
63. Allen DJ. Treatment of distal iliotibial band syndrome in a long distance runner with gait re-training emphasizing step rate manipulation. Int J Sports Phys Ther 2014;2:222–31.
64. Heiderscheit BC, Chumanov ES, Michalski MP, et al. Effects of step rate manipulation on joint mechanics during running. Med Sci Sports Exerc 2011;2:296–302.

Running Injuries
The Infrapatellar Fat Pad and Plica Injuries

Jenny McConnell, AM, DPT, B App Sci(Phty), Grad Dip Man Ther, M Biomed Eng[a,b]

KEYWORDS

- Hoffa pad • Nociceptive • OA pain • Knee biomechanics • Quadriceps inhibition

KEY POINTS

- The infrapatellar fat pad (IFP) is highly innervated and when inflamed is responsible for inferior, medial, retropatellar, and in some cases posterior knee pain.
- The IFP stabilizes the patella in extremes of knee motion (<20° and >100°).
- The IFP can be injured with rapid extension or hyperextension of the knee, such as over-extending the knee when running downhill.
- Inflammation of the IFP causes quadriceps atrophy.
- Inflammatory changes in the IFP seen on MRI are the consequence of trauma and degeneration, the commonest trauma being arthroscopy.

INTRODUCTION

Various intraarticular structures of the knee generate neurosensory signals that result in conscious pain perception. Pain is defined as an unpleasant sensory or emotional experience associated with actual or potential tissue damage (nociception).[1] Pain involves an individual's reaction to nociception, so it is very much a personal experience with a learned component. Pain can become memorized because pain mechanisms are not fixed (hard wired) but are plastic (soft wired).[1] Through neuroplasticity, hyperalgesia can be learned and unlearned, from both tissue-based and environmental afferent inputs.[2]

The tissue-based structures that can be the potential source of knee pain are the synovium, lateral retinaculum, subchondral bone, and the infrapatellar fat pad (IFP), with the articular cartilage because it is aneural, providing only an indirect source, perhaps either through synovial irritation or increasing subchondral bone stress.

There is, however, no correlation between the amount of articular cartilage degeneration and pain experienced by individuals with knee osteoarthritis (OA), for example.

Disclosures: None.
[a] McConnell Physiotherapy Group, 4 Bond St, Mosman, NSW 2088, Australia; [b] Centre for Sports Medicine Research and Education, University of Melbourne, Melbourne, Victoria, Australia
E-mail address: jennymcconnell@bigpond.com

The severity of OA knee pain is associated with bone marrow lesions (edema) with subarticular bone attrition,[3–5] synovitis/effusion, and degenerative meniscal tears, but it is not associated with presence of osteophytes or reduction in joint space.[6] Hill and colleagues[7] followed 270 subjects with tibiofemoral and patellofemoral (PF) OA for 30 months finding no correlation between baseline synovitis and baseline pain score but a decrease in synovitis at follow-up was correlated with a reduction in pain. These investigators found synovitis in 3 locations, namely, the superior, medial, and inferior patella, with infrapatellar synovitis being most strongly correlated with pain severity. The synovitis was not associated with cartilage loss in either the tibiofemoral or PF compartments.[7]

Free nerve endings (IVa) are present in the synovium,[8] so peripatellar synovitis is a possible source of knee pain. Despite the evidence supporting the synovium as a potential pain source, histologic changes in the synovium of patients with PF pain are only moderate.[9] However, there is evidence of histologic changes in the lateral retinaculum with increased numbers of myelinated and unmyelinated nerve fibers, neuroma formation, and nerve fibrosis being found in some patients with PF pain.[10–12] Additionally, increased intraosseous pressure of the patella has been found in patients with PF pain who complain of pain when sitting with a bent knee ("movie goers knee"), possibly secondary to a transient venous outflow obstruction.[10,13] However, the structure that until recently has largely been ignored by the orthopedic community, even though it was first identified as a potent source of pain by Hoffa in 1904, is the (IFP). Hoffa described the symptoms originating from the IFP as being "pain felt quite suddenly on the medial side of the joint; with the patient having difficulty bending and straightening the knee and the presence of knee joint swelling on both sides of the patella."[14] Consequently, the IFP is often referred to as Hoffa's fat pad, with most clinicians thinking of Hoffa's syndrome as a result of a direct blow to the knee. Superolateral fat pad edema is a frequent finding with patellar maltracking and may precede clinically significant chondrosis.[15] In a recent study by Matcuk and Cen,[15] a patient with patellar maltracking was placed in the Hoffa group (superolateral fat pad edema), if 1 of 3 conditions was met: lateral patellar displacement greater than -3.6 mm and Insall–Salvati ratio (ratio of patellar tendon length and patellar length) greater than 0.99; lateral patellar displacement of -3.6 mm or less and Insall–Salvati ratio greater than 1.23; or lateral patellar displacement of -3.6 mm or less, Insall–Salvati ratio of 1.23 or less, and lateral trochlear inclination of 16.5° or less. These findings had 91.6% sensitivity and 88.9% specificity for identifying the Hoffa group.

ANATOMY

The IFP is a highly vascular, richly innervated, intracapsular, extrasynovial structure, lined by synovium, filling the anterior knee compartment with between 21 to 39 mL of adipose tissue, although there is considerable individual volumetric variation.[16–18] The IFP covers the extraarticular part of the posterior patellar surface and merges superiorly with the peripatellar fold. Posteriorly, the IFP extends into ligamentum mucosum, which in many individuals is continuous with the anterior cruciate ligament (ACL), finally connecting to the intercondylar notch of the femur.[16,17] Inflammation of the pericruciate portion of the IFP causes posterior knee pain in athletes.[19]

The IFP also attaches to the proximal patellar tendon, inferior pole of the patella, transverse meniscal ligament, medial and lateral meniscal horns, and the retinaculum, as well as the periosteum of the tibia. The medial and lateral patellomeniscal ligaments appear as thickening of the edges of the IFP as it merges with the capsular synovium.[16,17]

VASCULARIZATION

The IFP is vascularized by a rich anastomotic network. Branches of the inferior genicular arteries run vertically through the IFP just posterior to the borders of the patellar tendon. Branches of the superomedial and superolateral genicular arteries wrap posteriorly around the distal half of the patella to enter the proximal aspect of the IFP and anastomose with the inferior genicular arteries. Two to 3 horizontal arteries connect the vertical arteries at the level of the femoral condyles, tibial plateau, or tibial tubercle.[16,17,20,21] A network of smaller arteries extending from the inferior genicular arteries infiltrate the remainder of the fat pad, although the central portion remains the least vascularized. In some individuals, a branch of the middle genicular artery, which runs through the ligamentum mucosum during embryonic development, persists as a robust connection between the arterial supplies of the ACL and the IFP. Without this middle genicular vascularization, the vascular network of the IFP sends smaller branches into the surrounding synovial lining as well as that of the cruciate ligaments.[16,20,22] The rich vascular supply found in the IFP supports the hypothesis that the IFP can aid in healing the ACL and other nearby structures, but also supports the hypothesis of IFP fibrosis after an injury.[22]

INNERVATION

The IFP is a potent source of knee pain owing to its rich innervation and relationship with the highly innervated synovium.[23] The innervation of the fat pad is linked with the entire knee joint structure, so the IFP may be affected by pathology in various knee joint components. The IFP is supplied by several nerves, including the terminal branch of the obturator nerve; branches of the femoral nerve, supplying the vastus medialis and vastus lateralis muscles; the lateral articular and recurrent peroneal branches of the common peroneal nerve; and the infrapatellar branch of the saphenous nerve and the posterior articular nerve, a branch of the posterior tibial nerve.[23]

Histologically nerves within the IFP stain positively for S-100, tyrosine hydroxylase, and nociceptive fibers, which contain substance P as well as type IVa free nerve endings, which are most dense in the central and lateral portions of the IFP and the surrounding synovium.[23,24] In fact, the IFP and medial retinaculum of PF pain patients contain a higher numbers of substance P nerve fibers than the same structures of individuals without PF pain.[25]

Knee pain has been induced experimentally by injecting hypertonic saline into the fat pad of asymptomatic individuals. All individuals complained of severe infrapatellar pain, with most also experiencing retropatellar pain and some reporting medial thigh, and even groin pain.[26] Experimentally inducing pain in the fat pad causes a decrease in vastus medialis obliquus and vastus lateralis activity.[27] Simulated acute knee joint pain leads to hyperalgesia and facilitated temporal summation in the IFP, as well as in the muscles located distant to the injection site, in subjects with no history of knee pain.[28] Injection or infusion of local anesthetic into the IFP after an operation or injury decreased patient use of opioids, decreased overall pain, and facilitated rehabilitation of the knee.[29]

To simulate early knee OA change, Clements and colleagues[30] injected monoiodoacetate into the right knee of 150 rats and after 21 days of weight-bearing asymmetry found marked inflammatory changes in the fat pad, concluding that the IFP contributed to the pain in the early stages of knee OA.

BIOMECHANICS

Although there has been debate about the role of the IFP, recent evidence of outcomes of patients 12 months after total knee arthroplasty has shown that the individuals where the IFP was preserved had significantly better Oxford Knee Score associated with rising from a chair, pain, limping, giving way, and pain interfering with work than those who had the IFP resected.[31] The role of the IFP is to stabilize the patella in the extremes of knee motion (that is less than 20° and >100° of knee flexion), increase tibial external rotation and facilitate distribution of synovial fluid.[18] A total resection of the IFP decreases PF contact area,[18] but has no effect in reducing PF pain. Excision of the IFP also results in a shortened patellar tendon after total knee arthroplasty. Edema in the IFP increases the volume of the anterior interval and leads to irritation of nearby tissue. Inflammatory changes in the IFP seen on MRI are most commonly the consequence of trauma and degeneration, with the commonest traumatic lesions after arthroscopy, where in 50% of cases fibrous scarring can still be present 12 months later.[32,33] Impingement of the fat pad with diffuse edema occurs after patellar dislocation, often mimicking a loose body.[34]

Clinical Features

Fat pad irritation is a poorly described and underdiagnosed condition. It is frequently confused with patellar tendinopathy and if acute in onset is associated with a rapid extension of knee such as overextending the knee when running downhill.[16,35] Patellar tendinopathy is often owing to an increased amount or volume of eccentric loading, such as increased hill or stair descent in running. Because the pain in both conditions is in the inferior patellar region, differential diagnosis can be difficult. Brukner and colleagues[36] found that found that 78% of college athletes diagnosed with patellar tendinopathy showed an increased uptake in the fat pad on T2-weighted MRI, suggestive of inflammation of the fat pad. It seems that the fat pad, rather than the patellar tendon, may be the source of the primary pathology of many athletes with a patellar tendinopathy diagnosis, particularly because the IFP also attaches to the proximal patellar tendon, or a combination of the 2 conditions may exist.

The patient's history may help to differentiate patellar tendinopathy from typical fat pad irritation. The patient with patellar tendinopathy must have a history of eccentric loading of the quadriceps muscle such as running downhill, whereas a patient with a fat pad irritation presents after a forceful extension maneuver. Both patient groups have inferior patellar pain; with patellar tendinopathy the pain is exacerbated by squatting, whereas pain with acute fat pad irritation is exacerbated by both flexion and extension maneuvers.[16,35] Thus, rehabilitation consisting of short arc quadriceps, straight leg raises, and non–weight-bearing knee extension exercises will increase fat pad symptoms The athlete can complain of pain during prolonged standing and can experience pain going up, as well as, down stairs. The athlete stands with hyperextended or "locked back" knees, but if the fat pad is acutely inflamed and extremely painful the patient will not be able to extend the knee. The fat pad seems to be fatter than the other asymptomatic side. On palpation, the inferior pole of the patella is embedded in underlying tissues. The patient may have focal tenderness of the inferior pole.[16] The symptoms are often exacerbated by knee extension and quadriceps contractions.[16]

The presence of pain decreases muscle activity, timing, and endurance as well as alters movement patterns.[27,28] However, because we know pain is very much a cortical experience, so extrinsic factors such as fear of pain, stress, and anxiety[37,38] can amplify the pain experience for the patient and the contribution of these factors must be understood if we are to satisfactorily improve the rehabilitation of individuals with PF pain. Fear of pain decreases vastus medialis obliquus activity, but does not decrease vastus lateralis activity, causing an increase in the dynamic valgus vector force, which results in further PF problems.

Athletes with hyperextended knees often have increased internal femoral rotation. Femoral internal rotation means that the gluteal muscles, maximus and medius posterior fibers, are elongated in standing, so these muscles may be inadequate in maintaining a stable pelvis during running, further increasing the dynamic valgus vector force and continuing the PF pain cycle.

As with all overuse knee problems, the clinician must be aware of the impact of the foot and the shoe, as well as the surface the athlete is running on, has on the symptoms, so a thorough examination of the landing pattern of the runner, the foot, and shoe type is essential when managing runners with inflamed fat pads.

Although not a common problem in runners, the infrapatellar plica, which is an inflammation of the ligamentum mucosum (an embryonic remnant), needs to be considered in the differential diagnoses of fat pad injuries. The ligamentum mucosum is one of several remnants of synovial membranes separating the embryonic knee into compartments. These gradually disappear, although the ligamentum mucosum remains in adulthood in 65% to 90% of knees and is mostly asymptomatic.[39,40] Normal ligamentum mucosum appear isointense to the IFP on T2-weighted MR.[41]

When symptomatic, the ligamentum mucosum becomes thickened and inflamed, and is referred to as an infrapatellar plica. The plica is rarely inflamed in runners but more commonly in elite cyclists, owing to high resistance repetitive knee flexion and extension movements. The patients report symptoms of popping and snapping with knee movement and have a positive Faber's test (palpation of the medial border of the patella in supine with the knee in a figure of 4 position will elicit pain). Unlike IFP pain, which is often exacerbated by an inferior tilt of the patella, pain from an inflamed plica is exacerbated by medial glide of the patella. Pathologic infrapatellar plicae have been shown to be hypointense on T2-weighted MR appearing along the ACL.[41]

Treatment

IFP problems are usually successfully managed with physical therapy. Physical therapy aims to unload abnormally inflamed tissue, both passively using tape and actively by improving the lower limb mechanics, which involves optimizing hip muscle control as well as foot function, which in turn, significantly decreases the patient's symptoms.

Unloading the inflamed soft tissue requires shortening of the inflamed tissue. With IFP problems, the inferior pole patella needs to be tilted out of the fat pad to decrease the repeated inflammation. One or 2 pieces of tape from the superior part of the patella may be sufficient to achieve this. If this procedure does not reduce the patient's symptoms, a further 2 pieces of tape need to be applied from the tibial tubercle to the medial and lateral joint lines, forming a V to unload the IFP further. The aim is to create a "muffin top" so that the fat pad is unloaded as much as possible. If the athlete is still experiencing some pain, the fat pad can be further unloaded by taping just distal to the popliteal fossa from posterior to anterior to pull the tibia forward (**Fig. 1**). Hug and colleagues[42] found that unloading tape significantly reduced muscle stress during contraction, as well as contraction of the muscle. Taping the knee is required until the runner is no longer experiencing symptoms. Patients should be taught how to

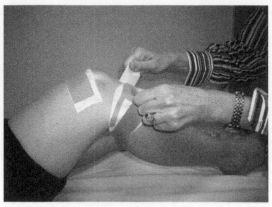

Fig. 1. The infrapatellar fat pad (IFP) is unloaded by tilting the inferior pole of the patella anteriorly (away from the fat pad), lifting the IFP tissue toward the patella, by taping from the tibial tubercle to the medial and lateral joint lines creating a "muffin top" and finally with the knee in 45° of flexion pulling the tibia forward.

tape themselves, so they can easily apply the tape before going for a run so they do not exacerbate their symptoms.

MUSCLE TRAINING

Muscle training needs to be precise for a long-term resolution of symptoms. Motor learning is induced by the performance of the actual movements and is modulated by attention, so in the beginning the runner has to focus on the correct technique of the training to optimize a change in the motor pattern.[43] Skill training, rather than strength training, demonstrates a strong correlation between changes in neurophysiological parameters and motor performance, reinforcing the concept that muscle training needs to be very specific to be effective.[44] Muscle training, therefore, is specific to limb position and joint angle, as well as the type, force, and velocity of contraction, so the runner with IFP symptoms needs to be given specific weight bearing exercises to improve lower limb loading, which in turn decreases fat pad irritation.[45–47] Thus, for the best outcome initially, the patient's muscle training program needs to be carefully monitored by the therapist.

Because weight bearing or closed chain training is more effective in promoting a more balanced initial quadriceps activation than open chain exercises and closed kinetic training allows simultaneous training not only of the vasti but also the gluteals and trunk muscles to control the limb position in weight bearing, athletes with IFP inflammation need to train their lower limb musculature in a position that simulates the stance phase of gait.[48,49] The patient stands with the asymptomatic leg closest to the wall at a distance of a fist away from the wall. The patient's whole body is turned 45° into the wall and the weight is transferred to the outside (symptomatic) leg. The knee of the leg closest to the wall is flexed to 60° with the knee touching, not pushing the wall, for balance purposes. The foot is off the ground. The hips are kept in neutral position so the thighs are parallel. The patient's weight is directed through the heel of the weight-bearing leg, the pelvis is slightly posteriorly tilted and the knee is just off lock (slightly flexed). The patient slightly externally rotates the standing leg without turning the foot, the pelvis, or the shoulders (**Fig. 2**). The patient should sustain the contraction for 15 to 20 seconds and repeat often during the day to improve gluteal

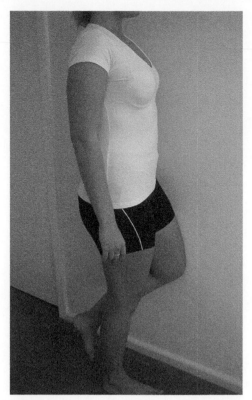

Fig. 2. Lower limb retraining simulating toe off in gait. The training is designed to improve the control of the weight-bearing limb.

and inner range quadriceps activation. The patient can progress this by flexing the hip of the non–weight-bearing leg to 45°. Again, the knee just touches the wall for balance while the patient externally rotates the standing leg without moving the foot, pelvis, or shoulders (**Fig. 3**). These positions improve the patient's control for the single support phase of walking and the strike phase of running. This exercise can be further progressed with added resistance from a rubberized band (Theraband), as well as standing on a pillow to change the stability of the surface.

If the patient has marked internal femoral rotation stretching of the anterior hip structures to increase the available external rotation may be required. The patient lies prone. The patient attempts to flatten the abducted and rotated hip by pushing along the length of the thigh and holding the stretch for 5 seconds. This action activates the gluteals in the inner range. Although this exercise is not functional, it may facilitate gluteus medius activity in someone who is finding it difficult to activate the muscle in weight bearing. If the athlete is finding it challenging to maintain lower limb control during running, then for a short period of time the gluteals may be taped to facilitate gluteal activation. Taping the gluteals enhances hip extension, which not only helps to decrease symptoms by improving proximal control, but may also improve running speed and efficiency.[50] Physical therapy consisting of tape to unload the fat pad and simple specific lower limb training has been shown to increase patellar varus alignment, increase patellar height, and alter medial drift of the patella, as well as decrease fat pad inflammation and volume.[51]

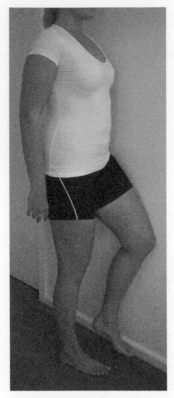

Fig. 3. Lower limb retraining midstance phase of gait. The non–weight-bearing leg is flexed to 45°, and the standing leg is slightly externally rotated to improve dynamic stability of the lower limb.

Injections

Injections of local anesthetic and corticosteroids have been used to treat IFP pain but with mixed results. One to 3 injections of hydrocortisone over a 4- to 6-week interval have led to improvements in IFP pain.[52,53] However, House and Connell[54] found that although 4 ultrasound-guided alcohol injections given weekly for fat pad impingement provided relief for some individuals, in others it did not, so treatment failure was correlated with and hence attributed to MRI of IFP scarring rather than IFP inflammation.

Patients after ACL reconstruction receiving bupivacaine into the IFP from an infusion pump have required fewer oral opioids than those without infusion pumps. However, intraarticular bupivacaine has been associated with increased chondrolysis, which would be counterproductive for treatment.[52]

Operative Treatment

Operative treatment includes fat pad excision, debridement of hypertrophic fibrosis, debridement of the anterior interval scarring, synovectomy, infrapatellar plica release, and denervation of the inferior patellar pole. The outcomes of these operative interventions are poor. Fat pad excision is often performed in a total knee arthroplasty but with limited success.[31,55] Arthroscopic debridement has been used to treat extension block owing to impingement of hypertrophic, fibrotic fat pad tissue (cyclops lesion) after an ACL reconstruction using a patellar tendon graft. However, 50% of patients were dissatisfied with the result and still experiencing symptoms 28 months later.[56] Open arthrotomy for scar tissue adhering the IFP to the anterior tibia (anterior interval scarring) has had moderate success with 85% of patients at the 5-year follow-up reporting they were pleased to have undergone the operation.[57]

SUMMARY

The IPFP is highly innervated and the probable source of most anterior knee pain. Knee pain inhibits quadriceps activity and fear of pain specifically inhibits vastus medialis obliquus. Taping to unload the IPFP significantly reduces pain, which allows the runner to continue his or her training. The athlete must, however, retrain the lower limb loading, which includes hip, knee, and foot musculature.

REFERENCES

1. Bogduk N, Twomey L. Clinical anatomy of the lumbar spine. Edinburgh (Untied Kingdom): Churchill Livingstone; 1991.
2. Hall T, Zusman M, Elvey R. Manually detected impediments during the straight leg raise test. Proceedings 9th Biennial Conference of the Manipulative Physiotherapists Association of Australia, Gold Coast. November 22–25, 1995. p. 48–53.
3. Torres L, Dunlop DD, Peterfy C, et al. The relationship between specific tissue lesions and pain severity in persons with knee osteoarthritis. Osteoarthritis Cartilage 2006;14(10):1033–40.
4. Cubukcu D, Sarsan A, Alkan H. Relationships between pain, function and radiographic findings in osteoarthritis of the knee: a cross-sectional study. Arthritis 2012;2012:984060.
5. Bedson J, Croft PR. The discordance between clinical and radiographic knee osteoarthritis: a systematic search and summary of the literature. BMC Musculoskelet Disord 2008;2(9):116.
6. Sengupta M, Zhang YQ, Niu JB, et al. High signal in knee osteophytes is not associated with knee pain. Osteoarthritis Cartilage 2006;14(5):413–7.
7. Hill CL, Hunter DJ, Niu J, et al. Synovitis detected on magnetic resonance imaging and its relation to pain and cartilage loss in knee osteoarthritis. Ann Rheum Dis 2007;66(12):1599–603.
8. Bierdert R, Stauffer E, Niklaus NF. Occurrence of free nerve endings in the soft tissue of the knee joint. A histologic investigation. Am J Sports Med 1992;20(4): 430–3.
9. Arnoldi CC. Patellar pain. Acta Orthop Scand 1991;62(Suppl 224):1–29. Surgery, Sports Traumatology and Arthroscopy 8:68–72.
10. Fulkerson JP, Tennant R, Jaivin JS, et al. Histological evidence of retinacular nerve injury associated with patellofemoral malalignment. Clin Orthop Relat Res 1985;197:196–205.
11. Vaatainen U, Lohmander LS, Thonar E, et al. Markers of cartilage and synovial metabolism in joint fluid and serum of patients with chondromalacia. Osteoarthritis Cartilage 1998;6(2):115–24.
12. Sanchis-Alfonso V, Rosello-Sastre E. Immunohistochemical analysis for neural markers of the lateral retinaculum in patients with isolated symptomatic patellofemoral malalignment. Am J Sports Med 2000;28(5):725–31.
13. Dye SF, Chew MH. The use of scintigraphy to detect increased osseous metabolic activity about the knee. J Bone Joint Surg Am 1993;75A(9):1388–406.
14. Hoffa A. The influence of the adipose tissue with regard to the pathology of the knee joint. JAMA 1904;43:795–6.

15. Matcuk GR, Cen SY. Superolateral Hoffa fat-pad edema and patellofemoral maltracking: predictive modeling. Am J Roentgenol 2014;203(2):207–12.
16. Dragoo JL, Johnson C, McConnell J. Evaluation and treatment of disorders of the infrapatellar fat pad. Sports Med 2012;42(1):51–67.
17. Gallagher J, Tierney P, Murray P, et al. The Infrapatellar fat pad: anatomy and clinical correlations. Knee Surg Sports Traumatol Arthrosc 2005;13(4):268–72.
18. Bohnsack M, Hurschler C, Demirtas T, et al. Infrapatellar fat pad pressure and volume changes of the anterior compartment during knee motion: possible clinical consequences to the anterior knee pain syndrome. Knee Surg Sports Traumatol Arthrosc 2005;13(2):135–41.
19. Skaf AY, Hernandez Filho G, Dirim B, et al. Pericruciate fat pad of the knee: anatomy and pericruciate fat pad inflammation: cadaveric and clinical study emphasizing MR imaging. Skeletal Radiol 2012;41(12):1591–6.
20. Kohn D, Deller S, Rudert M. Arterial blood supply of the infrapatellar fat pad. Anatomy and clinical consequences. Arch Orthop Trauma Surg 1995;114(2):72–5.
21. Scapinelli R. Vascular anatomy of the human cruciate ligaments and surrounding structures. Clin Anat 1997;10(3):151–62.
22. Dye SF, Vaupel GL, Dye CC. Conscious neurosensory mapping of the internal structures of the human knee without intraarticular anesthesia. Am J Sports Med 1998;26(6):773–7.
23. Kennedy JC, Alexander IJ, Hayes KC. Nerve supply of the human knee and its functional importance. Am J Sports Med 1982;10(6):329–35.
24. Wojtys EM, Beaman DN, Glover RA, et al. Innervation of the human knee joint by substance-P fibers. Arthroscopy 1990;6(4):254–63.
25. Witonski D, Wagrowska-Danielewicz M. Distribution of substance-P nerve fibers in the knee joint in patients with anterior knee pain syndrome: a preliminary report. Knee Surg Sports Traumatol Arthrosc 1999;7(3):177–83.
26. Bennell K, Hodges P, Mellor R, et al. The nature of anterior knee pain following injection of hypertonic saline into the infrapatellar fat pad. J Orthop Res 2004; 22(1):116–21.
27. Hodges PW, Mellor R, Crossley K, et al. Pain induced by injection of hypertonic saline into the infrapatellar fat pad and effect on coordination of the quadriceps muscles. Arthritis Rheum 2009;61(1):70–7.
28. Henriksen M, Klokker L, Bartholdy C, et al. The associations between pain sensitivity and knee muscle strength in healthy volunteers: a cross-sectional study. Pain Res Treat 2013;2013:787054.
29. Chew HF, Evans NA, Stanish WD. Patient controlled bupivacaine infusion into the infrapatellar fat pad after anterior cruciate ligament reconstruction. Arthroscopy 2003;19(5):500–5.
30. Clements KM, Ball AD, Jones HB, et al. Cellular and histopathological changes in the infrapatellar fat pad. Osteoarthritis Cartilage 2009;17(6):805–12.
31. Moverley R, Williams D, Bardakos N, et al. Removal of the infrapatellar fat pad during total knee arthroplasty: does it affect patient outcomes? Int Orthop 2014;38(12):2483–7.
32. Saddik D, McNally EG, Richardson M. MRI of Hoffa's fat pad. Skeletal Radiol 2004;33(8):433–44.
33. Tang G, Niitsu M, Ikeda K, et al. Fibrous scar in the infrapatellar fat pad after arthroscopy: MR imaging. Radiat Med 2000;18(1):1–5.
34. Apostolaki E, Cassar-Pullicino VN, Tyrrell PN, et al. MRI appearances of the infrapatellar fat pad in occult traumatic patellar dislocation. Clin Radiol 1999;54(11): 743–7.

35. McConnell J. Fat pad irritation - a mistaken patellar tendonitis. Sports Health 1991;9(4):7–9.
36. Brukner P, McConnell J, Bergman A, et al. Infrapatellar fat pad impingement: correlation between clinical and MR findings. Sports Health 2003;21(5):8–11.
37. Van de Kar LD, Blair ML. Forebrain pathways mediating stress-induced hormone secretion. Front Neuroendocrinol 1999;20(1):1–48.
38. Juhn SK, Li W, Kim JY, et al. Effect of stress-related hormones on inner ear fluid homeostasis and function. Am J Otol 1999;20(6):800–6.
39. Patel SJ, Kaplan PA, Dussault RG, et al. Anatomy and clinical significance of the horizontal cleft in the infrapatellar fat pad of the knee: MR imaging. AJR Am J Roentgenol 1998;170(6):1551–5.
40. Kosarek FJ, Helms CA. The MR appearance of the infrapatellar plica. AJR Am J Roentgenol 1999;172(2):481–4.
41. Demirag B, Osturk C, Karakayali M. Symptomatic infrapatellar plica. Knee Surg Sports Traumatol Arthrosc 2006;14(2):156–60.
42. Hug F, Ouellette A, Vicenzino B, et al. Deloading tape reduces muscle stress at rest and during contraction. Med Sci Sports Exerc 2014;46(12):2317.
43. Stefan K, Wyeislo M, Classen J. Modulation of associative human motor cortical plasticity by attention. J Neurophysiol 2004;92:66–72.
44. Jensen JL, Marstrand PC, Nielsen JB. Motor skill training and strength training are associated with different plastic changes in the central nervous system. J Appl Physiol 2005;99(4):1558–68.
45. Sale D, MacDougall D. Specificity of strength training: a review for coach & athlete. Can J Appl Sport Sci 1981;6(2):87–92.
46. Sale D. Influence of exercise and training on motor unit activation. Exerc Sport Sci Rev 1987;5:95–151.
47. Kitai T, Sale D. Specificity of joint angle in isometric training. Eur J Appl Physiol 1989;64:1500.
48. Stensdotter AK, Hodges PW, Mellor R, et al. Quadriceps activation in closed and in open kinetic chain exercise. Med Sci Sports Exerc 2003;35(12):2043–7.
49. Escamilla RF, Fleisig GS, Zheng N. Biomechanics of the knee during closed kinetic chain and open kinetic chain exercises. Med Sci Sports Exerc 1998; 30(4):556–69.
50. Kilbreath SL, Perkins S, Crosbie J, et al. Gluteal taping improves hip extension during stance phase of walking following stroke. Aust J Physiother 2006;52(1):53–6.
51. McConnell J, Read JW. Magnetic resonance imaging pre and 4 months post physiotherapy – a pilot study. Rheumatol Curr Res 2014. http://dx.doi.org/10.4172/2161-1149.S16-008.
52. Chu CR, Coyle CH, Chu CT, et al. In vivo effects of single intra-articular injection of 0.5% bupivacaine on articular cartilage. J Bone Joint Surg 2010;92(3):599–608.
53. Dragoo JL, Korootkova T, Kanwar R, et al. The effect of local anaesthetics administered via pain pump on chondrocyte viability. Am J Sports Med 2008;36(8):1484–8.
54. House CV, Connell DA. Therapeutic ablation of the infrapatellar fat pad under ultrasound guidance: A pilot study. Clin Radiol 2007;62(12):1198–201.
55. Macule F, Sastre S, Lasurt S, et al. Hoffa's fat pad resection in total knee arthroplasty. Acta Orthop Belg 2005;71(6):714–7.
56. Kim DH, Gill TJ, Millet PJ. Arthroscopic treatment of the arthrofibrotic knee. Arthroscopy 2004;20:187–94.
57. Millet PJ, Williams RJ, Wickiewicz TL. Open debridement and soft tissue release as a salvage procedure for the severely arthrofibrotic knee. Am J Sports Med 1999;27(5):552–61.

Exertional Leg Pain

Sathish Rajasekaran, MD[a,b,]*, Jonathan T. Finnoff, DO[c,d,e]

KEYWORDS

- Medial tibial stress syndrome • Stress fractures • Compartment syndromes
- Popliteal artery • Iliac artery • Nerve compression syndromes • Leg injuries
- Athletic injuries

KEY POINTS

- A detailed history, physical examination, and evidence-based approach to diagnostic testing are essential in the evaluation and management of exertional leg pain.
- The clinician should be aware of the possibility of more than 1 diagnosis to explain complex presentations of exertional leg pain.
- The physical examination is often normal at rest, and provocative maneuvers or exertional activities are often required to precipitate examination findings.

INTRODUCTION

Exertional leg pain (ELP) is defined as pain distal to the knee and proximal to the talocrural joint that is associated with exertion.[1]

The incidence of ELP in runners varies in the literature, with one retrospective study of 2002 running injuries reporting a rate of 12.8%, and another reporting that 82.4% of cross-country athletes had a history of ELP.[2] A further study noted that running more than 40 miles per week was associated with patients presenting with ELP.[3]

ELP is commonly categorized as having a musculoskeletal, vascular, or neurologic origin. This article focuses on medial tibial stress syndrome (MTSS), tibial bone stress injury (TBSI), chronic exertional compartment syndrome (CECS), arterial endofibrosis, popliteal artery entrapment syndrome (PAES), and entrapment neuropathies.[1,4]

Disclosure Statement: The authors have nothing to disclose.
[a] Department of Orthopaedics and Rehabilitation, University of Iowa Sports Medicine, 2701 Prairie Meadow Drive, Iowa City, IA 52242, USA; [b] Division of Physical Medicine and Rehabilitation, University of Alberta, 10230 111 Avenue Northwest, Edmonton, AB T5G 0B7, Canada; [c] Department of Physical Medicine and Rehabilitation, Mayo Clinic School of Medicine, 200 1st St SW, Rochester, MN 55905, USA; [d] Department of Physical Medicine and Rehabilitation, University of California Davis School of Medicine, 4860 Y Street, Sacramento, CA 95817, USA; [e] Mayo Clinic Sports Medicine Center, Mayo Clinic Square, 600 Hennepin Avenue, Suite 310, Minneapolis, MN 55403, USA
* Corresponding author. University of Iowa Sports Medicine, 2701 Prairie Meadow Drive, Iowa City, IA 52242.
E-mail address: sathish.k.rajasekaran@gmail.com

MEDIAL TIBIAL STRESS SYNDROME

The incidence of MTSS in runners is between 13.6% and 20.0%.[5] Other names for this condition include shin soreness, tibial stress syndrome, medial tibial syndrome, shin splints syndrome, and shin splints.[6] The most commonly accepted definition of MTSS is pain along the posteromedial border of the tibia that occurs during exercise, excluding pain from ischemic origin or signs of stress fracture.[7]

MTSS affects the posteromedial tibia, most commonly in the middle or distal third. The exact mechanism of injury is unclear, but studies show that patients with MTSS may be less adapted than control subjects to tibial load.[8] In addition, low tibial bone density has been noted in MTSS patients compared with healthy controls.[9] The decreased tibial bone density normalizes once the athlete recovers from MTSS.[10] Thus, tibial bones with decreased bone density may not tolerate the repeated loads experienced by athletes, resulting in MTSS, or repeated loads may themselves cause decreased bone density and lead to MTSS.

History and Physical Examination

MTSS should lead the differential diagnosis for running athletes with posteromedial tibial border pain.[6] The pain is usually located in the middle or distal third of the tibia. Patients will often report that symptoms initially were absent at rest, began with exertion, and subsided with continued exercise.[6] As the condition worsens, symptoms may not resolve during exercise.[6] Pain after exertion can also manifest, but in these cases it is essential to rule out TBSI.[11]

On examination, diffuse tenderness to palpation along the posteromedial distal two-thirds of the tibia is reportedly more sensitive than the pain on hopping or with percussion.[6] **Table 1** details intrinsic risk factors found to be associated with MTSS.[12] Foot pronation can be assessed using the navicular drop test (**Fig. 1**).

Table 1
Intrinsic risk factors found to be associated with the development of medial tibial stress syndrome in a systematic review and meta-analysis of the literature

	No. of MTSS	No. of Controls	MD [95% CI]	I^2 (%)	Overall Effect
Significant Difference					
BMI	187	264	0.79 [0.4, 1.2]	0.00	$P<.001$
Navicular drop	198	366	1.2 [0.5, 1.8]	40.19	$P<.001$
Ankle PF ROM	71	166	5.9 [3.6, 9.2]	0.00	$P<.001$
HIP ER	117	162	3.9 [1.8, 6.1]	0.00	$P<.001$
No Significant Difference					
Ankle DF ROM	173	308	−0.01 [−0.96, 0.93]	17.89	$P=.98$
Ankle eversion ROM	108	173	1.17 [−0.02, 2.36]	31.58	$P=.06$
Ankle inversion ROM	89	160	0.98 [−3.11, 5.07]	71.58	$P=.64$
Q-angle	132	214	−0.22 [−0.95, 0.50]	5.23	$P=.54$
Hip IR	117	162	0.18 [−5.37, 5.73]	83.74	$P=.95$

Abbreviations: BMI, body mass index; CI, confidence interval; DF, dorsiflexion; ER, external rotation; I^2, heterogeneity; IR, internal rotation; MD, mean difference; MTSS, medial tibial stress syndrome; PF, plantar flexion; ROM, range of motion.

Data from Magnusson HI, Westlin NE, Nyqvist F, et al. Abnormally decreased regional bone density in athletes with medial tibial stress syndrome. Am J Sports Med 2001;29(6):712–15.

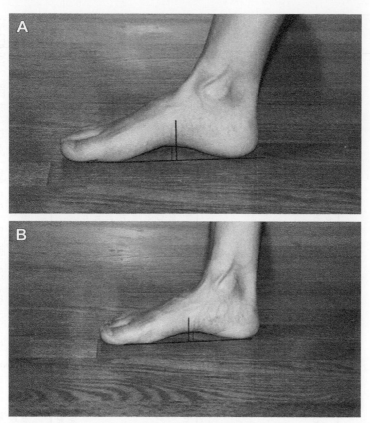

Fig. 1. Navicular drop test. (*A*) Unloaded foot. (*B*) Loaded foot. (*From* Reshef N, Guelich DR. Medial tibial stress syndrome. Clin Sports Med 2012;31(2):277; with permission.)

Clinicians should be aware of other causes of ELP that can mimic the presentation of MTSS, the most noteworthy being TBSI and CECS. Differentiating between these 3 conditions can most often be done by obtaining a detailed history and performing a thorough physical examination. In cases where uncertainty exits, diagnostic imaging and compartment pressure testing can help clarify the underlying cause.

Diagnostic Evaluation

Imaging is not indicated for cases of uncomplicated MTSS. However, when diagnostic uncertainty exists, imaging may be warranted to confirm the diagnosis of MTSS and exclude TBSI. The use of radiography in the diagnosis of MTSS is limited, but may help rule out other causes of ELP (**Table 2**).[13] The high false-positive rate of bone scintigraphy and its poor ability to differentiate between MTSS and TBSI may limit its utility in the assessment of MTSS.[13] MRI has been increasingly used over bone scintigraphy in the assessment of ELP (**Fig. 2**).[13] Not only has MRI been shown to accurately differentiate between MTSS and TBSI, it may also be used to guide treatment.[14] MRI also provides information regarding other potential causes of ELP, particularly when used after exertion.[1] The role of computed tomography (CT) in the assessment of MTSS is unclear at present.[13]

Table 2
Tibial stress imaging grading system and rehabilitation guidelines

Grade	Clinical Diagnosis	Radiography	Bone Scan	MRI	CT Scan	Rehabilitation
1	Medial tibial stress syndrome	Gray cortex sign; margin is indistinct, density lower	Linear increased activity in cortical region	Mild to moderate periosteal edema on T2-weighted images; marrow: normal on T1- and T2-weighted images	Soft-tissue mass adjacent to periosteal surface	2–3 wk nonimpact activity
2		Acute periosteal reaction, density differs from rest of cortex showing incomplete mineralization	Small focal region of increased activity	Grade 1+ marrow edema on T2-weighted images	Increased attenuation of yellow marrow	4–6 wk nonimpact activity
3	Tibial bone stress injury	Lucent areas in cortex, ill-defined foci at site of pain	Larger focal lesion with highly increased activity in the cortical region	Grade 2 + marrow edema on T1-weighted images	Increased hypattenuation (osteopenia), intracortical hypoattenuation (resorption activity), and subtle intracortical linear hypoattenuation (striation)	6–9 wk nonimpact activity
4		Fracture line present	Very large focal region of highly increased activity	Grade 3 + fracture line clearly visible	Hypoattenuating line	6 wk of cast, followed by 6 wk of nonimpact activity

Abbreviation: CT, computed tomography.
Adapted from Beck BR, Bergman AG, Miner M, et al. Tibial stress injury: relationship of radiographic, nuclear medicine bone scanning, MR imaging, and CT severity grades to clinical severity and time to healing. Radiology 2012;263(3):811–8; and Fredericson M, Bergman AG, Hoffman KL, et al. Tibial stress reaction in runners. Correlation of clinical symptoms and scintigraphy with a new magnetic resonance imaging grading system. Am J Sports Med 1995;23(4):472–81; with permission.

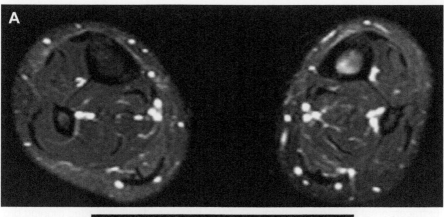
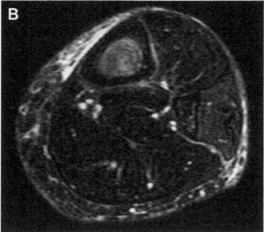

Fig. 2. (*A*) Axial T2-weighted MR image of the legs, showing bone marrow edema in the left leg of an athlete with medial tibial stress syndrome (MTSS). (*B*) Axial T2-weighted MR image of an athlete with MTSS showing periosteal edema on the anteromedial side of the tibia. (*From* Moen MH, Schmikli SL, Weir A, et al. A prospective study on MRI findings and prognostic factors in athletes with MTSS. Scand J Med Sci Sports 2014;24(1):206–7; with permission.)

Management

Initial treatment includes activity modification to avoid aggravating activities, and correction of modifiable risk factors (see **Table 1**). If the navicular drop test is positive, specific measures addressing overpronation (custom foot orthosis, shoe modifications, motion control footwear, therapeutic adhesive taping, or gait retraining) should be pursued.[15,16] The duration of rest from aggravating activity can be guided by MRI using the imaging criteria of Fredericson and colleagues[14] (see **Table 2**). If an MRI has not been completed, the patient should rest until pain-free during normal daily activities and nontender over the area; this typically requires 2 to 6 weeks of rest, but can take longer if the condition is more severe.[17]

The patient should progress from restricted to unrestricted activity in a systematic, gradual fashion. For example, the patient initially may exercise in a non–weight-bearing environment (eg, pool running) as long as he or she is pain-free. As their symptoms improve, patients may be transitioned to bicycling using a low gear and high cadence in a seated position. The next step in the progression can include higher-resistance seated or standing bicycling, or exercise on an elliptical machine. When they have no pain with these activities or with palpation over the previously tender area, patients can be transitioned to running. Running should begin on a treadmill so patients have absolute control over the pace, duration, and incline/decline of their run. If an antigravity treadmill is available, it can be used before the use of a conventional treadmill. However, clinicians should be aware that no studies have examined its use in the rehabilitation of MTSS, and a recent study noted a significant difference between the reported and measured body weight supported by the antigravity treadmill.[18] Duration should be increased before intensity, but should not be increased greater than 10% per week. Eventually patients can transition to running outside, preferably on a track rather than concrete or asphalt, and high-intensity running workouts (eg, intervals) and plyometrics can be incorporated into their training regimen.[17]

Extracorporeal shock-wave therapy (ESWT), when used with a graded running program, has been found to significantly decrease the time to full recovery compared with controls.[19] In recalcitrant cases where general conservative measures and those aimed at addressing patients' intrinsic risk factors (see **Table 1**) have failed, surgery can be considered.[6]

TIBIAL BONE STRESS INJURY

TBSI can involve the cortical (compact) bone located in the diaphysis of long bones, or cancellous bone (trabecular bone) located in the metaphysis and epiphysis of long bones. The term stress fracture has been supplanted by stress injury to acknowledge that TBSI can occur without a true fracture on imaging.[14] Although the incidence of TBSI in runners has not been elucidated, in a large cohort of bone stress injuries in athletes the prevalence of TBSI was 49.1%.[20]

Two distinct types of diaphyseal TBSI have been described. One affects the anterior tibial cortex while the other affects the posterior tibial cortex.[21] Anterior TBSI is proposed to occur secondary to tension strain, whereas posterior TBSI is due to compressive strain (**Fig. 3**).[21] Both can occur proximally or distally.[22] The exact pathophysiology of TBSI has not been elucidated, but it has been proposed that

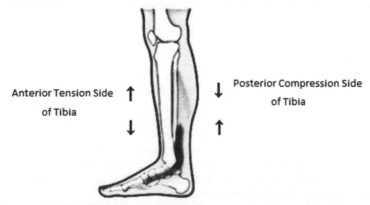

Anterior Tension Side of Tibia

Posterior Compression Side of Tibia

Fig. 3. Location of tibial diaphyseal stress fracture. (*From* Robertson GA, Wood AM. Return to sports after stress fractures of the tibial diaphysis: a systematic review. Br Med Bull 2015;114(1):2; with permission.)

microdamage occurs when the tibia is exposed to repetitive strain, resulting in a bone remodeling response (osteoclastic activity).[23] During this process whereby resorption precedes deposition (osteoblastic activity), the tibia is thought to be weakened, leading to a tibial stress reaction or fracture.[23] The overarching causation for TBSI can be dichotomized into fatigue and insufficiency types.[23] Fatigue stress injuries are related to overuse injuries in athletes with a normal bone mineral density.[23] Two studies suggested that decreased muscle mass and decreased tibial bone cross-sectional area may be predisposing factors.[24–26] Insufficiency types are related to a decreased bone mineral density, and may be more relevant in female athletes.[23,27] When eliciting details on history and during physical examination, the clinician can categorize suspected intrinsic and extrinsic risk factors under these 2 groupings.

History and Physical Examination

Athletes will characteristically present with localized pain of insidious onset, which worsens with weight-bearing activities.[14] The hallmark sign is pain after exertion, which progresses to pain during exertion. This aspect assists in differentiating TBSI from MTSS.[11,14] In severe cases, pain can occur at night.[23,28] While obtaining the history, recent changes in frequency, intensity, timing, and type of exercise training should be noted, as recent increases in these variables may lead to the development of TBSI.[14] In female athletes, risk factors for the female athlete triad should also be ascertained, and can be screened for using a 12-item screening tool.[29] The duration of running-shoe use should be noted, as it has been suggested that shoes older than 6 months can predispose a runner to TBSI.[30]

On examination, the region of discomfort is often tender to palpation and can be swollen.[14] In one study, a 128-Hz tuning fork was used to elicit pain by placing it on the anterior tibia (75% sensitive and 67% specific).[31] This study used bone scintigraphy within 30 days of the tuning fork test as the gold standard, which may have weakened the strength of its findings.[31] Limb alignment, muscle tone, and straight-leg raise range of motion should be assessed, as these may be risk factors for the development of TBSI.[32,33] Caution should be exercised when excluding the diagnosis of TBSI based on physical examination findings alone if the history is suggestive of TBSI. When TBSI is included in the differential diagnosis of ELP, further imaging is essential to make this diagnosis and classify the injury.[14]

Diagnostic Evaluation

Beck and colleagues[13] correlated radiography, bone scintigraphy, MRI, and CT in the assessment of TBSI (grade III–IV) using criteria from 4 previously published articles (see Table 2). Although radiography is often the first line of imaging and can reveal a fracture (Fig. 4), it has low sensitivity for TBSI.[13] Bone scintigraphy, previously thought to be the reference standard for assessing TBSI, is now discouraged in the assessment of TBSI because of its low specificity and inaccuracy in grading TBSI.[13,34] MRI has been proved to be superior to radiography and bone scintigraphy in the assessment of TBSI, providing more information on the extent and level of TBSI.[13,14,35–38] MRI can also be used to determine management in TBSI.[14] Although Gaeta and colleagues[22] have published a grading system for CT in the assessment of TBSI, its clinical role is limited by its low sensitivity. Thus, MRI is indicated in athletes with suspected TBSI whose initial radiographs are negative.[13]

Management

Current management strategies for TBSI are based on the Fredericson MRI criteria,[14] whereby grade III injuries are rehabilitated with 6 to 9 weeks of nonimpact activities,

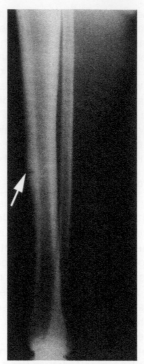

Fig. 4. Stress fracture revealed at presentation. Arrow indicates fracture line. (*From* Rettig AC, Shelbourne KD, McCarroll JR, et al. The natural history and treatment of delayed union stress fractures of the anterior cortex of the tibia. Am J Sports Med 1988;16(3):253; with permission.)

and grade IV injuries are immobilized for 6 weeks followed by 6 weeks of nonimpact activity. Robertson and Wood[21] systematically reviewed the literature investigating return to sport after diaphyseal TBSI, and found that posterior diaphyseal TBSI responded to shorter durations of nonoperative treatment (6–12 weeks), anterior TBSI required up to 6 months of nonoperative treatment and occasionally required surgery, and complete tibial fractures were treated in the same manner as an acute fracture. A Cochrane review assessing treatments for "stress fractures and stress reactions" noted a possible role for pneumatic bracing in the treatment of TBSI, leading to a quicker recovery.[39] The rehabilitation process should be guided by pain and the Fredericson criteria[14] (**Fig. 5**).[40] Surgical options can be explored with anterior TBSI in cases of delayed healing, in elite athletes, or in female athletes with a low bone mineral density and high-grade TBSI (found to have delayed recovery), as surgery may decrease recovery time.[21,40,41] Three surgical procedures have been described (intramedullary nailing, plating, and excision and drilling), with the former 2 having a pooled return-to-play rate of 100%, and the latter a rate of 92.5%.[21] Of the 3 surgical techniques, intramedullary nailing seems to be the procedure of choice for TBSI.[40]

Educating athletes and training staff on the symptoms of TBSI can shorten the time from symptom onset to diagnosis, given that a delay in diagnosis can worsen the athlete's prognosis.[21] A Cochrane database review suggested that shock-absorbing shoe inserts may reduce the incidence of TBSI.[39] Athletes should be screened for the female athlete triad and, when identified, treated appropriately. Vitamin D levels higher than 40 ng/mL (<50 ng/mL) may also help to prevent bone stress injuries.[42]

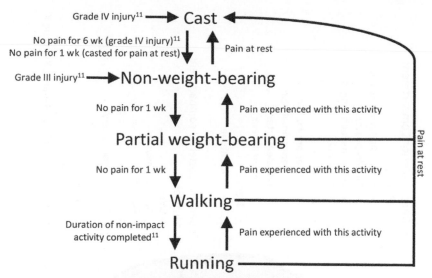

Fig. 5. Return-to-play guidelines for tibial bone stress injuries.

CHRONIC EXERTIONAL COMPARTMENT SYNDROME

In athletes presenting with undiagnosed leg pain, the incidence of CECS has been reported to be between 14% and 27%.[1] The mean age of presentation for CECS is between 26 and 28 years, with an equal distribution in males and females.[43–45] Ninety percent of diabetics with of mean age 48 years with nonvascular ELP have CECS in one study.[1] Although CECS affects the lower leg in approximately 95% of cases, it can also affect the forearm, thigh, and foot.[1]

CECS can occur in any of the 4 lower leg compartments (**Fig. 6**).[1] The deep posterior compartment may also have a fifth compartment, containing only the tibialis posterior. CECS is reported almost equally in the anterior compartment (40%–60%) and deep posterior compartment (32%–60%); less frequently in the lateral compartment (12%–35%), which can accompany CECS of the anterior compartment; and least frequently in the superficial posterior compartment (2%–20%).[1]

CECS was initially thought to occur secondarily to thickened compartment fascia, leading to a decrease in compliance.[46] This theory has more recently been called into question.[47,48] Other theories include reduced microcapillary capacity, venous congestion, increased interstitial volume secondary to creatine monohydrate supplementation, and stiff connective tissue in diabetic patients.[1] Although the underlying pathology of CECS is not clearly understood, it has been shown that intracompartmental volume increases after exertion with an associated increase in compartment pressure above that seen in normal patients.[1] The cause of the pain associated with this increase in intracompartmental pressure in CECS has also not been ascertained, but is postulated to occur secondarily to muscle or nerve deoxygenation, direct stimulation of fascial or periosteal sensory nerves, or release of local kinins.[1]

History and Physical Examination

Athletes with CECS will often describe symptom development after a specific volume (time, distance, or intensity) of exertion involving the lower legs and feet.[1] Symptoms can be localized to any or all of the compartments of the lower leg, and bilateral

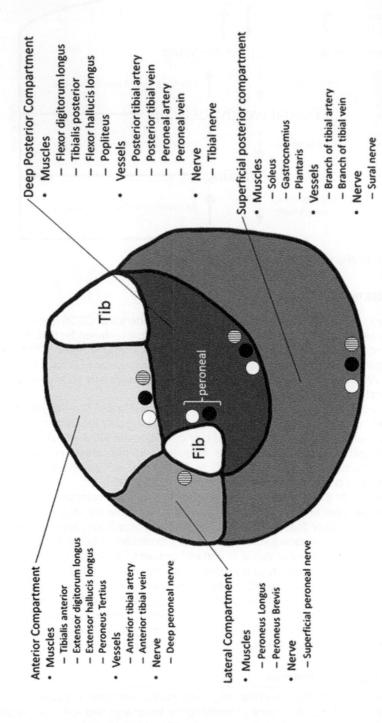

Fig. 6. Compartments of the leg. Black circles, arteries; striped circles, nerves; white circles, veins. Fib, fibula; Tib, tibia. (*From* Rajasekaran S, Kvinlaug K, Finnoff JT. Exertional leg pain in the athlete. PM R 2012;4(12):986; with permission.)

presentation is apparent in up to 82% of cases.[1] Patients characterize the pain as a fullness or cramp-like sensation of the affected compartment, which increases in intensity with exertion. Numbness, paresthesias, and weakness in the sensorimotor distribution of the nerves in the affected compartments are possible accompanying symptoms, which may occur when the athlete attempts to continue the precipitating activity after symptom onset.[1] Symptoms are described to cease immediately after or shortly after the precipitating activity is stopped, but over time the recovery time increases.[43] The volume of exercise required to precipitate symptoms also decreases with time, and some patients experience decreased athletic performance the day after symptom onset.[1] Though rare, CECS can develop into acute compartment syndrome, a limb-threatening surgical emergency.[49] Several similarities in patient population and demographics, and presenting symptoms, were noted between CECS and functional PAES, and it has been recommended that ankle brachial index (ABI) testing with ankle provocation maneuvers be conducted in this group to rule this alternative diagnosis in or out.[50]

The examination is completely normal at rest in CECS.[43] Following precipitating exercise, neurologic impairments in the affected sensorimotor nerve distribution may be appreciated, and passive stretching of muscles in the involved compartment may be painful.[1] Although fascial hernias have been described with CECS, their presence can also be seen in the asymptomatic population.[51,52]

Diagnostic Evaluation

French and Price[53] first described the use of needle manometry in CECS. Intracompartmental pressure testing continues to be a mainstay in the workup of CECS, and the preexertional and postexertional measurements published by Pedowitz and colleagues[44] are the criteria most commonly used to diagnose CECS (**Table 3**). Several different needle manometry devices have been described in the literature, but an international survey found the side-port needle manometer to be the most commonly used.[54,55] Two systematic reviews have noted several weaknesses in needle manometry technique and the diagnostic criteria used in the assessment of CECS.[55,56] Nevertheless, most clinicians continue to use this technique. A recent meta-analysis suggested that the Pedowitz criteria should be modified as follows to improve their sensitivity and specificity: preexercise greater than 14 mm Hg, 1 minute postexercise greater than 35 mm Hg, and 5 minutes postexercise greater than 23 mm Hg.[57] No clear exercise protocol exists for compartment pressure testing, but it has been suggested that patients should exercise until maximally tolerated symptoms are produced before postexercise compartment testing.[58]

Postexertional MRI has been noted to show increased signal intensity, but only 2 studies from the same institution reported validated diagnostic criteria in the assessment of anterior compartment CECS using an in-scanner exercise protocol (**Fig. 7**).[59,60] Although functional imaging (thallium scintigraphy, thallium single-photon emission CT, methoxyisobutylisonitrile, ^{99m}Tc-tetrofosmin single-photon

Table 3		
Modified Pedowitz criteria for the diagnosis of CECS[44]		
CECS is suggested if the patient meets 1 or more of the following criteria		
1		Preexercise pressure ≥15 mm Hg
2		1-min postexercise pressure ≥30 mm Hg
3		5-min postexercise pressure ≥20 mm Hg

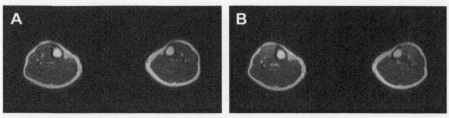

Fig. 7. (*A*) T2-weighted MR image of patient with chronic exertional compartment syndrome (CECS) at rest. (*B*) T2-weighted image of CECS patient following isometric dorsiflexion. Note increased T2 signal in anterior compartments in *B*. (*From* Ringler MD, Litwiller DV, Felmlee JP, et al. MRI accurately detects chronic exertional compartment syndrome: a validation study. Skeletal Radiol 2013;42(3):388; with permission.)

emission CT, and functional MRI) have been studied in the assessment of CECS, their clinical utility has not been proven.[61] Near-infrared spectroscopy has been reported to approach the accuracy of intracompartmental pressure testing, but quantitative diagnostic criteria need to be established to advocate for its use clinically.[61] A recent prospective pilot study showed that ultrasonography can detect a significant increase in anterior compartment thickness in CECS patients when compared with controls, but this technique requires further study before it can be recommended for clinical use.[47]

Management

If an athlete presenting with CECS only experiences symptoms with a specific exercise, he or she can be counseled to refrain from that activity, on the understanding that symptoms can recur with the same or similar exercises.[51] Forefoot running, first described by Kirby and McDermott,[62] was shown to be an effective treatment of anterior compartment CECS by Diebal and colleagues[63,64] in 2 published case series. In both studies, anterior compartment CECS patients were rehabilitated with a forefoot running technique, and demonstrated decreased symptoms and intracompartmental pressures.[63,64] A second nonsurgical treatment option involves injecting botulinum toxin A into the muscles of the affected compartments. Two case series have shown this to be an effective treatment in anterior and lateral leg compartment CECS.[65,66] Although not assessed in this case series, because reinnervation takes place over 6 to 9 months after injection, this treatment option may require repeat injections to maintain its efficacy.[65,66] Furthermore, a reduction in strength was also reported with this treatment option, which may limit its application in elite athletes.[66]

Surgery remains the mainstay in the treatment of CECS. Options include open and endoscopic fasciotomies, and fasciectomies. Although lower success rates have been published for fasciectomies, no direct comparison with fasciotomy or between open and endoscopic procedures has been undertaken.[67] In the treatment of anterior compartment CECS, success ranges between 81% and 100%. The lower range of success is associated with concomitant lateral compartment release.[68] The success rate for deep posterior compartment surgical release is between 30% and 65%, which may be due to the complex nature of the surgery and the possible presence of a fifth compartment.[69] Complication rates of up to 16% have been reported in the literature and include infection, hematomas, neurovascular injury, deep venous thrombosis, and lymphocele formation.[43,45] Although postsurgical guidelines may vary from center to center, general guidelines have been published (**Table 4**).[1]

Table 4	
Postoperative chronic exertional compartment syndrome return-to-play guidelines	
POD 1–2	Gentle active and passive range of motion, weight bearing as tolerated, institute measures to control edema, undertake basic activities of daily living, protect the healing incision at all times
POD 3–4	Achieve independence with activities of daily living and begin unassisted ambulation
Weeks 1–4	Add stair climbing and increase walking distance
Weeks 4–6	Begin nonimpact lower extremity aerobic exercise
Week 6+	Initiate unrestricted impact lower extremity activities

From Rajasekaran S, Kvinlaug K, Finnoff JT. Exertional leg pain in the athlete. PM R 2012;4(12): 985–1000; with permission.

EXTERNAL ILIAC ARTERY ENDOFIBROSIS

External iliac artery endofibrosis (EIAE) is the most common subtype (90%) of arterial endofibrosis.[70] EIAE can occur in any endurance sport involving repetitive hip flexion, but is most commonly seen in competitive cyclists, with a reported prevalence of up to 20%.[71] Most cases present unilaterally (85%) with preponderance on the left side. Although no studies have formally investigated the predominance of the left side, lower lumbar degenerative scoliosis has been shown to occur more commonly convex to the left side, and the convex side has been found to develop psoas hypertrophy, which is associated with EIAE.[72,73] Future studies are needed to determine whether there is any validity to this potential association. EIAE occurs at a younger age than that of atherosclerotic peripheral vascular disease.[74]

Fig. 8 depicts the common iliac artery dividing into the internal and external iliac artery (EIA) in the pelvis. The EIA courses distally in the anterior portion of the psoas muscle, and is anterior to the axis of rotation of the hip. This location leads to functional lengthening of the EIA during hip flexion.[71] Functional lengthening of the EIA may lead to arterial kinking during hip flexion, which may be further exacerbated by psoas hypertrophy or tethering by fibrous bands or arterial branches to the psoas muscle.[74] Repetitive hip flexion and EIA kinking associated with endurance sports are thought to cause turbulence in the EIA, leading to intimal hyperplasia and subsequent arterial stenosis.[1]

History and Physical Examination

EIAE, which often presents unilaterally on the left side, affects the muscles distal to the lesion site with the highest oxygen demand.[74] Patients may report pain, cramping, tightness, distension, or weakness in these muscles.[1] Symptoms are absent with submaximal effort, and are brought on with maximal or near-maximal exercise, and can be further worsened with activities requiring extreme hip flexion (eg, time-trial cycling).[1]

Examination findings are often normal at rest, but a bruit may be auscultated over the anterior hip.[75] Auscultation for a bruit should not be performed after exertion, as this is a normal finding in asymptomatic individuals.[75] Peach and colleagues[75] reported a positive predictive value of 79% for EIAE when 3 or more compartments of the involved limb are affected, a bruit is present at rest with the hip extended, and symptoms resolve within 5 minutes of exercise cessation. Schep and colleagues[76] developed a questionnaire to further assist the clinician in differentiating between vascular and nonvascular causes of ELP.

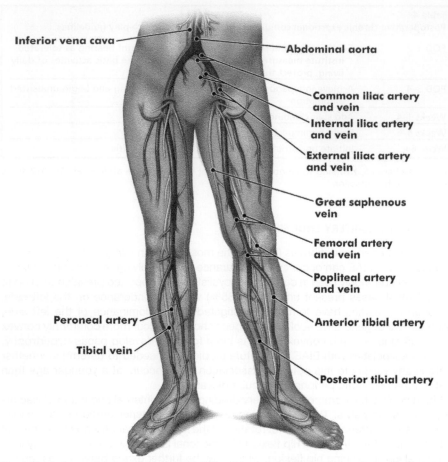

Inferior vena cava

Abdominal aorta

Common iliac artery and vein

Internal iliac artery and vein

External iliac artery and vein

Great saphenous vein

Femoral artery and vein

Popliteal artery and vein

Peroneal artery

Anterior tibial artery

Tibial vein

Posterior tibial artery

Fig. 8. Vascular anatomy of the lower limbs. (*Courtesy of* Mayo Foundation for Medical Education and Research, Rochester, MN, 2015; with permission. All rights reserved.)

Diagnostic Evaluation

An ABI can be used to differentiate between nonatherosclerotic vascular and nonvascular causes of ELP.[1] At rest, both groups will have a normal ABI (0.9–1.2), with the nonatherosclerotic vascular group demonstrating a decrease in ABI after exertion.[1] A 1-minute postexertion ABI of 0.66 or less is 90% sensitive and 87% specific for non-atherosclerotic vascular causes of ELP.[1] In patients with unilateral symptoms, as is often the case in EIAE, a resting difference in ankle systolic blood pressure of 23 mm Hg or a 1-minute postexercise ABI difference of 0.18 or greater can also suggest nonatherosclerotic vascular causes of ELP.[1]

If the ABI is positive or there is a high index of suspicion despite a negative ABI, a detailed duplex ultrasonographic assessment can identify vascular kinking and intravascular lesions (**Fig. 9**).[75] Magnetic resonance angiography (MRA) and digital subtraction angiography (**Fig. 10**) can also provide information regarding the location and severity of arterial stenosis and assist with presurgical planning.[75]

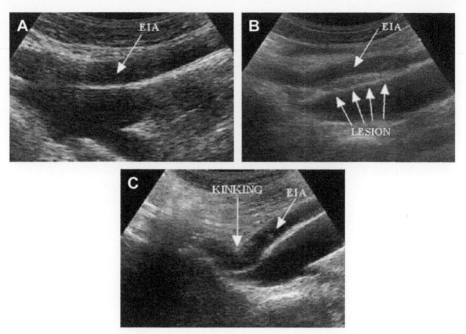

Fig. 9. Echo-Doppler imaging. (*A*) Normal external iliac artery with the hip extended. (*B*) Intravascular lesion located eccentrically on the dorsal side of the proximal external iliac artery lesion. (*C*) With the hips flexed, a kinking is demonstrated, which is identified by an abrupt change in the tangent of the artery. EIA, external iliac artery. (*From* Schep G, Schmikli SL, Bender MH, et al. Recognising vascular causes of leg complaints in endurance athletes. Part 1: validation of a decision algorithm. Int J Sports Med 2002;23(5):315; with permission.)

Management

The only definitive nonsurgical treatment described in the literature is cessation of the provoking sport.[75] If activity cessation is not possible, decreasing the volume of participation or exercising at submaximal levels can be pursued.[1] Up to 80% of symptoms in EIAE patients worsen if left untreated.[77] Acute thrombosis has been described in the literature in association with EIAE, so all patients should be educated on the presenting symptoms of thrombosis (pain at rest, and cold, cyanosed, and pulseless limb), and advised to seek immediate medical attention if any potential symptoms develop.[78]

Several surgical options are available for the treatment of EIAE, and are in part decided upon based on imaging findings (**Fig. 11**).[74,75] Percutaneous transluminal angioplasty and vascular stenting are advised against, as both have shown disappointing results in the treatment of EIAE.[75] General return-to-play guidelines have been published, which the clinician can use after surgical intervention for EIAE (**Table 5**).[1]

POPLITEAL ARTERY ENTRAPMENT SYNDROME

The incidence of PAES in the general population is unknown. At one center between 1987 and 2007, of the 854 patients treated for atypical claudication, 6.7% (57/854) were found to have PAES, 5.0% (43/854) of whom had functional PAES (PAES

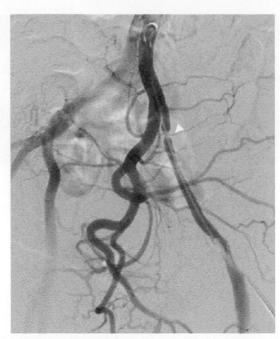

Fig. 10. Aortoiliac digital subtraction angiography in the right anterior oblique projection. Arrowhead indicates focal stenosis in the left external iliac artery. (*From* Maree AO, Ashequl Islam M, Snuderl M, et al. External iliac artery endofibrosis in an amateur runner: hemodynamic, angiographic, histopathological evaluation and percutaneous revascularization. Vasc Med 2007;12(3):204; with permission.)

type F; **Fig. 12**), and 1.6% (20/854) of whom had anatomic PAES (see **Fig. 12**).[50,79] In the same study, PAES type F was more commonly seen in females (77%) with a mean age of 26 years. Anatomic PAES was more commonly seen in males (71%) with a mean age of 46 years.[50] PAES type F occurs in athletic individuals, similarly to those who experience CECS, whereas anatomic PAES is more common in sedentary individuals.[50]

The popliteal artery and vein are branches from the femoral artery and vein (**Fig. 13**). In the popliteal fossa, they are bordered superolaterally by the biceps femoris tendon, superomedially by the semimembranosus muscle and semitendinosus tendon, inferomedially by the medial head of the gastrocnemius muscle, and inferolaterally by the lateral head of the gastrocnemius muscle. As the popliteal artery and vein exit the popliteal fossa with the tibial nerve, they course deep to the soleus and gastrocnemius muscles, and superficial to the popliteus muscle. PAES is classified into 7 types (see **Fig. 12**).

History and Physical Examination

In PAES type F, patients present with claudicatory symptoms in the anterior or posterior aspect of the leg. Associated signs and symptoms include paresthesias in the tibial nerve distribution in 40% of affected individuals, and calf swelling in 7%.[50] In anatomic PAES, the following symptoms may occur: claudication (50%), digital ischemia (43%), paresthesias in tibial nerve distribution (14%), and calf swelling (14%).[50] In PAES type V, venous occlusive symptoms (edema and vein dilation)

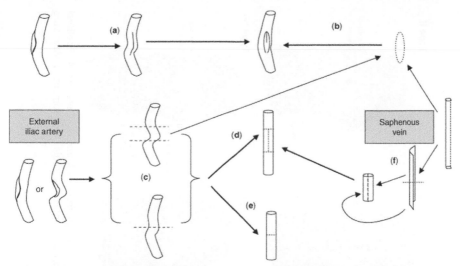

Fig. 11. Overview of the techniques used for surgery. Either the plaque is removed by a longitudinal incision (*a*) generally associated with a saphenous/arterial enlargement patch (*b*), or, depending on the length of the artery, the artery is shortened or not (*c*) followed by end-to-end anastomosis with (*d*) or without (*e*) interposition of a venous bypass. A sufficient diameter of the saphenous bypass is obtained by reconstructing side by side a conduit with 2 segments of the saphenous vein opened on one side (*f*). (*From* Abraham P, Bouye P, Quere I, et al. Past, present and future of arterial endofibrosis in athletes: a point of view. Sports Med 2004;34(7):422; with permission.)

may occur.[80] PAES type F occurs bilaterally in 14% of cases while anatomic PAES occurs bilaterally 56% of the time.[50,81] Several similarities in patient population and demographics, and presenting symptoms, were noted between functional PAES and CECS, and it has been recommended that compartment pressure testing be conducted in this group to rule this diagnosis in or out.[50]

As with many causes of ELP, the resting examination is often normal in PAES. A diminution of the tibial or dorsalis pedis pulse may be seen with passive ankle dorsiflexion or active ankle plantar flexion (lower specificity) with the knee extended.[1] In advanced cases, the tibial or dorsalis pedis pulse can be diminished or absent even without provocative maneuvers.[82]

Table 5	
Return-to-play guidelines after an open arterial revascularization procedure	
POD 1–2	Gentle active and passive range of motion, weight bearing as tolerated, institute measures to control edema, undertake basic activities of daily living
POD 3–4	Supervised walking
POD 5–6	Stairs
Weeks 2–4	Unsupervised walking, lifting <5 kg
Weeks 4–6	Low resistance, low-cadence cycling, low-resistance isotonic exercises
Week 6+	Unrestricted progressive resistance and aerobic conditioning

From Rajasekaran S, Kvinlaug K, Finnoff JT. Exertional leg pain in the athlete. PM R 2012;4(12):985–1000; with permission.

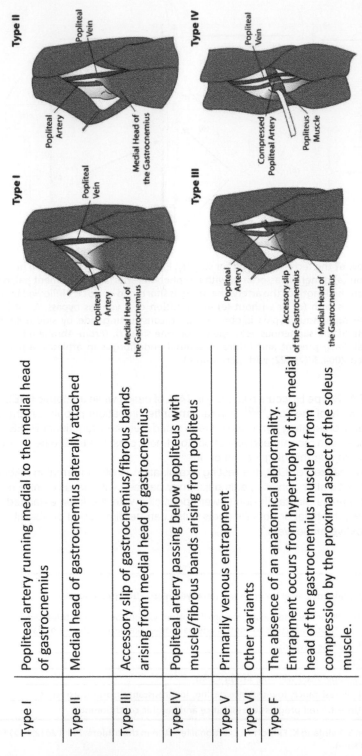

Type I	Popliteal artery running medial to the medial head of gastrocnemius
Type II	Medial head of gastrocnemius laterally attached
Type III	Accessory slip of gastrocnemius/fibrous bands arising from medial head of gastrocnemius
Type IV	Popliteal artery passing below popliteus with muscle/fibrous bands arising from popliteus
Type V	Primarily venous entrapment
Type VI	Other variants
Type F	The absence of an anatomical abnormality. Entrapment occurs from hypertrophy of the medial head of the gastrocnemius muscle or from compression by the proximal aspect of the soleus muscle.

Fig. 12. Popliteal Vascular Entrapment Forum classification of popliteal entrapment syndrome. (*Adapted from* di Marzo L, Cavallaro A. Popliteal vascular entrapment. World J Surg 2005;29(Suppl 1):S44; and Pillai J. A current interpretation of popliteal vascular entrapment. J Vasc Surg 2008;48(6 Suppl):62S; [discussion 5S]; with permission.)

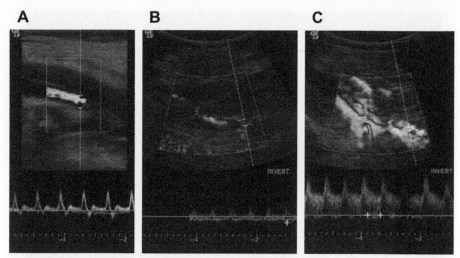

Fig. 13. Doppler findings with functional popliteal artery entrapment syndrome. (*A*) Popliteal artery longitudinal duplex scan in neutral position. (*B*) Same popliteal longitudinal scan with plantar flexion. (*C*) Reactive hyperemic response following resumption of normal position. (*From* Lane R, Nguyen T, Cuzzilla M, et al. Functional popliteal entrapment syndrome in the sportsperson. Eur J Vasc Endovasc Surg 2012;43(1):83; with permission.)

Diagnostic Evaluation

ABI testing as described for EIAE should be performed in the assessment of PAES.[1] In addition, the same ankle provocation maneuvers done on physical examination should be performed with ABI testing, looking for a reduction in ABI.[50] A systematic review noted that both conventional angiography and Doppler ultasonography (see **Fig. 13**) are commonly reported in the assessment of PAES. Both of these imaging modalities are limited by their inability to adequately evaluate the adjacent anatomy to determine the cause of PAES.[83] Therefore, when possible, the use of MRI with MRA (**Fig. 14**) or CT with CT angiography (**Fig. 15**) is recommended to image not only the popliteal artery and vein but also the adjacent soft-tissue anatomy, to evaluate abnormal muscular attachments or hypertrophy.[83] It is also important to note that there is a high false-positive rate with diagnostic imaging studies, which should be kept in mind when interpreting the results of such studies. One study reported a false-positive rate of 69% with Doppler ultrasonography and MRA.[84]

Management

Surgery is the definitive treatment of PAES.[50] Several surgical techniques have been described for anatomic PAES, most of which entail musculotendinous division or mobilization of the medial gastrocnemius attachments or body itself.[83] With functional PAES, surgery involves fasciotomy of the medial gastrocnemius, take-down of the soleus attachments to the tibia, and resection of the attachment band of the soleus to the fibula.[50] When the popliteal artery is found to be injured it is repaired with bypass surgery, as thromboendarterectomy is not recommended.[85] Success rates close to 100% have been reported for functional and anatomic PAES, with rates between 48% and 57% when the popliteal vein is also entrapped.[83] Unlike EIAE, endovascular therapy alone is not effective in the treatment of PAES, as it does not address the underlying soft-tissue entrapment. General return-to-play guidelines have been published, which the clinician can use after surgical intervention (see **Table 5**).[1]

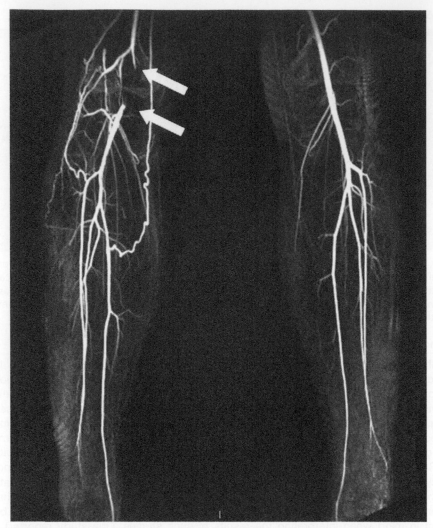

Fig. 14. Magnetic resonance angiography demonstrating popliteal artery occlusion (*arrows*) at the level of the medial head of the gastrocnemius with collateral flow, consistent with type I entrapment. (*From* Politano AD, Bhamidipati CM, Tracci MC, et al. Anatomic popliteal entrapment syndrome is often a difficult diagnosis. Vasc Endovascular Surg 2012;46(7):543; with permission.)

LOWER EXTREMITY NERVE ENTRAPMENT

Lower extremity nerve entrapment most commonly involves the saphenous nerve (SN), common peroneal nerve (CPN), superficial peroneal nerve (SPN), or deep peroneal nerve (DPN). The SN can become entrapped as it exits the adductor (Hunter's) canal, where it courses between the sartorius and gracilis tendons.[1] Surgeries of the lower leg have also been implicated in the development of SN entrapment.[1] Compression of the CPN most commonly occurs as it traverses the fibular neck in the peroneal tunnel.[1] In addition to external compression, the CPN can be injured in

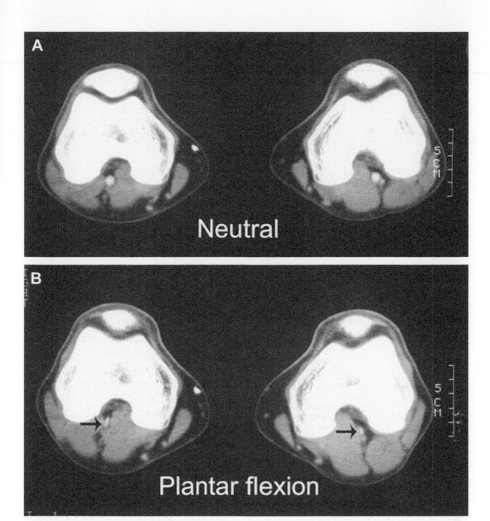

Fig. 15. Computed tomography (CT) angiogram with ankles in neutral (*A*) and plantar flexion (*B*), demonstrating bilateral external compression of the popliteal artery in *B*. Arrows indicate popliteal artery. (*Data from* Noorani A, Walsh SR, Cooper DG, et al. Entrapment syndromes. Eur J Vasc Endovasc Surg 2009;37(2):215.)

this region by exercises involving repetitive inversion and eversion of the ankle (eg, running) or following proximal tibiofibular joint dislocations.[1,40] SPN entrapment occurs as it pierces the lateral compartment crural fascia, and DPN entrapment occurs in the anterior tarsal tunnel (**Fig. 16**). CECS has been associated with entrapment of the SPN (lateral compartment) and DPN (anterior compartment).

History and Physical Examination

Patients presenting with lower extremity nerve entrapment may report pain at rest, but often report the development or worsening of symptoms during or after exertion.[1,40] **Fig. 17** details the SN, CPN, SPN, and DPN lower limb sensory innervation patterns reported by patients with numbness or paresthesias. As the SN has no motor

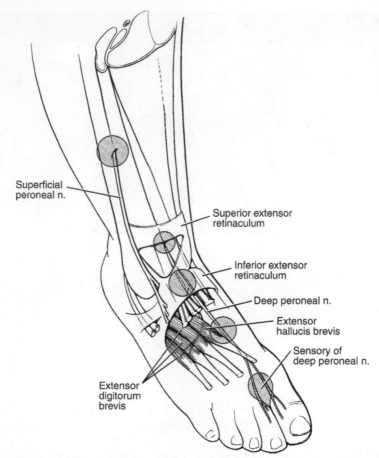

Superficial peroneal n.

Superior extensor retinaculum

Inferior extensor retinaculum

Deep peroneal n.

Extensor hallucis brevis

Sensory of deep peroneal n.

Extensor digitorum brevis

Fig. 16. Potential entrapment sites of superficial peroneal and deep peroneal nerves. (*Courtesy of* Mayo Foundation for Medical Education and Research, Rochester, MN, 2000; with permission. All rights reserved.)

innervation, patients with entrapment of this nerve present only with sensory symptoms. In CPN entrapment, weakness of ankle dorsiflexion, toe extension, and ankle eversion can be seen, whereas SPN entrapment can present with ankle eversion weakness and DPN entrapment with toe extension weakness.[1]

Preexertional and postexertional physical examinations are valuable in the assessment of leg nerve entrapment, as the preexertional examination is often normal. The examination should include a detailed sensory and motor examination of the lower limbs. If entrapment of the SN, CPN, SPN, or DPN is suspected, performing a Tinel test at and distal to the site of potential compression may be beneficial.

Diagnostic Evaluation

Electrodiagnostic studies are frequently ordered in the assessment of lower extremity nerve entrapment, but their clinical utility has been reported to be limited.[1] A recent article noted the added value of ultrasonography in the assessment of CPN.[86] On ultrasonography, nerve compression can be seen at any of the aforestated entrapment

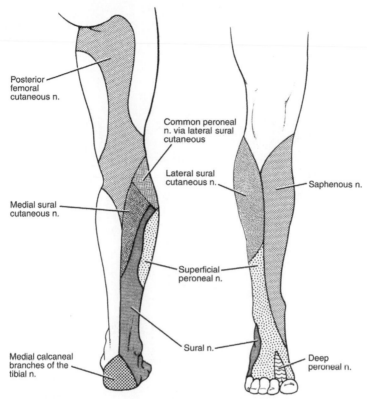

Fig. 17. Cutaneous innervation of the lower limb. (*Courtesy of* Mayo Foundation for Medical Education and Research, Rochester, MN, 2000; with permission. All rights reserved.)

sites of the SN, CPN, SPN, and DPN with dilation of the nerve proximal to this site.[1] In addition to visualizing nerve entrapment, ultrasonography may reveal contributing factors from adjacent tissues (eg, ganglion cysts, fibrous bands).[1] An ultrasound-guided nerve block at the suspected entrapment site can also be performed to obtain additional diagnostic information.[1] If nerve entrapment is suspected, but not ascertained with ultrasonography, an MRI may be ordered for a more global assessment of the region, or alternatively or concomitantly an MRI neurogram can be obtained to further assess the peripheral nerve.[87] As SPN and DPN can be associated with CECS, compartment pressure testing may need to be completed if the history is also suggestive of this diagnosis.[40]

Management

In patients with negative electrodiagnostic studies, or in the absence of axonal damage, conservative measures aimed at addressing the offending causes (eg, shoe modifications, running technique modifications, and neuromodulatory medications) can be pursued.[1] If an entrapment site is located and conservative management fails, an ultrasound-guided nerve block or hydrodissection of the entrapped nerve can be performed.[1] In cases where axonal damage is identified with electrodiagnostic testing, or if conservative measures and injections fail, neurolysis with or without fascial release (SPN and DPN) should be considered.[1]

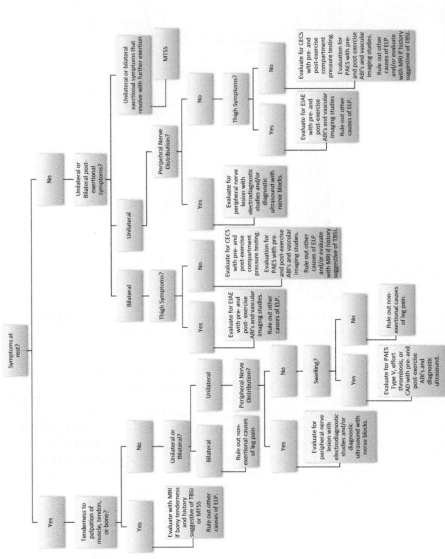

Fig. 18. Algorithm for the evaluation of patients with exertional leg pain (ELP). Patients who are symptomatic after treatment should be reassessed with this algorithm for other diagnoses. ABI, ankle brachial index; CAD, cystic adventitial disease; CECS, chronic exertional compartment syndrome; EIAE, external iliac artery endofibrosis; ELP, exertional leg pain; MRI, magnetic resonance imaging; MTSS, medial tibial stress syndrome; PAES, popliteal artery entrapment syndrome; TBSI, tibial bone stress injury. (*Adapted from* Rajasekaran S, Kvinlaug K, Finnoff JT. Exertional leg pain in the athlete. PM R

SUMMARY

ELP can be a challenging presentation for clinicians. A detailed history and physical examination, along with a thorough knowledge of specific diagnostic tests and the order in which to conduct such testing, is paramount in narrowing the differential diagnosis (**Fig. 18**). In select cases, more than 1 diagnosis may coexist; this may be suspected on initial presentation, but should definitely be considered if symptoms persist despite appropriate treatment.

REFERENCES

1. Rajasekaran S, Kvinlaug K, Finnoff JT. Exertional leg pain in the athlete. PM R 2012;4(12):985–1000.
2. Taunton JE, Ryan MB, Clement DB, et al. A retrospective case-control analysis of 2002 running injuries. Br J Sports Med 2002;36(2):95–101.
3. Reinking MF, Austin TM, Hayes AM. Risk factors for self-reported exercise-related leg pain in high school cross-country athletes. J Athl Train 2010;45(1):51–7.
4. Walter SD, Hart LE, McIntosh JM, et al. The Ontario cohort study of running-related injuries. Arch Intern Med 1989;149(11):2561–4.
5. Lopes AD, Hespanhol Junior LC, Yeung SS, et al. What are the main running-related musculoskeletal injuries? A systematic review. Sports Med 2012;42(10): 891–905.
6. Moen MH, Tol JL, Weir A, et al. Medial tibial stress syndrome: a critical review. Sports Med 2009;39(7):523–46.
7. Yates B, White S. The incidence and risk factors in the development of medial tibial stress syndrome among naval recruits. Am J Sports Med 2004;32(3): 772–80.
8. Franklyn M, Oakes B, Field B, et al. Section modulus is the optimum geometric predictor for stress fractures and medial tibial stress syndrome in both male and female athletes. Am J Sports Med 2008;36(6):1179–89.
9. Magnusson HI, Westlin NE, Nyqvist F, et al. Abnormally decreased regional bone density in athletes with medial tibial stress syndrome. Am J Sports Med 2001; 29(6):712–5.
10. Magnusson HI, Ahlborg HG, Karlsson C, et al. Low regional tibial bone density in athletes with medial tibial stress syndrome normalizes after recovery from symptoms. Am J Sports Med 2003;31(4):596–600.
11. Kortebein PM, Kaufman KR, Basford JR, et al. Medial tibial stress syndrome. Med Sci Sports Exerc 2000;32(3 Suppl):S27–33.
12. Hamstra-Wright KL, Bliven KC, Bay C. Risk factors for medial tibial stress syndrome in physically active individuals such as runners and military personnel: a systematic review and meta-analysis. Br J Sports Med 2015;49(6):362–9.
13. Beck BR, Bergman AG, Miner M, et al. Tibial stress injury: relationship of radiographic, nuclear medicine bone scanning, MR imaging, and CT severity grades to clinical severity and time to healing. Radiology 2012;263(3):811–8.
14. Fredericson M, Bergman AG, Hoffman KL, et al. Tibial stress reaction in runners. Correlation of clinical symptoms and scintigraphy with a new magnetic resonance imaging grading system. Am J Sports Med 1995;23(4):472–81.
15. Napier C, Cochrane CK, Taunton JE, et al. Gait modifications to change lower extremity gait biomechanics in runners: a systematic review. Br J Sports Med 2015. [Epub ahead of print].
16. Cheung RT, Chung RC, Ng GY. Efficacies of different external controls for excessive foot pronation: a meta-analysis. Br J Sports Med 2011;45(9):743–51.

17. Galbraith RM, Lavallee ME. Medial tibial stress syndrome: conservative treatment options. Curr Rev Musculoskelet Med 2009;2(3):127–33.
18. McNeill DK, de Heer HD, Bounds RG, et al. Accuracy of unloading with the anti-gravity treadmill. J Strength Cond Res 2015;29(3):863–8.
19. Moen MH, Rayer S, Schipper M, et al. Shockwave treatment for medial tibial stress syndrome in athletes; a prospective controlled study. Br J Sports Med 2012;46(4):253–7.
20. Matheson GO, Clement DB, McKenzie DC, et al. Stress fractures in athletes. A study of 320 cases. Am J Sports Med 1987;15(1):46–58.
21. Robertson GA, Wood AM. Return to sports after stress fractures of the tibial diaphysis: a systematic review. Br Med Bull 2015;114(1):95–111.
22. Gaeta M, Minutoli F, Scribano E, et al. CT and MR imaging findings in athletes with early tibial stress injuries: comparison with bone scintigraphy findings and emphasis on cortical abnormalities. Radiology 2005;235(2):553–61.
23. Harrast MA, Colonno D. Stress fractures in runners. Clin Sports Med 2010;29(3):399–416.
24. Bennell KL, Malcolm SA, Thomas SA, et al. The incidence and distribution of stress fractures in competitive track and field athletes. A twelve-month prospective study. Am J Sports Med 1996;24(2):211–7.
25. Bennell K, Crossley K, Jayarajan J, et al. Ground reaction forces and bone parameters in females with tibial stress fracture. Med Sci Sports Exerc 2004;36(3):397–404.
26. Crossley K, Bennell KL, Wrigley T, et al. Ground reaction forces, bone characteristics, and tibial stress fracture in male runners. Med Sci Sports Exerc 1999;31(8):1088–93.
27. Barrack MT, Gibbs JC, De Souza MJ, et al. Higher incidence of bone stress injuries with increasing female athlete triad-related risk factors: a prospective multisite study of exercising girls and women. Am J Sports Med 2014;42(4):949–58.
28. Brukner P. Exercise-related lower leg pain: bone. Med Sci Sports Exerc 2000;32(3 Suppl):S15–26.
29. Mencias T, Noon M, Hoch AZ. Female athlete triad screening in National Collegiate Athletic Association Division I athletes: is the preparticipation evaluation form effective? Clin J Sport Med 2012;22(2):122–5.
30. Gardner LI Jr, Dziados JE, Jones BH, et al. Prevention of lower extremity stress fractures: a controlled trial of a shock absorbent insole. Am J Public Health 1988;78(12):1563–7.
31. Lesho EP. Can tuning forks replace bone scans for identification of tibial stress fractures? Mil Med 1997;162(12):802–3.
32. Yagi S, Muneta T, Sekiya I. Incidence and risk factors for medial tibial stress syndrome and tibial stress fracture in high school runners. Knee Surg Sports Traumatol Arthrosc 2013;21(3):556–63.
33. RFt Pell, Khanuja HS, Cooley GR. Leg pain in the running athlete. J Am Acad Orthop Surg 2004;12(6):396–404.
34. Zwas ST, Elkanovitch R, Frank G. Interpretation and classification of bone scintigraphic findings in stress fractures. J Nucl Med 1987;28(4):452–7.
35. Ishibashi Y, Okamura Y, Otsuka H, et al. Comparison of scintigraphy and magnetic resonance imaging for stress injuries of bone. Clin J Sport Med 2002;12(2):79–84.
36. Aoki Y, Yasuda K, Tohyama H, et al. Magnetic resonance imaging in stress fractures and shin splints. Clin Orthop Relat Res 2004;(421):260–7.

37. Boniotti V, Del Giudice E, Fengoni E, et al. Imaging of bone micro-injuries. Radiol Med 2003;105(5–6):425–35.
38. Kiuru MJ, Pihlajamaki HK, Hietanen HJ, et al. MR imaging, bone scintigraphy, and radiography in bone stress injuries of the pelvis and the lower extremity. Acta Radiol 2002;43(2):207–12.
39. Rome K, Handoll HH, Ashford R. Interventions for preventing and treating stress fractures and stress reactions of bone of the lower limbs in young adults. Cochrane Database Syst Rev 2005;(2):CD000450.
40. Burrus MT, Werner BC, Starman JS, et al. Chronic leg pain in athletes. Am J Sports Med 2015;43(6):1538–47.
41. Nattiv A, Kennedy G, Barrack MT, et al. Correlation of MRI grading of bone stress injuries with clinical risk factors and return to play: a 5-year prospective study in collegiate track and field athletes. Am J Sports Med 2013;41(8):1930–41.
42. Shuler FD, Wingate MK, Moore GH, et al. Sports health benefits of vitamin D. Sports Health 2012;4(6):496–501.
43. Detmer DE, Sharpe K, Sufit RL, et al. Chronic compartment syndrome: diagnosis, management, and outcomes. Am J Sports Med 1985;13(3):162–70.
44. Pedowitz RA, Hargens AR, Mubarak SJ, et al. Modified criteria for the objective diagnosis of chronic compartment syndrome of the leg. Am J Sports Med 1990;18(1):35–40.
45. Waterman BR, Laughlin M, Kilcoyne K, et al. Surgical treatment of chronic exertional compartment syndrome of the leg: failure rates and postoperative disability in an active patient population. J Bone Joint Surg Am 2013;95(7):592–6.
46. Hurschler C, Vanderby R Jr, Martinez DA, et al. Mechanical and biochemical analyses of tibial compartment fascia in chronic compartment syndrome. Ann Biomed Eng 1994;22(3):272–9.
47. Rajasekaran S, Beavis C, Aly AR, et al. The utility of ultrasound in detecting anterior compartment thickness changes in chronic exertional compartment syndrome: a pilot study. Clin J Sport Med 2013;23(4):305–11.
48. Dahl M, Hansen P, Stal P, et al. Stiffness and thickness of fascia do not explain chronic exertional compartment syndrome. Clin Orthop Relat Res 2011;469(12):3495–500.
49. Popovic N, Bottoni C, Cassidy C. Unrecognized acute exertional compartment syndrome of the leg and treatment. Acta Orthop Belg 2011;77(2):265–9.
50. Turnipseed WD. Functional popliteal artery entrapment syndrome: A poorly understood and often missed diagnosis that is frequently mistreated. J Vasc Surg 2009;49(5):1189–95.
51. Fronek J, Mubarak SJ, Hargens AR, et al. Management of chronic exertional anterior compartment syndrome of the lower extremity. Clin Orthop Relat Res 1987;(220):217–27.
52. Nguyen JT, Nguyen JL, Wheatley MJ, et al. Muscle hernias of the leg: a case report and comprehensive review of the literature. Can J Plast Surg 2013;21(4):243–7.
53. French EB, Price WH. Anterior tibial pain. Br Med J 1962;2(5315):1290–6.
54. Hislop M, Tierney P. Intracompartmental pressure testing: results of an international survey of current clinical practice, highlighting the need for standardised protocols. Br J Sports Med 2011;45(12):956–8.
55. Aweid O, Del Buono A, Malliaras P, et al. Systematic review and recommendations for intracompartmental pressure monitoring in diagnosing chronic exertional compartment syndrome of the leg. Clin J Sport Med 2012;22(4):356–70.

56. Roberts A, Franklyn-Miller A. The validity of the diagnostic criteria used in chronic exertional compartment syndrome: a systematic review. Scand J Med Sci Sports 2011;22:585–95.
57. Roberts AJ, Krishnasamy P, Quayle JM, et al. Outcomes of surgery for chronic exertional compartment syndrome in a military population. J R Army Med Corps 2015;161(1):42–5.
58. Roscoe D, Roberts AJ, Hulse D. Intramuscular compartment pressure measurement in chronic exertional compartment syndrome: new and improved diagnostic criteria. Am J Sports Med 2015;43(2):392–8.
59. Litwiller DV, Amrami KK, Dahm DL, et al. Chronic exertional compartment syndrome of the lower extremities: improved screening using a novel dual birdcage coil and in-scanner exercise protocol. Skeletal Radiol 2007;36(11):1067–75.
60. Ringler MD, Litwiller DV, Felmlee JP, et al. MRI accurately detects chronic exertional compartment syndrome: a validation study. Skeletal Radiol 2013;42(3): 385–92.
61. McDonald S, Bearcroft P. Compartment syndromes. Semin Musculoskelet Radiol 2010;14(2):236–44.
62. Kirby RL, McDermott AG. Anterior tibial compartment pressures during running with rearfoot and forefoot landing styles. Arch Phys Med Rehabil 1983;64(7): 296–9.
63. Diebal AR, Gregory R, Alitz C, et al. Forefoot running improves pain and disability associated with chronic exertional compartment syndrome. Am J Sports Med 2012;40(5):1060–7.
64. Diebal AR, Gregory R, Alitz C, et al. Effects of forefoot running on chronic exertional compartment syndrome: a case series. Int J Sports Phys Ther 2011;6(4): 312–21.
65. Lecocq J, Isner-Horobeti ME. Treatment of exertional compartment syndrome leg with botulinum toxin A: a first open pilot study. J Rehabil Med 2008;40(Suppl 47): 111–2.
66. Isner-Horobeti ME, Dufour SP, Blaes C, et al. Intramuscular pressure before and after botulinum toxin in chronic exertional compartment syndrome of the leg: a preliminary study. Am J Sports Med 2013;41(11):2558–66.
67. Slimmon D, Bennell K, Brukner P, et al. Long-term outcome of fasciotomy with partial fasciectomy for chronic exertional compartment syndrome of the lower leg. Am J Sports Med 2002;30(4):581–8.
68. Packer JD, Day MS, Nguyen JT, et al. Functional outcomes and patient satisfaction after fasciotomy for chronic exertional compartment syndrome. Am J Sports Med 2013;41(2):430–6.
69. Winkes MB, Hoogeveen AR, Scheltinga MR. Is surgery effective for deep posterior compartment syndrome of the leg? A systematic review. Br J Sports Med 2014;48(22):1592–8.
70. Schep G, Bender MH, Kaandorp D, et al. Flow limitations in the iliac arteries in endurance athletes. Current knowledge and directions for the future. Int J Sports Med 1999;20(7):421–8.
71. Bruneau A, Le Faucheur A, Mahe G, et al. Endofibrosis in athletes: is a simple bedside exercise helpful or sufficient for the diagnosis? Clin J Sport Med 2009; 19(4):282–6.
72. de Vries AA, Mullender MG, Pluymakers WJ, et al. Spinal decompensation in degenerative lumbar scoliosis. Eur Spine J 2010;19(9):1540–4.

73. Kim H, Lee CK, Yeom JS, et al. Asymmetry of the cross-sectional area of paravertebral and psoas muscle in patients with degenerative scoliosis. Eur Spine J 2013;22(6):1332–8.
74. Abraham P, Bouye P, Quere I, et al. Past, present and future of arterial endofibrosis in athletes: a point of view. Sports Med 2004;34(7):419–25.
75. Peach G, Schep G, Palfreeman R, et al. Endofibrosis and kinking of the iliac arteries in athletes: a systematic review. Eur J Vasc Endovasc Surg 2012;43(2): 208–17.
76. Schep G, Schmikli SL, Bender MH, et al. Recognising vascular causes of leg complaints in endurance athletes. Part 1: validation of a decision algorithm. Int J Sports Med 2002;23(5):313–21.
77. Schep G, Bender MH, Schmikli SL, et al. Recognising vascular causes of leg complaints in endurance athletes. Part 2: the value of patient history, physical examination, cycling exercise test and echo-Doppler examination. Int J Sports Med 2002;23(5):322–8.
78. Bucci F, Ottaviani N, Plagnol P. Acute thrombosis of external iliac artery secondary to endofibrosis. Ann Vasc Surg 2011;25(5):698.e5–7.
79. Pillai J. A current interpretation of popliteal vascular entrapment. J Vasc Surg 2008;48(6 Suppl):61S–5S [discussion: 5S].
80. Angeli AA, Angeli DA, Aggeli CA, et al. Chronic lower leg swelling caused by isolated popliteal venous entrapment. J Vasc Surg 2011;54(3):851–3.
81. Rich NM, Collins GJ Jr, McDonald PT, et al. Popliteal vascular entrapment. Its increasing interest. Arch Surg 1979;114(12):1377–84.
82. di Marzo L, Cavallaro A, Sciacca V, et al. Natural history of entrapment of the popliteal artery. J Am Coll Surg 1994;178(6):553–6.
83. Sinha S, Houghton J, Holt PJ, et al. Popliteal entrapment syndrome. J Vasc Surg 2012;55(1):252–62.e30.
84. Chernoff DM, Walker AT, Khorasani R, et al. Asymptomatic functional popliteal artery entrapment: demonstration at MR imaging. Radiology 1995;195(1):176–80.
85. Lambert AW, Wilkins DC. Popliteal artery entrapment syndrome. Br J Surg 1999; 86(11):1365–70.
86. Visser LH, Hens V, Soethout M, et al. Diagnostic value of high-resolution sonography in common fibular neuropathy at the fibular head. Muscle Nerve 2013; 48(2):171–8.
87. Pineda D, Barroso F, Chaves H, et al. High resolution 3T magnetic resonance neurography of the peroneal nerve. Radiologia 2014;56(2):107–17 [in Spanish].

Foot and Ankle Injuries in Runners

Adam S. Tenforde, MD[a], Amy Yin, MD[b], Kenneth J. Hunt, MD[c],*

KEYWORDS

- Achilles tendinopathy • Plantar fasciitis • Ankle sprain • Posterior tibial tendinitis
- Stress fracture • Running athlete • Injury prevention

KEY POINTS

- Achilles tendinopathy is common and may require comprehensive assessment and management. A similar approach is required for most foot and ankle tendon-related diseases.
- Plantar fasciopathy is the most common cause of plantar foot pain in runners; interdigital neuromas, tarsal tunnel syndrome, and jogger's foot should also be considered.
- Although lateral ankle sprains are a common cause of ligament injury and ankle dysfunction, other joint conditions must be considered in chronic cases with refractory pain and dysfunction.
- Most foot and ankle conditions respond favorably to conservative management, including activity modification along with corrective exercises to restore strength and function.
- Preventive measures may reduce the risk for injury and are an emerging area for future investigation and research.

INTRODUCTION

Foot and ankle injuries are estimated to compose 31% of total running injuries sustained.[1] A systematic review of running injuries by Lopes[2] in 2012 revealed that Achilles tendinopathy, plantar fasciopathy, and ankle sprains are 3 of the top 5 most common running injuries. The complex anatomy and biomechanics of the foot and ankle underscore the importance of a careful and thorough history, examination, and workup to confirm a diagnosis and rule out concomitant conditions. The running athlete requires special consideration during rehabilitation and return to participation. This review encompasses common foot and ankle injuries in running athletes,

Authors have no conflicts of interest to disclose, and no funding was received in preparation of this review.

[a] Department of Physical Medicine and Rehabilitation, Spaulding Rehabilitation Hospital, Harvard University, 1575 Cambridge Street, Cambridge, MA 02138, USA; [b] Division of Physical Medicine and Rehabilitation, Department of Orthopaedic Surgery, Stanford University, 450 Broadway Street, Redwood City, CA 94063, USA; [c] Department of Orthopaedic Surgery, Stanford University, Stanford, CA 94063, USA
* Corresponding author. 450 Broadway Street, MC 6342, Redwood City, CA 94063.
E-mail address: kj.hunt@ucdenver.edu

Phys Med Rehabil Clin N Am 27 (2016) 121–137
http://dx.doi.org/10.1016/j.pmr.2015.08.007
1047-9651/16/$ – see front matter © 2016 Elsevier Inc. All rights reserved.

pmr.theclinics.com

including evaluation and management of these conditions. Although the majority of our focus is on the most common injuries, this comprehensive discussion covers the full spectrum of pathology from tendinopathies to bone, joint, and nerve disorders (**Table 1**).

ACHILLES TENDINOPATHY

The Achilles tendon is the largest tendon of the body and connects the soleus, and medial and lateral gastrocnemius muscles (collectively referred to as triceps surae) to the insertion on the calcaneus. Insertional fibers of the Achilles tendon are in continuity with the plantar aponeurosis. This musculotendinous group serves as the primary plantar flexor of the foot and ankle. The Achilles tendon is a common site of pain in runners and may be the second most common musculoskeletal injury, after medial tibial stress syndrome, with an incidence of 9.1% to 10.9%.[2] The lifetime risk in former elite male distance runners is 52%.[3] In addition to overuse from running, multiple intrinsic and extrinsic risk factors have been outlined that may contribute, including systemic disease, older age, sex, body composition, and biomechanics.[4]

Terminology becomes important in the assessment and management of Achilles tendon disorders. In the acute phase, Achilles tendinitis refers to inflammatory changes at the tendon level and may include the paratenon that surrounds the tendon. In the chronic phase, Achilles tendinosis represents a more chronic and degenerative process. Achilles tendinopathy is our preferred term to use for Achilles tendon pain, with recent proposed definition for tendon pathology on a continuum of 3 stages: "reactive tendinopathy, tendon disrepair (failed healing), and degenerative tendinopathy."[5]

Clinical Evaluation

The 2 most common sites of injury in runners include midportion Achilles tendinopathy (2–6 cm distal to the calcaneal insertion, a region of reduced vascularity[6]) and insertional Achilles tendinopathy (injury localized to the insertion of the Achilles tendon with calcaneus), although injuries to other regions including the myotendinous junction can occur.

Table 1 Categories of running injuries	
Category	**Diagnosis**
Tendinopathies	Achilles tendinopathy Posterior tibial tendon dysfunction Peroneal tendinopathy Flexor hallucis longus tendinopathy Anterior tibial tendinopathy
Ligament and fascia conditions	Plantar fasciopathy Inversion ankle sprain High ankle sprain (syndesmosis injury)
Bone conditions	Bone stress injuries
Joint disorders	Hallux rigidus Osteochondral defect of the talus Osteoarthritis
Nerve disorders	Interdigital neuralgia/Morton's neuroma Tarsal tunnel syndrome Superficial peroneal neuropathy Jogger's foot

Developing a systemic clinical evaluation is recommended to evaluate this injury and differentiate from other causes of heel pain. First, the runner should be asked to localize the site of maximal pain. Examination should include inspection of the tendon for differences in the general appearance of the Achilles tendon, including thickening or overlying erythema. The calcaneus should be evaluated for difference in size or prominence of the posterior aspect that may suggest presence of Haglund's deformity. On palpation, patients with unilateral Achilles tendinopathy may have differences in the quality of the tendon, such as thickening. Presence of crepitus, swelling, and tenderness localized to a fixed position with ankle range of motion (ROM) suggests active inflammation in the paratenon surrounding the Achilles tendon. Dorsiflexion ROM may be limited on the affected side. Dorsiflexion ROM assessment should include evaluation of ROM with knee in full extension and 90° of knee flexion to determine differences in ROM (the Silfverskiold test), with decreased ROM with full knee extension suggesting the presence of gastrocnemius tightness or contracture that may place the Achilles tendon in increased tension. Evaluation of strength should include requesting the patient perform a series of single leg calf raises and evaluating for pain during this maneuver, differences in heel height from side-to-side, and fatigue.

If there is concern for Achilles tendon rupture (based on patient history or presence of palpable gap of the tendon), the Thompson's test should be performed. To perform this maneuver, the patient lies prone and examiner squeezes the triceps surae distal to the knee. Passive foot plantar flexion suggests that the Achilles tendon is contiguous with the calcaneus and unlikely to have a full-thickness tear. If there is no foot plantarflexion with calf squeeze (be sure to compare with the contralateral side), there is concern for Achilles rupture. Extensor lag and a palpable gap at the rupture site are also signs of rupture. The calcaneal squeeze test is helpful to exclude the presence of a calcaneal BSI. This test is performed with the clinician pressing both medially and laterally onto the calcaneus and evaluates for pain localized to the calcaneus.

With regard to imaging, weight-bearing radiographs (lateral and axial views of the heel), may be helpful to evaluate for Haglund's deformity, calcific tendinopathy, or if the diagnosis is unclear. MRI is indicated primarily if there is concern for significant tear or rupture of the Achilles tendon or to evaluate for a BSI. Ultrasonography is a useful modality that can be helpful to qualify Achilles tendon injury.[7]

Differential Diagnosis

The differential diagnosis for heel pain in a runner includes Achilles tendinopathy, posterior ankle impingement, retrocalcaneal bursitis, symptomatic Haglund's deformity, BSI to the distal tibia, fibula, or calcaneus, peroneal tendinopathy, and hindfoot arthrosis.

Management

In the acute phase, initial management includes rest, activity modification, trial of heel lifts, and stretching the triceps surae. If the patient has significant pain with weight bearing, a brief period of immobilization in a boot can help to alleviate this, but long periods of time in a boot should be avoided owing to the risk of increased muscle atrophy. Local modalities including ice, massage, and ultrasound may reduce pain. Iontophoresis may also be considered to reduce local inflammation for acute presentation.[8] Nonsteroidal antiinflammatory medications (NSAIDs) are commonly prescribed for a short course of treatment, although the degree of true inflammation is questionable in more chronic conditions. Topical nitroglycerine does not have clear evidence to support its use.[9]

After achieving pain control, treatment should focus on strengthening the integrity of the Achilles tendon and triceps surae. Alfredson and colleagues[10] demonstrated efficacy of eccentric loading protocol for addressing pain and strength in patients with Achilles tendinopathy. In this landmark study, 15 subjects with unilateral midportion Achilles tendinopathy completed a 12-week session of single leg eccentric loading program with progressive weight loading. Subjects who completed this protocol of 3 sets of 15 repetitions with both knees bent and straight twice per day had normalization of strength, reduction of pain, and all returned to running over 12 weeks.[10] A larger study using Alfredson's protocol in athletes with a 5-year follow-up reported that most individuals experienced gains in function, although nearly one-half of subjects pursued other therapies and most reported mild pain.[11] For insertional Achilles tendinopathy, the authors recommend a modified version of Alfredson's protocol with eccentric load calf raises that do not include heel drop.[12]

Additionally, rehabilitation exercises that address function of the full kinetic chain are important given studies that suggest biomechanical factors may contribute to Achilles tendinopathy including reduced activity of tibialis anterior, rectus femoris,[13] gluteus medius, and gluteus maximus.[14] Foot intrinsic strengthening and restoring proprioception is important for this condition, as with any foot and ankle disorder.

Treatment for chronic refractory Achilles tendinopathy may include injection of platelet-rich plasma (PRP) at the affected site. PRP injection has shown benefit for Achilles tendinopathy in symptomatic patients based on published case series.[15,16] However, 1 randomized control trial in chronic patients who were treated with eccentric exercise, a PRP compared with a saline injection did not result in improved management of this condition.[17,18]

Operative management for this condition may include debridement of degenerative tendon and repair of remaining healthy tendon. In cases of recalcitrant insertional Achilles tendinopathy, removal of an associated Haglund's deformity and retrocalcaneal bursectomy can be beneficial. In individuals over 50 years of age or with severe tendon degeneration, the augmenting the repair with ipsilateral flexor hallucis longus (FHL) transfer may provide additional benefit.[19,20]

PLANTAR FASCIOPATHY

The plantar fascia serves as both a static and dynamic stabilizer for the medial longitudinal arch of the foot and consists of lateral, medial, and central bands.[21] The central band spans the medial tubercle of the calcaneus to the 5 toes of the foot. The term plantar fasciopathy reflects that this condition may include acute inflammation or chronic degenerative changes, both of which result in significant pain and limitations during running activity.

Clinical Evaluation

A runner typically reports a sensation of pain over the plantar aspect of the foot, typically worse with initial morning ambulation and improved during the course of a run, with worsening pain after discontinuation of activity. Duration of symptoms helps to classify the phase of injury and guide management.[22]

The runner commonly exhibits tenderness to palpation over the medial calcaneal tubercle and along the plantar fascia. Thus, the plantar fascia should be palpated for presence of crepitus, thickening, or swelling. The Achilles tendon contributes fibers in continuity with the plantar fascia and should also be evaluated by palpation for presence of pain. Ankle ROM is important to assess, as described, using the Silfverskiold test. Passive extension of the toes places the plantar fascia and medial longitudinal arch on stretch and may elicit pain (Windlass test). Tinel's sign, or shooting pains elicited by tapping over the tarsal tunnel, may help to identify tarsal tunnel syndrome as a contributor to pain. The calcaneal squeeze test should be performed to evaluate for signs of a calcaneal BSI. The calcaneal fat pad should be examined for evidence of atrophy or tenderness to palpation, because this may suggest fat pad atrophy. Weight-bearing radiograph of the foot and ankle is valuable to assess for presence of tension esophytes or calcifications, and can help exclude fracture or stress injury of the calcaneus. In a runner with acute onset of plantar foot pain with suspicion for significant tearing, MRI can be helpful to further evaluate for plantar fascia tear or rupture. New ultrasound techniques are emerging as a tool for dynamic evaluation of hindfoot structures including evaluating the plantar fascia.[23]

Differential Diagnosis

Personal and family history of rheumatologic conditions, including seronegative spondyloarthropathies, should be queried, because enthesopathy of the foot may mimic plantar fasciopathy. Additionally, a history of low back pain or radicular symptoms is important to elicit and consider as lumbosacral referred pain patterns can result in plantar foot pain. Other conditions on the differential diagnosis for plantar foot pain include sesamoiditis (inflammation and irritation of the sesamoid bones that lie on the plantar aspect of the hallux) and metatarsalgia, or pain localized to the metatarsal heads. These conditions are usually differentiated from plantar fasciopathy by its more forefoot location. Further discussion is beyond the scope of this article, but can be found elsewhere in the literature.[24]

Management

The vast majority of cases of plantar fasciopathy respond to conservative treatment. A passive plantar foot stretching program has been shown to improve pain compared with active Achilles tendon stretching exercises for chronic plantar fasciopathy with good long-term effects.[25,26] In this stretching protocol, the runner should be instructed to use 1 hand to passively extend the toes toward the shin until a stretching sensation is achieved, with the other hand palpating the medial longitudinal arch to ensure the plantar fascia structure is being stretched, held for 10 seconds for 10 total repetitions and performed 3 times daily.[25,26] A recent, randomized, controlled trial demonstrated high load strength training resulted in less pain at 3 months and similar outcomes at 1 year compared with the passive plantar foot stretching program.[27] The high load strength training program consisted of performing single leg calf raises with the toes supported under a towel to aid in Windlass mechanism. The program started with 3 sets of 12 repetitions and advanced to added weight with 5 sets of 8 repetitions, performed every other day. The strength training program has added advantage of being performed less frequently than passive plantar stretching and may be reasonable initial therapy for most runners. Foot orthosis can also be beneficial.[28]

Other treatment may include use of low-dye or calcaneal taping, accommodative foot orthosis, acupuncture, manual therapy, night splints, iontophoresis, and extracorporeal shockwave therapy. Treatment may also include injections, including corticosteroid medication, PRP, or botulinum toxin. Corticosteroid injections have been shown to provide pain relief for 1 month[29,30] and may be more effective under ultrasound guidance.[31] However, complications for corticosteroid injection include heel fat pad atrophy, nerve damage, and risk for rupture of the plantar fascia that result in biomechanical changes in the Windlass mechanism. Thus, corticosteroid injections should be used with caution, and the number limited. PRP and botulinum toxin injections may provide greater duration of benefits. PRP has been shown to provide durable benefits up to 24 months when compared with corticosteroids.[32] Botulinum toxin has been shown to provide pain relief at 3 months after treatment.[33] Because studies on management of plantar fasciopathy have been primarily performed in nonathlete populations, the effectiveness of these treatments in runners is unknown.

ANKLE SPRAINS

Acute ankle sprains are a common injury in runners, especially those who run on uneven terrain. One study found that nearly one-third of female and one-quarter of male high school-aged runners have a history of ankle sprain.[34] Lateral (ie, inversion) ankle sprains are most common and result from damage a combination of the anterior talofibular ligament, calcaneofibular ligament, and posterior tibiofibular ligament. High ankle sprains (ie, eversion or external rotation) are less common and result in injury to the syndesmotic ligaments and/or deltoid.

Clinical Evaluation

A careful history should be obtained regarding injury mechanism, history of ankle sprain, or feelings of instability and prior rehabilitation completed. Physical findings from a comprehensive examination allow for grading of ankle sprain severity, and may be used to guide appropriate management and return to play[35–37] (**Table 2**).

The clinician should evaluate for the presence of swelling, discoloration, and pain with ambulation. The clinician should systematically palpate the full length of the tibia, fibula, and over the anterior inferior tibiofibular ligament to evaluate for evidence of syndesmotic injury or high ankle sprain. The anterior talofibular ligament, calcaneofibular ligament, and posterior tibiofibular ligament should each be palpated for tenderness. Additionally, the fifth metatarsal, and the cuboid and tarsal navicular should be assessed for bony tenderness. Single leg balance can be assessed for general proprioception and neuromuscular control of the lower extremity. The peroneal tendons

Table 2 Severity of ankle sprain	
Grade	**Signs and Symptoms**
First degree (mild)	Ligament strain with or without some ligament fibers torn Mild tenderness and swelling No laxity or residual instability Full function Full strength
Second degree (moderate)	Incomplete ligament tear Moderate pain and swelling Mild laxity and instability Slight reduction in function Possible decrease in strength Potential loss of proprioception
Third degree (severe)	Complete ligament tear Severe pain and swelling Gross instability and laxity Potential complete loss of function Potential complete loss of strength Potential complete loss of proprioception

Grading criteria modified from Wolfe (2001),[37] original reference.[35]

should be evaluated for subluxation, tendinosis, and/or weakness. Anterior drawer test and talar tilt tests are compared with the asymptomatic side for differences in total translation and laxity to assess for the integrity of the anterior talofibular and calcaneofibular ligaments, respectively.

A weight-bearing radiograph of the ankle should be obtained based on the Ottawa Ankle Rules for acute presentation[38] or based on concern for high ankle sprain, syndesmotic injury, or associated fracture.

Differential Diagnosis

Differential diagnosis for acute low lateral ankle sprain should include consideration for high ankle sprain involving the syndesmosis and associated fracture, such as a Maisonneuve fracture, because this would urgently change management decision making. There are 5 concomitant injuries that should be considered in patients who have not made expected progress during their course of injury rehabilitation after an inversion sprain. These include (1) peroneal tendinopathy or tear, (2) osteochondral lesion of the talar dome, (3) fracture of the anterior process of the calcaneus, (4) neuritis of the superficial peroneal nerve or sural nerve, and (5) lateral malleolar fracture.

Management

Initial management for inversion ankle sprain begins with PRICE: protection, rest, icing, compression, and elevation. This can be accomplished with use of a walking boot for runners with painful ambulation, or a stirrup ankle brace. The authors advocate a short period in a walking boot until pain free (usually 7–10 days) followed by transition to functional bracing. NSAIDs can be initiated 24 hours after the injury. Initial rehabilitation goals include resolution of edema and restoring painless ROM of the ankle. Postural control is impaired after both acute and chronic lateral ankle trauma, and balance exercises have been shown to help address this impairment.[39] Additionally, reduced muscle activity of the hip, knee, and ankle has been observed in patients with chronic ankle instability.[40] Therefore, advanced ankle rehabilitation protocols should include strengthening both intrinsic and extrinsic muscles of the foot and ankle along with addressing neuromuscular control and evaluation of the full kinetic chain. Although an optimal protocol for injury rehabilitation and prevention has not been defined, we recommend applying concepts of foot core paradigm for management of this injury.[41] For patients with recurrent ankle sprains ($\geq$3 total), or persistent anatomic and functional instability despite appropriate conservative care, referral to an orthopedist for evaluation and surgical reconstruction of the lateral ligaments may be considered.

BONE STRESS INJURIES

Bone stress injuries (BSI) are a common form of overuse injury in runners, developing when the bone fails to respond to submaximal forces from running and resulting in structural damage and pain.[42] The biological and biomechanical risk factors are discussed elsewhere.[43,44] Most anatomic locations for injury in the foot are considered high risk owing to biomechanical forces that increase likelihood of malunion, nonunion, or progression to full fracture.[42]

Clinical Evaluation

The runner should be queried for risk factors, including history of prior fracture or BSI; changes in training volume, intensity, or technique; and screening for female athlete triad risk factors, including disordered eating, low energy availability, late menarche (defined as first menstrual period at age ≥15 years), menstrual dysfunction (including periods >35 days apart or <10 periods in 12 months), and a history of low bone mineral density.[45]

Physical examination helps to localize bone pain and differentiate from other soft tissue etiologies of pain. On examination, evaluate general alignment of the foot, because cavovarus foot type may increase the risk of injury.[46] Assess for presence of pain with weight bearing, including the single leg hop test. Focal swelling or erythema, tenderness to palpation, and pain with indirect percussion can also be clinical signs of BSI.

Radiographs can demonstrate evidence of cortical hypertrophy to suggest healing response or radiolucency may be visible in the setting of a high grade BSI. When clinical suspicion is high and radiographs are equivocal or when determining a specific timeline for recovery is needed, the authors recommend use of MRI to further evaluate for presence of a BSI and value in grading severity of the injury to help with guide return to play.[47] Other forms of advanced imaging may be required to evaluate BSI depending on clinical context. For example, computed tomography scans may be helpful to assess navicular BSI because surgical decision making is based in large part on whether the fracture is complete or incomplete.

Differential Diagnosis

Differential diagnosis of BSI varies by location and must be differentiated from other forms of injury, including soft tissue injuries such as chronic tendinopathy, arthropathy, joint instability, rheumatologic, or even oncologic pathology.

Management

BSI can occur in virtually any bone of the foot (although they are rare in the phalanges). Locations considered high risk include the tarsal navicular, base of the fifth metatarsal (Jones fracture), talus, base of the second metatarsal, sesamoids, and medial malleolus.[48] Common low-risk factures in the foot and ankle include the calcaneus, and the second through fifth metatarsals (excluding the base of the second metatarsal and metaphysis of the fifth metatarsal).[49] Initial management for all BSI includes immobilization or shoe modifications to achieve pain free ambulation. High-risk fracture sites typically require surgical decision making or use of immobilizer boot or cast with crutches to maintain a non–weight-bearing status, often for 6 or more weeks to facilitate bony healing. Repeat clinical evaluation is needed to ensure the patient is pain free before advancing weight bearing and initiation of cross-training and aerobic activity. It is appropriate to refer the runner to a foot and ankle orthopedic surgeon when managing injuries in high-risk locations to optimize management decisions. In female runners, current evaluation for female athlete triad risk factors and management of this condition is critical to ensure the overall health of female runners.[45] Both males and females must meet Institute of Medicine calcium and vitamin D guidelines to assist in fracture healing and prevention, including calcium targets of 1300 mg for ages 9 to 18 years old (both sexes) and 1000 mg ages 19 to 50 in females and ages 19 to 70 in males and vitamin D targets of 600 IU daily for ages 9 to 70.[50] Footwear and training regimens must be evaluated for possible contribution as well.

POSTERIOR TIBIAL TENDON DYSFUNCTION

Although not as common as Achilles tendinopathy, posterior tibial tendon dysfunction is another potential cause of posteromedial ankle pain in runners. The posterior tibial tendon runs from the deep posterior compartment of the leg down to insert extensively on multiple areas of the foot, including the navicular tuberosity, middle cuneiform, and second through fourth metatarsals, although variants have been described.[51] The posterior tibial tendon acts as a shock absorber during heel strike, stabilizes the foot during midstance, and aids in force generation in heel lift and toe off. Thus, dysfunction of the posterior tibial tendon can cause significant changes in biomechanics and, thus, runner performance and health.

Posterior tibial tendon dysfunction was classically discussed in 3 stages by Johnson and Strom,[52] and later refined into a 4-stage classification system.[53] The acute phase may include significant synovial inflammation within the tibialis posterior tendon sheath and/or paratenon. In later stages, this may progress to involve degenerative changes manifesting as thickening of the tendon, adhesion formation, and stenosing of the tendon. With progression of posterior tibial tendon dysfunction, a painful flatfoot deformity may develop.

Clinical Evaluation

A runner usually presents with slow progressive onset of swelling and pain along the path of the posterior tibial tendon, and possibly extends more proximally to the myotendinous junction. The pain is initially aggravated by running and progresses to include normal ambulation.

Clinical examination should involve inspection and palpation of the entire path of the tendon, both distally to the navicular tuberosity and proximally to the posterior tibial muscle. Swelling and tenderness are commonly present in injured runners. Functional testing may include evaluating ability to perform heel raises both in single and double stance, and pain and/or weakness with resisted inversion of a plantarflexed foot. The double-limb heel rise test can also be useful to evaluate posterior tibial tendon function. For this test, the asymptomatic side goes into ankle plantarflexion and the other foot is lifted off the floor. The normal foot remains inverted whereas the affected side stays in hindfoot valgus in the setting of posterior tibial tendon dysfunction. Resisted inversion should be tested for weakness or reproduction of pain.

Radiographs may be helpful to evaluate for bony abnormalities including presence of os trigonum. Ultrasonography is useful in evaluation of the posterior tibial tendon and may be helpful to demonstrate inflammation of the tendon and/or paratenon as well as heterogenicity or disruption of the tendon fiber, indicating degenerative changes or tears. Neovascularization may be evaluated with use of Doppler imaging with ultrasonography. MRI may also be considered, especially to evaluate abnormalities in the surrounding structures, such as in the spring and deltoid ligament complex.

Differential Diagnosis

Differential diagnosis for posterior tibial tendon dysfunction is similar to Achilles tendinopathy, and includes bone stress injuries of the distal tibia, fibula, or calcaneus, retrocalcaneal bursitis, posterior ankle impingement, and tendinopathies of the toe flexors. Rheumatologic disease may also contribute and should be considered with presentation of significant posterior tibial tendon inflammation or an unusual presentation. Os trigonum can cause posterior ankle pain and may be visualized on lateral radiographs of the ankle.

Management

Treatment for acute posterior tibial tendinitis includes activity modification, including immobilization with a walking boot and/or relative rest from repetitive loading activities, ice, NSAIDs, and iontophoresis.[54] Use of an arch support orthotic to decrease pronation may be helpful as well. In a study of 47 patients with posterior tibial tendon dysfunction, Alvarez and colleagues (2006)[55] used a structured nonoperative protocol in patients with stage I and II posterior tibial tendon dysfunction including use of a foot orthosis or short articulated ankle foot orthosis, and a rehabilitation consisting of aggressive high repetition plantarflexion exercises and heel cord stretches. After 10 physical therapy visits over 4 months, 39 (83%) had successful subjective and functional outcome.[55] Thus, functional restoration should then be the focus of treatment, to include addressing both muscle weakness and imbalance as well as tightness of the triceps surae.

Historical treatment for posterior tibial dysfunction include corticosteroid injections, which carry significant risk of complications, with tendon rupture a significant concern with steroid exposure.[56] These authors do not recommend the use of steroid injections for posterior tibial tendinopathy and Achilles tendinopathy given that these are high weight-bearing tendons and are at increased risk of rupture with injection. In contrast with Achilles tendinopathy, we are unaware of published studies evaluating the use of PRP in posterior tibial tendon dysfunction. Surgical management may be considered in severe and refractory cases.

PERONEAL TENDINOPATHY

The peroneus longus and brevis tendons course from the lateral compartment of the leg, then via a common synovial sheath runs posterior to the lateral malleolus, and finally insert onto the base of the first metatarsal and the tuberosity of the fifth metatarsal, respectively. The peroneal muscles serve as primary everters of the foot. Peroneal tendinopathy is often seen in runners and may be especially common for those with chronic ankle instability.[57]

Clinical Evaluation

Runners with peroneal tendinopathy most often present with chronic lateral ankle pain posterior or distal to the lateral malleoli, which may be accompanied by radiating pain proximally along the lateral aspect of the leg. If there is associated peroneal subluxation or dislocation, there may be a sensation of snapping or popping when bringing the foot into plantar flexion. Although some runners may report a history of sharp and acute pop in the setting of an ankle sprain, often this is not the case.

Evaluation should begin with inspection, which may note swelling and warmth along the peroneal tendon. Alignment of the foot should also be assessed given the association of a cavovarus foot with increased rates of peroneal tendon disorder.[58] Palpation of the tendon may note pain and palpable tendon thickening. The peroneus longus may be differentiated from brevis when asking the runner to plantarflex the great toe given the insertion of peroneus longus. The examiner should also palpate for the presence of subluxation of the peroneal tendon over the lateral malleolus. Provocative maneuvers that may reproduce symptoms include passive inversion of a plantarflexed foot or resisted eversion of a dorsiflexed foot.

With regard to radiographic studies, radiographs are helpful to evaluate for the presence of fracture or anatomic variants including os perineum. Ultrasound may be useful to elucidate signs of inflammation along the tendon and tendon sheath. Irregularity and tears of the tendon could also be evaluated, with reported accuracy of 90% (sensitivity, 100%; specificity, 85%) for diagnosis of peroneal tendon tear.[59] Dynamic testing under ultrasound guidance to visualize tendon subluxation and dislocation can also be performed. MRI may also be helpful to characterize extent of peroneal tendinopathy and/or tear.

Differential Diagnosis

The differential diagnosis of peroneal tendinopathy includes lateral ankle sprain and fibular fracture in the acute setting, whereas in chronic cases clinicians should consider peroneal subluxation or dislocation and os perineum syndrome.

Management

Peroneal tendinopathy usually responds well to conservative management, including a short period of immobilization, relative rest, lateral heel wedge, and physical therapy. Given the role of hindfoot cavovarus in peroneal tendinopathy, an accommodative custom foot orthotic should be considered.[60] The role of injection of biological agents in peroneal tendinopathy is unclear, given there has only been 1 published pilot study investigating ultrasound guided PRP injection as a treatment for peroneal (among others) tendinopathy.[61] Surgical debridement with tenosynovectomy and repair may be considered after a period of at least 3 to 6 months of nonoperative management.[62]

OTHER TENDINOPATHIES
Flexor Hallucis Longus Tendinopathy

FHL tendinopathy is more common in classical ballet dancers,[63] although this injury may occur with running athletes performing repetitive forceful push off. Pain from FHL tendinopathy can occur anywhere along the course of the FHL, from the posterior aspect of the fibula down to the base of the distal phalanx of the hallux, although the pain may localize to the posteromedial ankle. Clinical examination may also note swelling, tenderness, and crepitus, with pain elicited by resisted plantar flexion of the hallux. Conservative management of FHL tendinopathy should include assessment of training errors and biomechanical deficits along the kinetic chain that contribute to increased FHL stress during push-off while running.

Anterior Tibial Tendinopathy

Anterior tibial tendinopathy may cause anterior leg or ankle pain in a runner. Weakness and pain with dorsiflexion is the primary clinical finding, and pain along the anterior tibial tendon with resisted dorsiflexion can be helpful to distinguish this condition from pain originating from the tibiotalar joint. There is no consensus on the management of anterior tibial tendinopathy and/or tear. Conservative management is reasonable for tendinopathy without significant tear, although surgical management seems to provide good outcomes for many patients with anterior tibial tendon rupture.[64]

JOINT PATHOLOGIES

There are a variety of joint pathologies that may contribute to pain in a runner. Given the prevalence of osteoarthritis, degenerative joint conditions should be considered for older runners. Hallux rigidus or osteoarthritis of the first metatarsalphalangeal joint is a common cause of forefoot pain. Runners may present with pain, crepitus, and stiffness with running and/or walking. Clinicians should start with evaluating for swelling and/or bony deformity over the dorsum of the first metatarsalphalangeal joint. ROM may be limited for both dorsiflexion and plantar flexion, whereas pain with plantar flexion may be associated with bone spur over the dorsum of the first metatarsophalangeal joint. Pain with palpation and with the "grind test," where the examiner applies axial compression onto the phalanx into the metatarsal head, are strongly supportive of this diagnosis. Radiographic evaluation can demonstrate characteristic findings of osteoarthritis changes, including joint space narrowing, osteophyte formation, and subchondral sclerosis and cyst formation. Initial conservative management includes PRICE as well as shoe modifications. Although injection of corticosteroids may provide temporary relief, the role of injectable viscosupplementation and biological agents have not been demonstrated in the literature for management of hallux rigidus. Wide toe-box shoes can help to alleviate pressure on the toe, and use of a rigid Morton extension or full-length carbon fiber orthosis can provide support to the medial column of the foot and symptom relief.[65] Surgical options include cheilectomy or arthrodesis.[24,66]

Osteochondral Lesions

Osteochondral lesions and defects of the foot and ankle are a potential cause of joint pain. A history of trauma is noted in 80% of medial and 100% of lateral talar osteochondral lesions[67,68] and should be suspected in those with history of ankle sprain with delayed healing and/or with a history of ankle instability or injury. Patients may present with pain and swelling of the ankle, and symptoms may be aggravated by weight bearing. Physical examination may demonstrate evidence of joint effusion and pain with palpation over the talus. Although radiographs may visualize a talus fracture, MRI may be useful with negative plain films. Nonoperative treatment with non–weight-bearing status and immobilization with a walking boot may be tried, although operative treatment is often required. Excision, curettage, and drilling was reported to be effective in management of osteochondral lesions of the talus by systemic review.[69] Others have proposed a role for use of regenerative techniques, such as autologous chondrocytes implantation or bone marrow–derived stem cell transplantation, in the treatment of osteochondral lesions of the talus.[70]

NERVE CONDITIONS

Disorders affecting the nerves that innervate the foot also affect runners. Nerve disorders should be included in the differential for most of the injuries discussed so far, particularly in cases that do not improve as anticipated.

A prevalent nerve disorder is interdigital neuralgia/neuroma, which is classically described as irritation and inflammation of the interdigital nerve to the toes as it passes below the transverse ligament of the metatarsal heads. Interdigital neuromas most commonly occur between the third and fourth metatarsals (referred to as a Morton's neuroma), although they can occur in other locations. This condition is common in the sixth decade of life and has a greater prevalence in women.[71] Patients typically present with pain or paresthesias in the metatarsal heads and/or the neighboring toes, which is aggravated by weight bearing and wearing heels or shoes with narrow toe boxes. In contrast, metatarsalgia tends to be worse when barefoot. Often, patients may describe this as a sensation of having "pebble" in their shoe. Radiographs are usually normal, but help to identify any other abnormalities. Although MRI is the primary diagnostic imaging tool, ultrasonography in the hands of an experienced provider can yield high sensitivity (100%) and specificity (83.3%) for the evaluation of a Morton's neuroma.[72] Management of an interdigital neuroma usually include offloading strategies, such as avoiding high heels, wearing shoes with a larger toe box, prefabricated metatarsal relief pads/bar, and/or use of custom foot orthoses. Injection with anesthetic and steroids can be both diagnostic and therapeutic. Sclerosing alcohol therapy under ultrasound guidance is highly controversial and lacks sufficient evidence to be recommended.[73] If symptoms do not improve with conservative management, surgical excision may be considered.

Additional neuropathies relevant for runners include tarsal tunnel syndrome, superficial peroneal neuropathy, and jogger's foot. Injury to the posterior tibial nerve as it courses beneath the flexor retinaculum on the medial side of the ankle is termed tarsal tunnel syndrome and may result in pain and paresthesias into the medial foot. The superficial peroneal nerve courses over the lateral aspect of the foot and can be injured with lateral foot and ankle injuries, including lateral ankle sprains. Jogger's foot is caused by irritation of the medial plantar nerve causing pain and paresthesias along the medial arch of the foot.[74] Tinel's sign along the tarsal tunnel, superficial peroneal nerve, or over the medial plantar nerve, may help with clinical evaluation. Additionally, nerve conduction studies and electromyography may help to localize the lesion and grade severity, although false negatives may occur in tarsal tunnel syndrome.[75] Although tarsal tunnel syndrome may ultimately require decompression surgery in certain patients,[75] superficial peroneal neuropathy and Jogger's foot usually can usually be managed conservatively with rehabilitation protocol, including anti-inflammatory medications, a running biomechanics evaluation, and assessment for proper footwear.[74]

INJURY PREVENTION AND MANAGEMENT

Many of the foot and ankle overuse running injury conditions are likely to recur without appropriate rehabilitation efforts to reduce risk for future injury. A foot–core paradigm was recently proposed that discusses the role of intrinsic, extrinsic, and neuromuscular training to address foot conditions.[41] Although custom foot orthotics or other shoe modifications may have a role for initial management of running injuries by changing the biomechanical forces through the foot, we acknowledge that compensatory changes may occur and result in unintended loading of other tissues and joints by altering the kinetic chain with continued use. Modifying foot function through rehabilitative exercises is an exciting and largely unexplored area for future research and advancement in management and prevention of overuse injuries in runners.

SUMMARY

Foot and ankle conditions are common causes of overuse injuries in runners. Similar to most overuse injuries, activity modification with corrective physical therapy program to restore strength and function are key to the management of most conditions. The role of prevention specifically optimizing foot and ankle function along with full kinetic chain assessment to optimize biomechanics of running form and foot strike patterns may be an effective strategy for injury prevention and requires further investigation given the high cumulative prevalence of overuse injuries in the running population.

REFERENCES

1. Epperly T, Fields KB. Running epidemiology. New York: McGraw-Hill; 2014.
2. Lopes AD, Hespanhol Junior LC, Yeung SS, et al. What are the main running-related musculoskeletal injuries? A systematic review. Sports Med 2012;42(10): 891–905.
3. Zafar MS, Mahmood A, Maffulli N. Basic science and clinical aspects of Achilles tendinopathy. Sports Med Arthrosc 2009;17(3):190–7.
4. Magnan B, Bondi M, Pierantoni S, et al. The pathogenesis of Achilles tendinopathy: a systematic review. Foot Ankle Surg 2014;20(3):154–9.

5. Cook JL, Purdam CR. Is tendon pathology a continuum? A pathology model to explain the clinical presentation of load-induced tendinopathy. Br J Sports Med 2009;43(6):409–16.

6. Carr AJ, Norris SH. The blood supply of the calcaneal tendon. J Bone Joint Surg Br 1989;71(1):100–1.

7. Paavola M, Paakkala T, Kannus P, et al. Ultrasonography in the differential diagnosis of Achilles tendon injuries and related disorders. A comparison between pre-operative ultrasonography and surgical findings. Acta Radiol 1998;39(6):612–9.

8. Neeter C, Thomee R, Silbernagel KG, et al. Iontophoresis with or without dexamethazone in the treatment of acute Achilles tendon pain. Scand J Med Sci Sports 2003;13(6):376–82.

9. Kane TP, Ismail M, Calder JD. Topical glyceryl trinitrate and noninsertional Achilles tendinopathy: a clinical and cellular investigation. Am J Sports Med 2008;36(6):1160–3.

10. Alfredson H, Pietila T, Jonsson P, et al. Heavy-load eccentric calf muscle training for the treatment of chronic Achilles tendinosis. Am J Sports Med 1998;26(3):360–6.

11. van der Plas A, de Jonge S, de Vos RJ, et al. A 5-year follow-up study of Alfredson's heel-drop exercise programme in chronic midportion Achilles tendinopathy. Br J Sports Med 2012;46(3):214–8.

12. Jonsson P, Alfredson H, Sunding K, et al. New regimen for eccentric calf-muscle training in patients with chronic insertional Achilles tendinopathy: results of a pilot study. Br J Sports Med 2008;42(9):746–9.

13. Azevedo LB, Lambert MI, Vaughan CL, et al. Biomechanical variables associated with Achilles tendinopathy in runners. Br J Sports Med 2009;43(4):288–92.

14. Franettovich Smith MM, Honeywill C, Wyndow N, et al. Neuromotor control of gluteal muscles in runners with Achilles tendinopathy. Med Sci Sports Exerc 2014;46(3):594–9.

15. Gaweda K, Tarczynska M, Krzyzanowski W. Treatment of Achilles tendinopathy with platelet-rich plasma. Int J Sports Med 2010;31(8):577–83.

16. Owens RF Jr, Ginnetti J, Conti SF, et al. Clinical and magnetic resonance imaging outcomes following platelet rich plasma injection for chronic midsubstance Achilles tendinopathy. Foot Ankle Int 2011;32(11):1032–9.

17. de Vos RJ, Weir A, van Schie HT, et al. Platelet-rich plasma injection for chronic Achilles tendinopathy: a randomized controlled trial. JAMA 2010;303(2):144–9.

18. de Jonge S, de Vos RJ, Weir A, et al. One-year follow-up of platelet-rich plasma treatment in chronic Achilles tendinopathy: a double-blind randomized placebo-controlled trial. Am J Sports Med 2011;39(8):1623–9.

19. Schon LC, Shores JL, Faro FD, et al. Flexor hallucis longus tendon transfer in treatment of Achilles tendinosis. J Bone Joint Surg Am 2013;95(1):54–60.

20. Hunt KJ, Cohen BE, Davis WH, et al. Surgical treatment of insertional Achilles tendinopathy with or without flexor hallucis longus tendon transfer: a prospective, randomized study. Foot Ankle Int 2015;36(9):998–1005.

21. Hicks JH. The mechanics of the foot. II. The plantar aponeurosis and the arch. J Anat 1954;88(1):25–30.

22. Berbrayer D, Fredericson M. Update on evidence-based treatments for plantar fasciopathy. PM R 2014;6(2):159–69.

23. Hoffman DF, Grothe HL, Bianchi S. Sonographic evaluation of hindfoot disorders. J Ultrasound 2014;17(2):141–50.

24. Hunt KJ, McCormick JJ, Anderson RB. Management of forefoot injuries in the athlete. Oper Tech Foot Ankle 2010;18:34–45.

25. Digiovanni BF, Nawoczenski DA, Malay DP, et al. Plantar fascia-specific stretching exercise improves outcomes in patients with chronic plantar fasciitis. A prospective clinical trial with two-year follow-up. J Bone Joint Surg Am 2006;88(8): 1775–81.
26. DiGiovanni BF, Nawoczenski DA, Lintal ME, et al. Tissue-specific plantar fascia-stretching exercise enhances outcomes in patients with chronic heel pain. A prospective, randomized study. J Bone Joint Surg Am 2003;85-A(7):1270–7.
27. Rathleff MS, Molgaard CM, Fredberg U, et al. High-load strength training improves outcome in patients with plantar fasciitis: a randomized controlled trial with 12-month follow-up. Scand J Med Sci Sports 2015;25(3):e292–300.
28. Lee SY, McKeon P, Hertel J. Does the use of orthoses improve self-reported pain and function measures in patients with plantar fasciitis? A meta-analysis. Phys Ther Sport 2009;10(1):12–8.
29. Crawford F, Atkins D, Young P, et al. Steroid injection for heel pain: evidence of short-term effectiveness. A randomized controlled trial. Rheumatology 1999; 38(10):974–7.
30. McMillan AM, Landorf KB, Gilheany MF, et al. Ultrasound guided corticosteroid injection for plantar fasciitis: randomised controlled trial. BMJ 2012;344:e3260.
31. Li Z, Xia C, Yu A, et al. Ultrasound- versus palpation-guided injection of corticosteroid for plantar fasciitis: a meta-analysis. PLoS One 2014;9(3):e92671.
32. Monto RR. Platelet-rich plasma efficacy versus corticosteroid injection treatment for chronic severe plantar fasciitis. Foot Ankle Int 2014;35(4):313–8.
33. Huang YC, Wei SH, Wang HK, et al. Ultrasonographic guided botulinum toxin type A treatment for plantar fasciitis: an outcome-based investigation for treating pain and gait changes. J Rehabil Med 2010;42(2):136–40.
34. Tenforde AS, Sayres LC, McCurdy ML, et al. Overuse injuries in high school runners: lifetime prevalence and prevention strategies. PM R 2011;3(2):125–31 [quiz: 131].
35. Lateral ankle pain. Park Ridge (IL): American College of Foot and Ankle Surgeons; 1997. preferred practice guideline no. 1/97.
36. Safran MR, Benedetti RS, Bartolozzi AR 3rd, et al. Lateral ankle sprains: a comprehensive review: part 1: etiology, pathoanatomy, histopathogenesis, and diagnosis. Med Sci Sports Exerc 1999;31(7 Suppl):S429–37.
37. Wolfe MW, Uhl TL, Mattacola CG, et al. Management of ankle sprains. Am Fam Physician 2001;63(1):93–104.
38. Stiell IG, Greenberg GH, McKnight RD, et al. A study to develop clinical decision rules for the use of radiography in acute ankle injuries. Ann Emerg Med 1992; 21(4):384–90.
39. Wikstrom EA, Naik S, Lodha N, et al. Balance capabilities after lateral ankle trauma and intervention: a meta-analysis. Med Sci Sports Exerc 2009;41(6):1287–95.
40. Feger MA, Donovan L, Hart JM, et al. Lower extremity muscle activation during functional exercises in patients with and without chronic ankle instability. PM R 2014;6(7):602–11 [quiz: 611].
41. McKeon PO, Hertel J, Bramble D, et al. The foot core system: a new paradigm for understanding intrinsic foot muscle function. Br J Sports Med 2015;49(5):290.
42. Warden SJ, Davis IS, Fredericson M. Management and prevention of bone stress injuries in long-distance runners. J Orthop Sports Phys Ther 2014;44(10):749–65.
43. Tenforde AS, Kraus E, Fredericson M. Bone stress injuries in runners. Phys Med Rehabil Clin N Am, in press.
44. Kim B, Nattiv A. Health considerations in the female runner. Phys Med Rehabil Clin N Am, in press.

45. De Souza MJ, Nattiv A, Joy E, et al. 2014 Female Athlete Triad Coalition Consensus Statement on Treatment and Return to Play of the Female Athlete Triad: 1st International Conference held in San Francisco, California, May 2012 and 2nd International Conference held in Indianapolis, Indiana, May 2013. Br J Sports Med 2014;48(4):289.

46. Lee KT, Kim KC, Park YU, et al. Radiographic evaluation of foot structure following fifth metatarsal stress fracture. Foot Ankle Int 2011;32(8):796–801.

47. Nattiv A, Kennedy G, Barrack MT, et al. Correlation of MRI grading of bone stress injuries with clinical risk factors and return to play: a 5-year prospective study in collegiate track and field athletes. Am J Sports Med 2013;41(8): 1930–41.

48. Boden BP, Osbahr DC. High-risk stress fractures: evaluation and treatment. J Am Acad Orthop Surg 2000;8(6):344–53.

49. Boden BP, Osbahr DC, Jimenez C. Low-risk stress fractures. Am J Sports Med 2001;29(1):100–11.

50. Institute of Medicine (2010). Dietary reference intakes for calcium and vitamin D. National Academy of Sciences; November 2010, Report Brief. Available at: https://iom.nationalacademies.org/~/media/Files/Report%20Files/2010/Dietary-Reference-Intakes-for-Calcium-and-Vitamin-D/Vitamin%20D%20and%20Calcium%202010%20Report%20Brief.pdf. Accessed March 1, 2015.

51. Bloome DM, Marymont JV, Varner KE. Variations on the insertion of the posterior tibialis tendon: a cadaveric study. Foot Ankle Int 2003;24(10):780–3.

52. Johnson KA, Strom DE. Tibialis posterior tendon dysfunction. Clin Orthop Relat Res 1989;(239):196–206.

53. Bluman EM, Title CI, Myerson MS. Posterior tibial tendon rupture: a refined classification system. Foot Ankle Clin 2007;12(2):233–49, v.

54. Giza E, Cush G, Schon LC. The flexible flatfoot in the adult. Foot Ankle Clin 2007; 12(2):251–71, vi.

55. Alvarez RG, Marini A, Schmitt C, et al. Stage I and II posterior tibial tendon dysfunction treated by a structured nonoperative management protocol: an orthosis and exercise program. Foot Ankle Int 2006;27(1):2–8.

56. Holmes GB Jr, Mann RA. Possible epidemiological factors associated with rupture of the posterior tibial tendon. Foot Ankle 1992;13(2):70–9.

57. DiGiovanni BF, Fraga CJ, Cohen BE, et al. Associated injuries found in chronic lateral ankle instability. Foot Ankle Int 2000;21(10):809–15.

58. Manoli A 2nd, Graham B. The subtle cavus foot, "the underpronator". Foot Ankle Int 2005;26(3):256–63.

59. Grant TH, Kelikian AS, Jereb SE, et al. Ultrasound diagnosis of peroneal tendon tears. A surgical correlation. J Bone Joint Surg Am 2005;87(8):1788–94.

60. Deben SE, Pomeroy GC. Subtle cavus foot: diagnosis and management. J Am Acad Orthop Surg 2014;22(8):512–20.

61. Dallaudiere B, Pesquer L, Meyer P, et al. Intratendinous injection of platelet-rich plasma under US guidance to treat tendinopathy: a long-term pilot study. J Vasc Interv Radiol 2014;25(5):717–23.

62. Heckman DS, Gluck GS, Parekh SG. Tendon disorders of the foot and ankle, part 1: peroneal tendon disorders. Am J Sports Med 2009;37(3):614–25.

63. Hamilton WG, Geppert MJ, Thompson FM. Pain in the posterior aspect of the ankle in dancers. Differential diagnosis and operative treatment. J Bone Joint Surg Am 1996;78(10):1491–500.

64. Christman-Skieller C, Merz MK, Tansey JP. A systematic review of tibialis anterior tendon rupture treatments and outcomes. Am J Orthop 2015;44(4):E94–9.

65. Sammarco VJ, Nichols R. Orthotic management for disorders of the hallux. Foot Ankle Clin 2005;10(1):191–209.
66. Geldwert JJ, Rock GD, McGrath MP, et al. Cheilectomy: still a useful technique for grade I and grade II hallux limitus/rigidus. J Foot Surg 1992;31(2):154–9.
67. Flick AB, Gould N. Osteochondritis dissecans of the talus (transchondral fractures of the talus): review of the literature and new surgical approach for medial dome lesions. Foot Ankle 1985;5(4):165–85.
68. Tol JL, Struijs PA, Bossuyt PM, et al. Treatment strategies in osteochondral defects of the talar dome: a systematic review. Foot Ankle Int 2000;21(2):119–26.
69. Verhagen RA, Struijs PA, Bossuyt PM, et al. Systematic review of treatment strategies for osteochondral defects of the talar dome. Foot Ankle Clin 2003;8(2): 233–42, viii–ix.
70. Buda R, Vannini F, Castagnini F, et al. Regenerative treatment in osteochondral lesions of the talus: autologous chondrocyte implantation versus one-step bone marrow derived cells transplantation. Int Orthop 2015;39(5):893–900.
71. Peters PG, Adams SB Jr, Schon LC. Interdigital neuralgia. Foot Ankle Clin 2011; 16(2):305–15.
72. Sobiesk GA, Wertheimer SJ, Schulz R, et al. Sonographic evaluation of interdigital neuromas. J Foot Ankle Surg 1997;36(5):364–6.
73. Espinosa N, Seybold JD, Jankauskas L, et al. Alcohol sclerosing therapy is not an effective treatment for interdigital neuroma. Foot Ankle Int 2011;32(6):576–80.
74. Rask MR. Medial plantar neurapraxia (jogger's foot): report of 3 cases. Clin Orthop Relat Res 1978;(134):193–5.
75. Ahmad M, Tsang K, Mackenney PJ, et al. Tarsal tunnel syndrome: a literature review. Foot Ankle Surg 2012;18(3):149–52.

Bone Stress Injuries in Runners

Adam S. Tenforde, MD[a], Emily Kraus, MD[b], Michael Fredericson, MD[c],*

KEYWORDS

- Stress fractures • Runners • Female athlete triad • Track and field • Cross-country

KEY POINTS

- Bone stress injuries (BSIs) are a common form of injury in runners of both sexes.
- Both biological and biomechanical risk factors may contribute to BSI.
- History and physical examination are helpful to diagnose BSI, and MRI may be useful for radiographic confirmation and grading BSI.
- Prevention strategies include screening for risk factors during preparticipation evaluation, promoting optimal nutrition, and encouraging appropriate bone loading activities, including ball sports.

INTRODUCTION

Bone stress injuries (BSIs) in runners result from the failure of skeleton to withstand repetitive, submaximal forces from running. BSI can range in severity, with early injuries showing radiographic findings of periosteal edema with varying degrees of marrow edema and more advanced stress fractures showing evidence of a fracture line. Stress fractures account for up to 20% of injuries seen in sports medicine clinic.[1]

Studies suggest the annual incidence of BSI may be greater than 20% in runners and that BSI is a common cause of injury in track and field athletes.[2,3] Early identification of a BSI is important in management, because delay in diagnosis or continued running may result in a higher-grade BSI that requires longer healing time.[4,5] This article discusses the incidence and distribution of BSI in runners. It reviews biological and biomechanical risk factors for BSI, with a focus on risk factors that can be

Conflicts of interest: The authors have no conflicts of interest to disclose, and no funding was received in the preparation of this review.
[a] Department of Physical Medicine and Rehabilitation, Harvard Medical School, Spaulding Rehabilitation Hospital, Spaulding National Running Center, 1575 Cambridge St., Cambridge, MA 02138, USA; [b] Division of Physical Medicine and Rehabilitation, Department of Orthopaedic Surgery, Stanford University, 450 Broadway Street, MC 6120, Redwood City, CA 94063, USA; [c] Division of Physical Medicine and Rehabilitation, Department of Orthopaedic Surgery, Stanford University, 450 Broadway Street, Pavilion A, 2nd Floor MC 6120, Redwood City, CA 94063, USA
* Corresponding author.
E-mail address: mfred2@stanford.edu

efficiently evaluated in the clinic setting. It discusses evaluation and management of BSI by anatomic location and grade of injury by MRI. In addition, it reviews evidence for prevention of BSI in runners.

SUMMARY/DISCUSSION
Incidence and Distribution

The incidence of BSI varies by age and sex. In a study comparing high school sports, female and male athletes participating in cross-country had the first and third highest incidences of injuries at 10.62 and 5.42 per 100,000 athletic exposures, respectively.[6] In a separate investigation, adolescent runners of both sexes sustained stress fractures at a similar rate of approximately 4% to 5% annually.[7] Elite collegiate runners may sustain BSIs at a rate exceeding 20% per year.[2] Common sites for BSI include the tibia, fibula, metatarsals, tarsals, calcaneus, and femur.

RISK FACTORS

Risk factors for BSI can be divided into biological and biomechanical risk factors (**Table 1**). Genetics are reported to modulate fracture risk.[8] Medications, including steroids, anticonvulsants, antidepressants, and antacids, may impair bone health. Nutritional deficiencies in calcium and vitamin D increase risk for BSI.[9–11] Female athletes seem to be at greater risk for BSI than male athletes.[12] Sex-specific differences include the female athlete triad (hereafter referred to as the triad), defined as the interrelationship of energy availability, menstrual function, and bone mineral density (BMD).[13] Each aspect occurs on a continuum of health with the most severe form of the triad represented by low energy availability with an eating disorder, functional hypothalamic amenorrhea, and osteoporosis.[13] A female runner may have 1 or more components of the triad, and greater number of triad risk factors has been associated with increased risk for BSI in female athletes.[14]

In both sexes, prior fracture has been found to be a risk factor for development of BSI in runners.[7,9,15] Lower whole body bone mineral content values increase risk for BSI in female runners aged 18 to 26 years.[9] In adolescent female runners, the combination of menstrual irregularities with fracture history was associated with low bone density.[16] The largest study to date in male runners identified lower BMD as an independent risk factor for increased time for healing from a BSI.[4] In addition, athletes with

Table 1	
Risk factors for BSI	
Biological Factors	**Biomechanical Factors**
Female sex	Training patterns, including volume or changes in intensity
Genetics	Bone characteristics (thinner cortex, lower bone mineral density)
Medications (including anticonvulsants, steroids, antidepressants, antacids)	Anatomic considerations (leg length discrepancy, lean mass, foot type, smaller calf cross-sectional area)
Female athlete triad (low energy availability, menstrual dysfunction, and low bone mineral density)	
Other dietary contributors (insufficient calcium and vitamin D)	—

trabecular sites of fracture, including the sacrum, pelvis, and femoral neck, had lower BMDs in the lumbar spine and proximal femur than runners with fractures in cortical sites. In addition to bone density, bone geometric properties may predispose to BSIs, including a thinner cortex of tibia in triathletes[17] and smaller tibial cross-sectional area in runners.[18]

Biomechanical factors can also contribute to BSI. Static alignment and anatomic issues may contribute, including leg length discrepancy,[3,19,20] smaller calf girth,[3] and cavus[19,21] or planus type foot.[22] Dynamic biomechanical loading patterns experienced during running may also contribute to injury. These characteristics have been evaluated primarily in female patients who sustain BSI in the tibia and include greater average vertical loading,[23,24] higher peak acceleration,[25] and greater peak free mass.[26] Higher peak hip adduction, knee internal rotation, knee abduction, tibial internal rotation, and rear foot eversion may also contribute.[24,27] Running volumes greater than 32 km (20 miles) per week increase risk for BSI.[7,22]

EVALUATION
Clinical Evaluation

Clinicians should complete a full history and physical examination in runners who present for evaluation of a BSI. A complete running history should be obtained (including changes in running volume, shoe type and duration of use, frequency of racing, and change in foot strike pattern strategy). In female runners, screening for triad risk factors is important, including dietary restriction behaviors, daily servings of foods rich in calcium and vitamin D, menstrual dysfunction, history of fractures, and personal/family history of low BMD.[28] Medications including hormones (oral contraceptive pills, estrogen, progesterone) and historical or current use of medications that influence bone health, including steroids and antacids, should be recorded.

During physical examination, the characteristics of a BSI include focal bony tenderness and pain with direct and/or indirect percussion. Single-leg hop test may be attempted to elicit pain depending on the clinical context. In more advanced cases, local swelling or skin color changes may be noted.

Specific forms of BSI may require additional aspects of the physical examination. In our clinical experience, and based on available research, we recommend clinicians consider the following for specific examination findings based on location of pain.

Sacral/pelvic location
In addition to focal tenderness, sacroiliac joint provocative maneuvers may elicit pain, including thigh thrust; pelvic distraction; pelvic compression; and flexion, abduction, and external rotation of hip (FABER maneuver). Evaluation for a leg length discrepancy may be valuable to correct for biomechanical risk factors contributing to injury.[20]

Femoral neck
Pain may be provoked with hip internal rotation. In addition, evaluate for the presence of femoral acetabular impingement with flexion adduction and internal rotation (FADIR maneuver) because this has been associated with femoral neck BSI.[29]

Lesser trochanter
The clinical evaluation is similar to evaluation for a femoral neck BSI. This injury is typically associated with iliopsoas tendinopathy and is a potentially high-risk injury because it can progress to full fracture.[30]

Femoral shaft
Fulcrum test may localize pain at the site of injury.[31]

Calcaneus
Calcaneal squeeze test may elicit pain and help differentiate from other causes of heel pain, including retrocalcaneal bursitis.

ANATOMY AND IMAGING

The anatomic locations for BSI can be divided into high-risk, moderate-risk, and low-risk locations based on time to heal and risk for nonunion (**Table 2**). **Table 2** is based on a modified version of previously published high-risk[32] and low-risk classifications,[33] including a moderate-risk category that may be more challenging to address given biological and biomechanical forces that can contribute to risk for impaired bone healing.

MRI is commonly used to evaluate BSI because of the value in grading severity of injury and use of nonionizing radiation. Multiple grading systems have been developed.[4,5,34] Two MRI imaging grades are shown in **Table 3**, including the initial proposed criteria by Fredericson and colleagues[5] that have been most recently updated by Nattiv and colleagues.[4]

MANAGEMENT
Activity Modification and Aerobic Activity

After the initial healing phase to achieve pain-free ambulation and no pain with provocative maneuvers on physical examination, most athletes initiate a nonimpact loading activity to maintain fitness and strength, including deep water running. Athletes should be counseled to maintain good caloric intake to meet the metabolic demands of cross-training and not inadvertently restrict caloric intake, which may risk delayed healing response. Use of an antigravity treadmill may allow for progressive impact loading to maintain fitness while allowing healing of lower extremity BSIs.[35] We outlined a protocol used at Stanford University for athletes recovering from BSIs using an antigravity treadmill that can modulate forces encountered in the lower extremities to allow for progressive weight bearing.[35]

Ensure Adequate Intake of Calcium and Vitamin D

All athletes with BSIs should be assessed to ensure adequate calcium and vitamin D intake, preferably through diet. Target values published by the Institute of Medicine based on age and sex in 2010 are as follows[36]:

- 600 IU of vitamin D daily is recommended for ages 9 to 70 years
- 800 IU of vitamin D daily is recommended for ages 71 years or older
- 1300 mg of calcium daily for ages 9 to 18 years

Table 2
Anatomical location and risk of BSI

Low Risk[33]	Medium Risk	High Risk[32]
Posteromedial tibia	Pelvis (sacrum and pubic rami)*	Femoral neck
Fibula/lateral malleolus	Femoral shaft	Patella
Calcaneus	Proximal tibia	Anterior tibial diaphysis
Diaphysis of second to fourth metatarsals	Cuboid	Medial malleolus
	Cuneiform	Talus (lateral process)

* The pelvis is a controversial anatomical location for determining risk for bone stress injury, but recent research by Nattiv and colleagues[4] showed that time to full return to play is longer in trabecular BSIs.

Table 3		
MRI grading systems		
	MRI Grading Scales for BSIs	
MRI Grade	Nattiv et al,[4] 2013	Fredericson et al,[5] 1995
1	Mild marrow or periosteal edema on T2; T1 normal	Mild to moderate periosteal edema on T2; normal marrow on T2 and T1
2	Moderate marrow or periosteal edema plus positive T2	Moderate to severe periosteal edema on T2; marrow edema on T2 but not T1
3	Severe marrow or periosteal edema on T2 and T1	Moderate to severe periosteal edema on T2; marrow edema on T2 and T1
4	Severe marrow or periosteal edema on T2 and T1 plus fracture line on T2 or T1	Moderate to severe periosteal edema on T2; marrow edema on T2 and T1; fracture line present

- 1000 mg of calcium daily for women aged 19 to 50 years and men aged 19 to 70 years
- 1200 mg of calcium daily for women aged 51 years and older and for men 71 years and older

Clinicians who suspect low energy availability should refer the runner for a complete nutritional assessment with a registered dietitian. This assessment is best accomplished with a dietician who has sports nutrition background and takes into account sports participation demands, caloric intake, and energy availability, in addition to other important nutrients of bone health. Given the prevalence of vitamin D deficiency, we recommend screening athletes who sustain a BSI by measuring 25-OH vitamin D level and providing supplemental vitamin D if needed to ensure that the runner is not vitamin D deficient. Further studies are needed to assess the relationship with BSIs and vitamin D.

Female Runners: Screening and Management of the Triad

In female runners, screening for the triad is critical for addressing risk factors for BSI and identifying health risks in this population. The Female Athlete Triad Coalition statement in 2014 outlined a risk factor assessment score that can be used to help in treatment and return-to-play guidelines in female athletes.[28] The key component to management of the triad is to ensure adequate energy availability, allow for ovulatory menstrual cycles, and maintain bone mass.[13] In addition to preventing disruptions to training from management of BSIs, female athletes may be motivated by research that suggests that performance improves in athletes who maintain ovulatory function with adequate nutrition.[37] A full description of the evaluation and management of the female athlete triad is described elsewhere.[38] One important consideration is to ensure that female runners understand that adequate energy availability (defined as the difference between energy intake and estimated energy expenditure standardized to fat-free mass per day[39]) should be maintained both during the healing process and on return to full running. Inadvertent low energy availability may occur if a female runner does not consume adequate calories to meet the metabolic demands of aerobic cross-training activities.

Evaluation of Bone Health in Male Runners

For male runners with diagnosed BSIs in trabecular sites, including the pelvis, sacrum, and femoral neck, practitioners should consider work-up for impaired bone health, including dual-energy X-ray absorptiometry (DXA) to measure BMD and initial endocrine work-up. Athletes with higher-grade BSI assessed by MRI and lower BMD values may have a longer healing time before return to sports.[4] BMD values from DXA in athletes less than 50 years of age should be interpreted using age, ethnicity, and male-sex reference values (Z-scores). The American College of Sports Medicine defines Z-score less than −1 as low bone mass in female athletes participating in weight-bearing sports,[13] although criteria have not been defined for male athletes. The International Society for Clinical Densitometry defines Z-scores less than −2 as low bone mass for age in both sexes.[40]

RECOMMENDATIONS BY ANATOMIC SITE

Some of the most common locations for injury and management recommendations are discussed here.

HIGH-RISK LOCATIONS
Femoral Neck and Lesser Trochanter

Femoral neck BSI are considered high risk because of complications that may occur with nonunion, particularly on the tension side of the bone. Tension-side fractures may be managed with bed rest, as long as widening of the cortical fracture is not observed on serial imaging.[41] Fractures adjacent to the lesser trochanter may also progress to femoral neck stress fractures if non–weight-bearing precautions are not followed during initial management.[30] For compression side fractures and lesser trochanteric fractures, we recommend use of crutches to maintain non–weight-bearing status, with clinical evaluation and repeat imaging to ensure bony healing. Runners can be advanced to cross-training exercises when pain free on examination and cortical bridging on radiographs. Consultation with an orthopedic surgeon should be sought early for tension-side injuries or failure to achieve interval bony healing on repeat radiographs. Complete healing is typically expected by 2 to 3 months.[1]

Anterior Tibial Cortex

Radiographs may include presence of the so-called dreaded black line, visualized as horizontal radiolucency localized to the tension side of the tibia. Clinicians should obtain repeat radiographs to ensure bony bridging and healing before progressing to weight-bearing status. Nonsurgical outcomes in management have been described as unsatisfying[42]; in the setting of nonunion, an intramedullary rod may be necessary.

Medial Malleolus

Fractures involving the medial malleolus are important to identify given that this structure contributes to the ankle mortise. A published case series of athletes managed surgically who had radiographic evidence of fracture line had good outcomes[43]; however, we recommend an initial trial of immobilization unless there was significant displacement of the fracture or involvement of the talocrural joint.

Base of Second Metatarsal

Fractures at the base of the second metatarsal are considered high risk, especially if the fracture extends to the Lisfranc joint (metatarsal-cuneiform joint). A minimum of 4 weeks' immobilization is recommended[44,45] and repeat radiographs and clinical examination are advised to ensure that the runner is pain free before advancing weight bearing. Morton toe (defined as second toe extending past the great toe) may be observed on examination and be an associated biomechanical risk factor for this injury because of increased force transmitted through the second ray of the foot. Custom foot orthosis with metatarsal pad beneath the second metatarsal may address these biomechanical forces to reduce risk for future injury.

Fifth Metatarsal Diaphysis Fractures

Also known as Jones fracture, this injury is considered high risk because of relative avascularity of the bone distal to the tuberosity, which may result in nonunion.[46] A review of nonoperative versus surgical management described current quality of evidence as low, although the investigators concluded that better results were observed with surgery.[42] Use of a CAM walker boot may offload this site most effectively to promote initial healing.[47] Surgical management, including intramedullary screw fixation and bone grafting, has been shown to result in predictable healing and return to play by as early as 12 weeks.[48]

Tarsal Navicular

Examination findings may include presence of tenderness over the navicular tuberosity or navicular-cuneiform joint. Maintaining strict non–weight-bearing status initially to promote healing may result in the best clinical outcome.[49] Computed tomography may be a helpful imaging modality when assessing for healing response in the setting of a chronic injury. Saxena and colleagues[50] proposed a grading system for navicular BSI, and higher-grade injuries treated with surgery may have more favorable outcomes, especially if there is radiographic evidence of avascular necrosis, cystic changes, or sclerosis.

Sesamoids

The sesamoids consist of a fibular and tibial sesamoid bone. Because of the loading demands, BSI at this location may have delayed healing response. Use of cushioned orthosis with accommodative insole to offload the sesamoid is helpful to reduce biomechanical stress and promote healing. Note that bipartite sesamoid with sesamoiditis may radiographically appear as a split sesamoid. Plain radiographs of the contralateral asymptomatic foot can sometimes show this normal anatomic variant.

MODERATE RISK
Sacrum and Pelvis

Most injuries in the sacrum have radiographic evidence of high-grade BSI. Crutches and other assistive devices to ensure pain-free mobility are important early in the clinical course and can be discontinued with pain-free ambulation. Runners usually return to full running activity around 12 weeks.[51]

Tarsals Cuboid and Cuneiform

Given their location, both cuboid and cuneiform BSIs can be difficult to heal given the biomechanical forces and loads encountered through the foot. Management includes immobilization if needed to ensure pain-free ambulation, followed by progression to a neutral shoe and physical therapy to address strength and other biomechanical deficits that may have contributed to injury.

Femoral Shaft

Injuries without evidence of displacement or cortical break tend to heal and allow return to running within 8 to 12 weeks.[1]

LOW RISK
Tibia

Injuries are typically located at the distal third posterior medial aspect of the tibia. Clinical features suggestive of more severe injuries include focal pain, tenderness elicited with direct or indirect palpation, and associated MRI grading criteria can predict length of recovery ranging from 3 to 12 weeks.[5]

Fibula

Easy to examine given the surface bony anatomy, these injuries tend to heal quickly and allow prompt return to running when asymptomatic.[1]

Calcaneus

Heel pain in an athlete may be a clue to the presence of an injury involving the calcaneus. The calcaneal squeeze test is helpful for eliciting bony pain. Given that the bone has significant trabecular content, screening for female athlete triad risk factors is particularly important. We recommend initial use of a walking boot and possibly use of crutches to ensure pain-free mobility.

Metatarsals

With exception of the base of the second metatarsal and fractures involving the metaphysis of the fifth metatarsal, fractures involving the shaft of metatarsals 2 to 4 are considered low risk and have good healing response. In lower grade BSI (injury without presence of fracture line), use of a metatarsal pad and firm-sole shoe may allow the athlete to ambulate without pain.[1] With the presence of a fracture line, repeat radiographs at 4 weeks are recommended to document evidence of bony bridging and cortical hypertrophy over the fracture site, along with a pain-free examination before advancing to cross-training and starting a return-to-running progression. Most injuries heal within 6 to 8 weeks to allow return to ground running.

PREVENTION
Participation in Ball Sports During Adolescence

We have proposed prehabilitation strategies, including ball sports (basketball and soccer) and related activities, during adolescence for 2 years to reduce BSI risk.[52] These findings are based on prior research showing that military recruits and runners who participated in ball sports during youth have reduced risk for stress fractures.[7,53,54]

Adequate Calcium and Vitamin D Intake

Calcium and vitamin D intake may reduce risk for BSI. We recommend meeting daily calcium and vitamin D intake levels published by the Institute of Medicine to optimize bone health.[36] The role of calcium and vitamin D in fracture prevention has previously been described. Nieves and colleagues[10] showed that female runners consuming 800 mg of calcium daily have 6-fold increased risk for stress fractures compared with those with intakes of 1500 mg daily. In this investigation, each cup of milk reduced prospective fractures by 62%, highlighting other aspects of nutrition as contributing to risk reduction.[10] Lappe and colleagues[55] found a 20% reduction in female navy recruits who were randomly assigned to supplemental calcium 2000 mg and vitamin D 800 IU daily during 8-week basic training.

Preparticipation Physical Examination Screening

During preparticipation screening, all athletes should be asked about prior fracture history and screened for triad risk factors. Female runners should be educated on the importance of normal menstrual periods during training. Work-up for menstrual dysfunction should be considered early to address this important aspect of female runner health.

SUMMARY

BSI is a common form of overuse injury in runners of both sexes. Clinicians should consider these injuries on the differential diagnosis for musculoskeletal complaints in runners. Early and effective management of the injury can help facilitate return to sport, and addressing underlying risk factors may prevent future injury. Early screening for triad risk factors, optimizing nutrition, and encouraging participation in higher-impact activities, including ball sports during adolescence, may reduce the burden of these injuries in runners and promote overall bone health.

REFERENCES

1. Fredericson M, Jennings F, Beaulieu C, et al. Stress fractures in athletes. Top Magn Reson Imaging 2006;17(5):309–25.
2. Tenforde AS, Nattiv A, Barrack MT, et al. Distribution of bone stress injuries in elite male and female collegiate endurance runners. Med Sci Sports Exerc 2015; 47(5S):905.
3. Bennell KL, Malcolm SA, Thomas SA, et al. Risk factors for stress fractures in track and field athletes. A twelve-month prospective study. Am J Sports Med 1996;24(6):810–8.
4. Nattiv A, Kennedy G, Barrack MT, et al. Correlation of MRI grading of bone stress injuries with clinical risk factors and return to play: a 5-year prospective study in collegiate track and field athletes. Am J Sports Med 2013;41(8):1930–41.
5. Fredericson M, Bergman AG, Hoffman KL, et al. Tibial stress reaction in runners. Correlation of clinical symptoms and scintigraphy with a new magnetic resonance imaging grading system. Am J Sports Med 1995;23(4):472–81.
6. Changstrom BG, Brou L, Khodaee M, et al. Epidemiology of stress fracture injuries among US high school athletes, 2005-2006 through 2012-2013. Am J Sports Med 2015;43(1):26–33.
7. Tenforde AS, Sayres LC, Liz McCurdy M, et al. Identifying sex-specific risk factors for stress fractures in adolescent runners. Med Sci Sports Exerc 2013;45(10): 1843–51.
8. Estrada K, Styrkarsdottir U, Evangelou E, et al. Genome-wide meta-analysis identifies 56 bone mineral density loci and reveals 14 loci associated with risk of fracture. Nat Genet 2012;44(5):491–501.
9. Kelsey JL, Bachrach LK, Procter-Gray E, et al. Risk factors for stress fracture among young female cross-country runners. Med Sci Sports Exerc 2007;39(9): 1457–63.
10. Nieves JW, Melsop K, Curtis M, et al. Nutritional factors that influence change in bone density and stress fracture risk among young female cross-country runners. PM R 2010;2(8):740–50 [quiz: 794].
11. Ruohola JP, Laaksi I, Ylikomi T, et al. Association between serum 25(OH)D concentrations and bone stress fractures in Finnish young men. J Bone Miner Res 2006;21(9):1483–8.
12. Wentz L, Liu PY, Haymes E, et al. Females have a greater incidence of stress fractures than males in both military and athletic populations: a systemic review. Mil Med 2011;176(4):420–30.
13. Nattiv A, Loucks AB, Manore MM, et al. American College of Sports Medicine position stand. The female athlete triad. Med Sci Sports Exerc 2007;39(10):1867–82.
14. Barrack MT, Gibbs JC, De Souza MJ, et al. Higher incidence of bone stress injuries with increasing female athlete triad-related risk factors: a prospective multisite study of exercising girls and women. Am J Sports Med 2014;42(4):949–58.

15. Touhy J, Nattiv A, Streja L. A prospective analysis of tibial stress fracture incidence, distribution and risk factors in collegiate track athletes. Clin J Sport Med 2008;18(2):186.
16. Tenforde AS, Sainani KL, Sayres LC, et al. Identifying sex-specific risk factors for low bone mineral density in adolescent runners. Am J Sports Med 2015;43(6):1494–504.
17. Newsham-West RJ, Lyons B, Milburn PD. Regional bone geometry of the tibia in triathletes and stress reactions–an observational study. J Sci Med Sport 2014; 17(2):150–4.
18. Crossley K, Bennell KL, Wrigley T, et al. Ground reaction forces, bone characteristics, and tibial stress fracture in male runners. Med Sci Sports Exerc 1999;31(8): 1088–93.
19. Korpelainen R, Orava S, Karpakka J, et al. Risk factors for recurrent stress fractures in athletes. Am J Sports Med 2001;29(3):304–10.
20. Friberg O. Leg length asymmetry in stress fractures. A clinical and radiological study. J Sports Med Phys Fitness 1982;22(4):485–8.
21. Simkin A, Leichter I, Giladi M, et al. Combined effect of foot arch structure and an orthotic device on stress fractures. Foot Ankle 1989;10(1):25–9.
22. Sullivan D, Warren RF, Pavlov H, et al. Stress fractures in 51 runners. Clin Orthop Relat Res 1984;187:188–92.
23. Milner CE, Ferber R, Pollard CD, et al. Biomechanical factors associated with tibial stress fracture in female runners. Med Sci Sports Exerc 2006;38(2):323–8.
24. Pohl MB, Mullineaux DR, Milner CE, et al. Biomechanical predictors of retrospective tibial stress fractures in runners. J Biomech 2008;41(6):1160–5.
25. Davis IS, Milner CE, Hamill J. Does increased loading during running lead to tibial stress fractures? A prospective study. Med Sci Sports Exerc 2004;36:S58.
26. Milner CE, Davis IS, Hamill J. Free moment as a predictor of tibial stress fracture in distance runners. J Biomech 2006;39(15):2819–25.
27. Milner CE, Davis IS, Hamill J. Is dynamic hip and knee malalignment associated with tibial stress fracture in female distance runners? Med Sci Sports Exerc 2005; 37(5s):S346.
28. De Souza MJ, Nattiv A, Joy E, et al. 2014 Female Athlete Triad Coalition consensus statement on treatment and return to play of the female athlete triad: 1st International Conference held in San Francisco, California, May 2012 and 2nd International Conference held in Indianapolis, Indiana, May 2013. Br J Sports Med 2014;48(4):289.
29. Goldin M, Anderson CN, Fredericson M, et al. Femoral neck stress fractures and imaging features of femoroacetabular impingement. PM R 2015;7(6):584–92.
30. Nguyen JT, Peterson JS, Biswal S, et al. Stress-related injuries around the lesser trochanter in long-distance runners. AJR Am J Roentgenol 2008;190(6):1616–20.
31. Johnson AW, Weiss CB Jr, Wheeler DL. Stress fractures of the femoral shaft in athletes–more common than expected. A new clinical test. Am J Sports Med 1994;22(2):248–56.
32. Boden BP, Osbahr DC. High-risk stress fractures: evaluation and treatment. J Am Acad Orthop Surg 2000;8(6):344–53.
33. Boden BP, Osbahr DC, Jimenez C. Low-risk stress fractures. Am J Sports Med 2001;29(1):100–11.
34. Arendt E, Agel J, Heikes C, et al. Stress injuries to bone in college athletes: a retrospective review of experience at a single institution. Am J Sports Med 2003;31(6):959–68.
35. Tenforde AS, Watanabe LM, Moreno TJ, et al. Use of an antigravity treadmill for rehabilitation of a pelvic stress injury. PM R 2012;4(8):629–31.

36. Institute of Medicine. Dietary reference intakes for calcium and vitamin D. National Academy of Sciences; November 2010, Report Brief. 2010. Available at: http://wwwiomedu/~/media/Files/Report Files/2010/Dietary-Reference-Intakes-for-Calcium-and-Vitamin-D/Vitamin D and Calcium 2010 Report Briefpdf. Available at: May 30, 2015.
37. Vanheest JL, Rodgers CD, Mahoney CE, et al. Ovarian suppression impairs sport performance in junior elite female swimmers. Med Sci Sports Exerc 2014;46(1):156–66.
38. Kim B, Nattiv A. Health considerations in the female runner. Phys Med Rehabil Clin North Am, in press.
39. Loucks AB. Low energy availability in the marathon and other endurance sports. Sports Med 2007;37(4–5):348–52.
40. Lewiecki EM, Gordon CM, Baim S, et al. International Society for Clinical Densitometry 2007 adult and pediatric official positions. Bone 2008;43(6):1115–21.
41. Fullerton LR Jr, Snowdy HA. Femoral neck stress fractures. Am J Sports Med 1988;16(4):365–77.
42. Mallee WH, Weel H, van Dijk CN, et al. Surgical versus conservative treatment for high-risk stress fractures of the lower leg (anterior tibial cortex, navicular and fifth metatarsal base): a systematic review. Br J Sports Med 2015;49(6):370–6.
43. Shelbourne KD, Fisher DA, Rettig AC, et al. Stress fractures of the medial malleolus. Am J Sports Med 1988;16(1):60–3.
44. Brukner PD, Bennell KL. Stress fractures in runners. J Back Musculoskeletal Rehabil 1995;5(4):341–51.
45. Micheli LJ, Sohn RS, Solomon R. Stress fractures of the second metatarsal involving Lisfranc's joint in ballet dancers. A new overuse injury of the foot. J Bone Jt Surg Am 1985;67(9):1372–5.
46. Lehman RC, Torg JS, Pavlov H, et al. Fractures of the base of the fifth metatarsal distal to the tuberosity: a review. Foot Ankle 1987;7(4):245–52.
47. Hunt KJ, Goeb Y, Esparza R, et al. Site-specific loading at the fifth metatarsal base in rehabilitative devices: implications for Jones fracture treatment. PM R 2014;6(11):1022–9 [quiz: 1029].
48. Hunt KJ, Anderson RB. Treatment of Jones fracture nonunions and refractures in the elite athlete: outcomes of intramedullary screw fixation with bone grafting. Am J Sports Med 2011;39(9):1948–54.
49. Torg JS, Pavlov H, Cooley LH, et al. Stress fractures of the tarsal navicular. A retrospective review of twenty-one cases. J Bone Jt Surg Am 1982;64(5):700–12.
50. Saxena A, Fullem B, Hannaford D. Results of treatment of 22 navicular stress fractures and a new proposed radiographic classification system. J Foot Ankle Surg 2000;39(2):96–103.
51. Fredericson M, Salamancha L, Beaulieu C. Sacral stress fractures: tracking down nonspecific pain in distance runners. Phys Sportsmed 2003;31(2):31–42.
52. Tenforde AS, Lynn Sainani K, Carter Sayres L, et al. Participation in ball sports may represent a prehabilitation strategy to prevent future stress fractures and promote bone health in young athletes. PM R 2015;7(2):222–5.
53. Milgrom C, Simkin A, Eldad A, et al. Using bone's adaptation ability to lower the incidence of stress fractures. Am J Sports Med 2000;28(2):245–51.
54. Fredericson M, Ngo J, Cobb K. Effects of ball sports on future risk of stress fracture in runners. Clin J Sport Med 2005;15(3):136–41.
55. Lappe J, Cullen D, Haynatzki G, et al. Calcium and vitamin D supplementation decreases incidence of stress fractures in female navy recruits. J Bone Miner Res 2008;23(5):741–9.

Health Considerations in Female Runners

Brian Y. Kim, MD, MS[a,b,*], Aurelia Nattiv, MD[a,b,c]

KEYWORDS

- Female athlete triad • Running • Nutrition • Bone health • Energy availability

KEY POINTS

- The adolescent years represent a vulnerable period because nutritional inadequacies and suboptimal bone accrual may have long-lasting consequences.
- Adequate intakes of calcium, vitamin D, and iron are of particular importance in female runners to optimize bone health and hematopoiesis.
- Female runners should strive to maintain an energy availability of 45 kcal/kg fat-free mass per day to avoid the downstream neurometabolic effects of menstrual dysfunction and low bone density.
- Recently released consensus guidelines and risk assessment tools may be helpful in stratifying individuals based on their risk of bone stress injury and other Triad-related sequelae.
- Nonpharmacologic therapy, such as nutritional intervention and activity modification, remains the mainstay of treatment of Triad-related conditions, with pharmacologic options reserved for severe or recalcitrant cases.

INTRODUCTION

The 1928 Summer Olympic Games marked the debut of female competition at the highest level of track and field. However, the historic occasion was marred by sensationalized accounts of female runners strewn across the finish line in prostration after completing the 800-m run. Such attitudes were informed by cultural norms and pseudoscience, and severely limited women's participation in athletics well into the second half of the twentieth century. The International Olympic Committee (IOC) would not allow women to compete at distances greater than 200 m for another 32 years. A major obstacle was overcome in 1972 with the passage of Title IX, which set a precedent

Conflicts of Interest: None.
[a] Division of Sports Medicine and Non-Operative Orthopaedics, Department of Family Medicine, David Geffen School of Medicine at UCLA, Los Angeles, CA, USA; [b] Department of Intercollegiate Athletics, UCLA, Los Angeles, CA, USA; [c] Department of Orthopaedic Surgery, David Geffen School of Medicine at UCLA, Los Angeles, CA, USA
* Corresponding author. UCLA Department of Family Medicine, Division of Sports Medicine and Non-operative Orthopaedics, Room 50-080 Center for Health Sciences, 10833 Le Conte Avenue, Los Angeles, California 90095, USA.
E-mail address: bykim@mednet.ucla.edu

Phys Med Rehabil Clin N Am 27 (2016) 151–178
http://dx.doi.org/10.1016/j.pmr.2015.08.011
1047-9651/16/$ – see front matter © 2016 Elsevier Inc. All rights reserved.

for the provision of equal opportunities for women and men in sport. However, major sporting bodies like the Amateur Athletic Union and the IOC were slow to offer tangible opportunities for female sports participation, particularly in distance running. Despite the slow start, female participation in running has increased greatly over the past few decades. In 2013, more than 40% of marathon finishers in the United States were female, compared with just 10% in 1980.[1] At the 2012 Summer Olympic Games, women comprised nearly 50% of track and field athletes and outnumbered men in the marathon by 118 to 105.[2] Girls at the youth level constitute the fastest-growing group of participants in organized sport, from 300,000 in 1972 to 3.2 million today.[3] In terms of participation, women compare favorably with men at both the National Collegiate Athletic Association (NCAA) and high school levels (**Table 1**), and track and field remains the most popular sport for high school girls, with nearly 500,000 participants in 2013 to 2014.[3] Although coeducational participation may now be the norm in many sports, the sporting worlds of women and men remain distinct. Women of all ages continue to compete with dated societal ideals of form and behavior. At the professional level, female athletes generally garner fewer accolades and less lucrative compensation in the form of contracts, prize earnings, and endorsements than male counterparts. These issues exist alongside a biological and hormonal milieu that varies markedly over different life stages, posing additional challenges for active women. With these considerations, this article offers a perspective on health considerations in female runners, focusing on the importance of nutrition and medical concerns related to the female athlete triad (Triad).

GROWTH AND DEVELOPMENT

Young female athletes face formidable challenges, including increased nutritional requirements, myths about ideal body types that may foster disordered eating (DE), and the need to reconcile advice from a variety of sources, including coaches, trainers, peers, parents, and increasingly the media. An imbalance between the demands of sport and those of normal development can be a source of stress among young athletes, and can persist into adulthood.[4] Hence, this article initially considers the growth and maturation of active girls.

Menarche

Widely considered the central event in pubescence, menarche is heralded by the onset of pulsatile gonadotropin-releasing hormone release and its downstream mediators: luteinizing hormone (LH), follicle-stimulating hormone, and estrogen. The

Table 1			
Participation in running sports in the United States 2013 to 2014			
	Cross-country	Outdoor Track	Indoor Track
Female (HS)	218,121	478,885	66,126
Male (HS)	252,547	580,321	73,650
Female (NCAA)	15,922	27,752	25,876
Male (NCAA)	14,218	27,514	24,785

Abbreviation: HS, high school.
  Data from National Federation of State High School Associations 2013-14 High School Athletics Participation Survey. 2014. Available at: http://www.nfhs.org/ParticipationStatics/PDF/2013-14_Participation_Survey_PDF.pdf. Accessed June 22, 2015; and NCAA Sports Sponsorship and Participation Rates Report 2013-2014. 2014. Available at: http://www.ncaapublications.com/productdownloads/PR1314.pdf. Accessed June 22, 2015.

mean age at menarche in the United States has recently been reported at 12.3 to 12.4 years,[5,6] and there is considerable agreement that this represents an earlier onset compared with previous reports.[5–8] The mechanisms underlying this trend are not clear, but may be related to changes in relative weight, ethnic composition, chemical exposure, and insulin resistance over time.[6,8,9] Although cross-sectional and retrospective studies have suggested a delayed onset of menarche in athletes, there is likely considerable bias in these observations, because late-maturing girls in sport seem to be over-represented as they pass from childhood through adolescence.[4,10,11]

Adolescent Growth Spurt

The growth spurt in girls is an early pubertal event, occurring soon after the initiation of breast development.[12] Peak height velocity (PHV) occurs at 10.8 to 11.3 years, or about 2 years earlier than in boys, but can vary significantly based on pubertal timing (ie, earlier, average, or later).[13] Age at PHV is not strongly correlated with adult stature.[13,14] In most cases, height velocity in girls slows dramatically by 14 or 15 years, whereas some boys grow beyond 18 years.[13] Sport participation itself does not seem to have an appreciable effect on vertical growth in healthy children.[15]

Changes in Body Composition

Sex differences in fat-free mass (FFM), fat mass (FM), and body fat percentage (BF%) during childhood become more clearly defined during adolescence. By the end of high school, girls have nearly twice the BF% of boys,[16] a proportion that seems to persist even at the level of elite adult runners.[17] Maximum increases in FFM occur at age 13 years in girls, preceding boys by about 2 years.[18] Unlike height, body composition can be influenced by athletic training, with increases in FFM and decreases in FM seen in athletes compared with nonathletes.[4] Weight is low for height in female distance runners (compared with nonrunners) at all ages, although it is difficult to separate effects of training from changes related to normal growth and maturation.[19,20]

Skeletal Maturity

The adolescent years represent a brief but critical window of opportunity for bone accumulation.[21] Puberty-associated increases in growth hormone and insulin-like growth factor-1 mediate this process, as well as the actions of hormones, such as dehydroepiandrosterone, estrogen, and leptin.[22,23] Bone acquisition is maximal in the years surrounding PHV, or about 11 to 15 years of age,[24] during which 33% to 46% of adult bone content is accrued.[25] Healthy adolescents of normal weight engaging in impact activities, such as soccer, generally have higher bone mineral density (BMD) than swimmers and athletes engaging in non–weight-bearing sports.[26] However, long-term participation in competitive endurance running may attenuate these gains in adolescent athletes,[27] particularly at the spine.[28] Longitudinal data show that in healthy girls bone mass accumulation declines markedly by age 16 years,[24] highlighting early adolescence as a vulnerable period during which interruptions in normal bone accumulation may have far-reaching consequences.[21]

Strength and Performance Measures

Before age 14 years, boys and girls differ marginally in their performance on a variety of motor tasks, including running speed. With puberty, dramatic differences in neuromuscular agility and explosiveness emerge, largely as a result of a plateau in the motor performance improvements of girls.[29] Aerobic performance trends similarly, whereby improvements in maximal oxygen uptake (Vo_{2max}) increase linearly from age 7 years to

PHV, then plateau in girls, but not in boys.[16] However, the magnitude of these differences seems to be mitigated in the endurance-trained population.[30]

Preadolescence and Adolescence: A Vulnerable Period

The adolescent growth spurt represents a period of increased vulnerability to overuse injuries. Laboratory studies have shown that growth cartilage present during rapid phases of growth is less resistant to tensile, shear, and compressive forces than either mature bone or less mature prepubescent bone.[31–33] Dissociation between bone matrix formation and bone mineralization during the growth spurt also results in diminished bone strength.[34,35] Stress fractures seem to occur more frequently during the adolescent spurt as well,[36] although prospective studies are lacking. Numerous cases of stress-related lower extremity physeal injuries involving young athletes have been reported in the literature, primarily from running-related activities.[37] These injuries may result in leg-length discrepancy or angular malalignment of the affected leg,[38] setting up the potential for long-term disability. The potential for catastrophic injury is highlighted by case reports of severe femoral neck stress fractures in female adolescent athletes.[39–41]

NUTRITIONAL CONSIDERATIONS

Nutrition is of paramount importance to female runners. Low energy intake (EI) can result in menstrual dysfunction, suboptimal BMD, increased risk of illness, and prolonged recovery from illness.[42] Guidelines for macronutrient intake in adult athletes can be found in **Table 2**. Of special consideration, vegetarian athletes may be at risk for low intakes of energy, protein, fat, and key micronutrients, such as iron, calcium, vitamin D, riboflavin, zinc, and vitamin B_{12}. Consultation with a sports dietitian is recommended to avoid deficiencies.[42]

Patterns of Intake in Female Runners

Across a variety of sports, female athletes reportedly consume about 30% less energy and carbohydrate (CHO) per kilogram of body weight than male athletes in the same sport.[43] Some investigators have attributed the large discrepancies between reported EI and measured energy expenditure of female endurance athletes with stable body weights to under-reporting of EI. However, under-reporting does not account for the widely observed neurometabolic effects of chronic energy deficiency in female

Table 2 Recommended macronutrient intake in adult athletes	
Carbohydrates	
General recommendations	6–10 g/kg BW/d
During moderate-intensity exercise >1 h	0.5–1.0 g/kg BW/h
After exercise	1–1.5 g/kg BW within 30 min and again every 2h for 4–6 h
Protein	1.2–1.7 g/kg BW/d
Fat	1–2 g/kg BW/d or 20%–35% of total EI

Abbreviations: BW, body weight; EI, energy intake.
Data from American Dietetic Association, Dietitians of Canada, American College of Sports Medicine, et al. American College of Sports Medicine position stand. Nutrition and athletic performance. Med Sci Sports Exerc 2009;41:709–31; and Rodriguez NR, DiMarco NM, Langley S, et al. Position of the American Dietetic Association, Dietitians of Canada, and the American College of Sports Medicine: nutrition and athletic performance. J Am Diet Assoc 2009;109:509–27.

endurance athletes.[44] Edwards and colleagues,[45] in a study of female endurance runners using 7-day food diaries and doubly labeled water, documented energy deficit in 9 of 9 subjects, with a mean deficit of 32%. An even greater proportion of female athletes (76%) were energy deficient in a larger heterogeneous study of endurance runners.[46] Similar results have been found among groups of adolescent,[47] NCAA,[48,49] and elite distance runners.[50,51] Deficits in protein (PRO) intake seem to be far less common.[49]

Several investigators have related suboptimal EI in female runners with menstrual abnormalities, including luteal phase dysfunction (LPD) and amenorrhea.[46,52,53] Amenorrheic runners have also been found to have lower resting metabolic rate (RMR) than matched, eumenorrheic counterparts, indicating an adaptive syndrome to conserve energy.[54,55] Suboptimal fat intake, although less common than CHO deficiency, has been observed in runners with suboptimal EI,[49,53] menstrual dysfunction,[53] and stress fractures.[56] In addition, suboptimal EI may be associated with certain patterns of cognitive dietary restraint.[48]

Defining Low Energy Availability

The determination of energy status is an imperfect science. One preferred index of energy status, energy availability (EA), is defined as EI minus exercise energy expenditure (EEE) divided by kilograms of FFM.[44] In controlled laboratory settings, this index has been significantly associated with changes in reproductive and metabolic hormone concentrations[57,58] and markers of bone formation and resorption.[59] **Table 3** outlines methods of assessing variables in the calculation of EA. Physically active women should strive for an EA of at least 45 kcal/kg FFM/d to ensure adequate energy for normal physiologic functions.[44,60,61] Many controlled experiments have identified 30 kcal/kg FFM/d as a critical threshold of EA,[57–59] associated with detrimental changes in reproductive function and bone metabolism.[57]

Intentional Versus Unintentional Underfueling

Unintentional underfueling may occur in athletes who do not realize that they need to increase their EI to match increased EEE from training activity; this commonly occurs in high school cross-country runners.[63] These athletes typically do not have psychological reasons that interfere with their ability to comprehend the need to increase EI. In contrast, intentional underfueling occurs when athletes restrict their EI to improve

Table 3
Methods of assessing variables in the calculation of EA*

EI	EEE	FFM
3-d food log	Metabolic equivalent of task[62]	Dual-energy X-ray absorptiometry
4-d food log	Heart rate monitoring	Air displacement plethysmography
7-d food log	Accelerometry	Bioelectrical impedance
24-h recall	—	Skin fold caliper measurement
Food frequency questionnaire	—	—

$$* \text{ EA} = \frac{EI(kcal) - EEE(kcal)}{kg \text{ of } FFM}$$

Abbreviations: EA, energy availability; EEE, exercise energy expenditure; EI, energy intake; FFM, fat-free mass.

Data from De Souza MJ, Nattiv A, Joy E, et al. 2014 Female Athlete Triad Coalition consensus statement on treatment and return to play of the female athlete triad: 1st International Conference held in San Francisco, California, May 2012 and 2nd International Conference held in Indianapolis, Indiana, May 2013. Br J Sports Med 2014;48:289; with permission.

appearance, fit preconceived ideals of body image, or enhance athletic performance; this can occur in the presence or absence of DE. In a study by Manore and colleagues,[64] 62% of female athletes endorsed a desire to lose at least 2.3 kg (5 pounds), compared with 23% of male athletes. These athletes may show behaviors such as binge eating, purging, diuretic/laxative abuse, use of diet supplements, or compulsive exercise in excess of normal training. Although athletes seldom meet the criteria for a clinical eating disorder (ED), many show signs of DE and may strive to achieve extremely low weight. In runners, motivating forces typically include the desire to achieve a body type consistent with societal pressures and/or perceived sport-specific ideals.[65]

Performance Considerations

A preponderance of research in endurance athletes has shown the short-term performance benefits of moderate-CHO to high-CHO diets, including the ability to fend off overtraining syndrome.[66–69] Regarding fueling during endurance training, the American College of Sports Medicine (ACSM) recommends ingestion of 0.7 g/kg/h of CHO during exercise in a 6% to 8% solution, particularly for events greater than 1 hour.[42] This intake translates to about 42 g of CHO, or 620 to 1000 mL (21–34 ounces) of sports beverage, per hour in a 60-kg athlete. These recommendations are supported by 2 recent meta-analyses that confirmed the performance benefits of CHO supplementation in this range for endurance performance.[70,71] In high-level runners, an individualized nutritional strategy should be developed that is designed to deliver CHO at a rate that is commensurate with exercise intensity as well as the duration of the event.[72] After exercise, the goal is to provide adequate fluids, electrolytes, energy, and CHO to accelerate glycogen resynthesis and promote an anabolic hormone profile to hasten recovery. A CHO intake of approximately 1.0 to 1.5 g/kg body weight (BW) during the first 30 minutes, and again every 2 hours for 4 to 6 hours, seems adequate to accomplish this goal.[42,73–75]

Many runners and coaches attempt to alter body composition to improve performance. Although average body composition measures of athletes in various sports are commonly reported in the literature, these values cannot be extrapolated to individuals. Specific body composition ranges may be a useful tool for clinicians monitoring high-risk athletes, but they have little relevance to performance. A multidisciplinary team, including the athlete, coach, dietitian, and physician, should work together to optimize EA, and to recognize athletes with low body mass indices (BMIs) and/or low BWs as at risk for the Triad consequences. Although low BF% is not independently associated with menstrual dysfunction, low BMD, or stress fractures, it should be considered as a consequence of inadequate EI, and/or excessive exercise, and addressed accordingly.[61] Weight loss, if desired, should take place in the off-season or before the competitive season with the support of a sports dietitian. Findings that should raise concerns are changes in menstrual status, recurrent illness or injury, or any signs of DE.[65]

Micronutrient Intake

Athletes who maintain a negative energy balance put themselves at risk for deficiencies in micronutrients, of which iron, calcium, and vitamin D are particularly relevant for female runners. Recommended intakes of these nutrients are summarized in **Table 4**.

Iron

Iron performs a vital role in hemoglobin synthesis and oxygen transport. Women are at greater risk of iron deficiency (ID) compared with men because of menstrual losses

Table 4
Recommended intakes for iron, calcium, and vitamin D in females

Age (y)	Iron (mg/d)	Calcium (mg/d)	Vitamin D (IU/d)[a]
9–13	8	1300	600
14–18	15	1300	600
19–30	18	1000	600
31–50	18	1000	600
51–70	8	1200	600
>70	8	1200	800
Pregnant or Lactating	**Iron (mg/d)**	**Calcium (mg/d)**	**Vitamin D (IU/d)[a]**
14–18	27 (pregnant) 10 (lactating)	1300	600
19–50	27 (pregnant) 9 (lactating)	1000	600

Abbreviation: IU, international unit.
[a] Goals for vitamin D intake are based on dietary recommendations and are independent of the individual's sun exposure.
Data from Refs.[76–78]

and decreased iron intake. In the United States, the prevalence of iron deficiency anemia (IDA) is 3% to 5% and iron deficiency without anemia (IDNA) is 16% in women of childbearing age.[79] Athletes may be at particular risk because of increased losses caused by gastrointestinal (GI) bleeding, and reduced absorption caused by subclinical inflammation.[80–83] Bioavailability of iron depends on several factors, including the individual's iron status, the form of iron consumed (heme vs nonheme), and the presence of inhibitors, such as bran, polyphenols, and antacids.[65,84] Meat consumption is a strong determinant of iron status[85] and good sources of heme iron include lean meat, poultry, and seafood.[86] Nonheme iron, found in white beans, lentils, spinach, and iron-enriched foods, is not as readily absorbed by the body. In a study of female runners, individuals consuming a modified vegetarian diet (<100 g red meat per week) showed 30% less iron bioavailability than those consuming a regular diet.[87] In general, athletes with low EI (<2000 kcal/d) have been shown to be at increased risk for poor iron status.[88] Koehler and colleagues,[89] in a group of elite female athletes, found a mean iron intake of 13.8 ± 4.1 mg/d, with 63% below the recommended daily amount. In another study, a group of active women had poorer indices of iron status compared with sedentary controls, despite higher dietary iron intake.[82] Female distance runners, even at the elite level,[90] may be at particular risk for suboptimal iron status.[90–93] Iron overload, typically resulting from chronic, high-dose supplementation, has been reported in runners, but is uncommon and more commonly observed in men.[94]

Calcium

Adequate calcium status is important for optimal bone health. Disruptions in bone homeostasis lead to the gradual weakening of bone and may accelerate the onset of low bone mass or osteoporosis. Adequate calcium intake during childhood is paramount for peak bone mass, which is attained by about age 25 years.[95] Suboptimal calcium intake is common in female athletes, especially in those for whom a drive for thinness leads to calorie restriction.[96–99] Barrack and colleagues,[49] in a study of female NCAA runners, reported intakes less than 1000 mg/d in 26% of subjects. Milk and milk products contribute substantially to calcium intake in the United States.

Nieves and colleagues[100] and Kelsey and colleagues[101] found that, in young female runners, higher intakes of calcium, skim milk, and dairy products are associated with lower rates of stress fracture. Removing dairy products from the diet requires careful replacement with other food sources of calcium, including fortified foods.[86] Although calcium supplements are widely available, recent evidence suggests a possible increased risk of cardiovascular events in postmenopausal women taking calcium supplements of 1 g/d.[102,103] Until further studies examine this association, we recommend that most calcium intake should come from dietary sources.

Vitamin D

Adequate vitamin D status is important for health, preventing growth retardation and skeletal deformities during childhood, and decreasing the risk of osteoporosis and fracture later in life. Vitamin D deficiency causes muscle weakness.[104–106] Vitamin D can be obtained from the diet, but few foods, apart from oily fish such as salmon, naturally contain vitamin D.[86,107] A study of collegiate runners found that nearly 80% failed to meet recommendations for vitamin D intake,[49] and those who did usually relied on supplements (Barrack MT, personal communication, 2015). Sunlight is a major contributor to vitamin D status, with 5 to 10 minutes of exposure to the arms and legs (depending on time of day, season, latitude, use of sunscreen, and skin pigmentation) resulting in the production of about 3000 international units (IU).[107] Because of the angle of the sun, little or no vitamin D can be produced from November to February in areas above about 35° north latitude (eg, Los Angeles; Charlotte, NC).[107] There is no consensus on optimal levels of vitamin D, although levels less than 20 ng/mL generally indicate deficiency. Levels between 20 and 29 ng/mL may indicate an insufficiency, and values greater than or equal to 30 ng/mL are generally considered adequate.[108] Studies in athletes are few, but vary considerably with population, location, and the time of year.[109–113] In a study of endurance runners, Willis and colleagues[114] found 30% of subjects to be insufficient, although none were frankly deficient (<20 ng/mL). Low levels have been associated with stress fracture risk in female military recruits,[115] although studies in athletes are lacking. More prospective studies are needed to evaluate the role of calcium and vitamin D intake in the prevention of bone stress injuries in athletes, particularly those participating in sports with greater incidences, such as distance running.[116]

THE FEMALE ATHLETE TRIAD

The Triad encompasses 3 components: (1) low EA with or without DE, (2) menstrual dysfunction, and (3) low BMD.[60,61] Over the past few decades, increased understanding of the Triad has clarified the mechanisms correlating inadequate EI with hypoestrogenemia, decreased BMD, and subsequent increased fracture risk.[60,117] Although early descriptions focused on the pathologic end points of the Triad (ED, amenorrhea, and osteoporosis), recent studies have increased recognition of subclinical disorders, such as DE, subclinical menstrual disturbances,[52,118] low bone density, and bone stress injuries.[119,120] Other medical complications of the Triad include endocrine, GI, renal, and neuropsychiatric manifestations.[60]

Energy Availability

Chronic energy deficit disrupts hypothalamic neuroendocrine function in women, negatively affecting menstrual function and bone turnover.[57,59,121] As a result, RMR is decreased, accounting for the ability of amenorrheic athletes to maintain weight stability.[60,61] Muscular function may be negatively affected as well, because short-term energy deficit of just 5 days has been shown to reduce postabsorptive myofibrillar protein synthesis.[122] Rates of bone formation are also suppressed within 5 days of decreasing EA from 45 to less than or equal to 30 kcal/kg FFM/d, and bone resorption may increase when EA is reduced enough to suppress estradiol.[59] In a large sample of trained, exercising women, EA was also able to distinguish amenorrheic from eumenorrheic athletes.[123] Hence, experts have recommended that exercising women should maintain an EA of at least 45 kcal/kg FFM/d to avoid the aforementioned clinical sequelae.[44,60,61] Views regarding body image may be useful in the assessment of the runner, because a drive for thinness has been shown to be a proxy indicator of underlying energy deficiency.[124] Monitoring athletes periodically during the year is prudent as well, because EA may change throughout the course of a season.[125] It is worth noting that, contrary to popular belief, the stress of exercise itself, independent of EA, does not alter LH pulsatility in women.[58]

Menstrual Status

Amenorrhea is the absence of menstrual cycles for more than 3 months and oligomenorrhea is characterized by menstrual cycles occurring at intervals longer than 35 days. Subclinical disturbances, such as LPD and anovulatory cycling, may have no perceptible symptoms.[60] A diagnosis of functional hypothalamic amenorrhea (FHA) secondary to low EA in athletes is a diagnosis of exclusion and must follow an evaluation to rule out pregnancy and endocrinopathies. The prevalence of secondary amenorrhea, which varies widely with sport, weight, and training volume,[126] has been reported to be as high as 65% in some studies of distance runners,[127] compared with 2% to 5% in the general population.[128–130] Amenorrhea in distance runners has been associated with increases in training mileage and decreases in BW, but not body fat per se,[131] and seems to be less prevalent with increasing age.[132,133] Subclinical menstrual disorders can be present in eumenorrheic athletes, with LPD or anovulation found in 78% of eumenorrheic recreational runners in at least 1 menstrual cycle out of 3.[52]

Effects on Bone

Low BMD can be diagnosed via dual-energy X-ray absorptiometry (DXA) based on guidelines from the International Society of Clinical Densitometry[134,135] and the ACSM.[60] Exercise has beneficial effects on bone mineral accumulation during childhood and early adolescence,[21,136–139] with 10% to 40% higher bone mass gains observed in physically active adolescents compared with sedentary individuals.[21,136,138] However, the hypoestrogenic state that underlies menstrual dysfunction has adverse effects on bone, with lower BMD values seen in amenorrheic versus eumenorrheic athletes.[140–144] DE is also associated with low BMD independently of menstrual irregularity in runners,[117] and dietary restraint may be the DE behavior most associated with negative bone health effects in young runners.[145,146] One systematic review of female athletes found the prevalence of osteopenia and osteoporosis in excess of what would be expected in a normal population distribution.[147] In a study by Barrack and colleagues,[148] nearly 40% of a sample of female adolescent runners had a Z-score less than −1 on DXA, which was approximately twice the proportion reported in a previous study of athletes representing multiple sports.[149] Female adolescent runners, in particular, seem to show a suppressed bone mineral accrual pattern that may put them at risk for suboptimal peak bone mass.[27] Tenforde and colleagues,[150] in their cross-sectional study of adolescent runners, found that female runners with a BMI less than or equal to 17.5 kg/m^2, or both menstrual irregularity and a history of fracture, were significantly more likely to have low bone mass. For adolescent boys, those with a BMI less than or equal to 17.5 kg/m^2 and the belief that thinness improves performance were significantly more likely to have low bone mass. In young runners who display low BMD at baseline, catch-up accrual may be difficult,[151] highlighting the importance of adequate EA and neuroendocrine function during the adolescent years.

Relationship to Stress Fractures

Bone stress injury (BSI) results from chronic repetitive mechanical stress and exists on a spectrum from mild stress reaction to cortical fracture. BSIs represent a significant burden for female runners, with a reported incidence of up to 21% in competitive track athletes,[56] and increased risk compared with male counterparts.[152,153] Numerous studies have documented the relationship between amenorrhea and low bone mass and the risk for stress fractures.[56,154–159] Bennell and colleagues,[56] in a study of track athletes, found late age at menarche to be one of the strongest predictors of stress fracture risk. Recent findings by Barrack and colleagues,[160] showing the cumulative risk conferred by multiple triad-related risk factors on bone health and susceptibility to fracture, have shown the important role that risk stratification may have in decreasing risk for injury. In this study, the highest risk was seen with a combination of greater than 12 h/wk of exercise, participating in a leanness sport/activity, and evidence of dietary restraint, which conferred a 46% risk of incurring a BSI (odds ratio, 8.7; 95% confidence interval, 2.7–28.3). Tenforde and colleagues[161] also reported that the combination of late age at menarche, prior fracture, participation in dance/gymnastics, and BMI less than 19 kg/m^2 conferred the greatest risk of BSI in a study of adolescent runners. Female athletes diagnosed with BSI who are found to have menstrual irregularity should also be screened for DE and low BMD.[60] A detailed discussion of BSI is beyond the scope of this review.

Screening

Screening for the Triad requires an understanding of the relationships among its components, the spectrum within each component, and rates of movement along each spectrum (**Fig. 1**).[61] The preparticipation physical and annual health examinations provide optimal screening opportunities,[162–164] but other occasions may present when athletes are evaluated for issues such as menstrual dysfunction, BSI, or recurrent injury or illness. Athletes who present with one component of the Triad should be assessed for the others.[61,164] A recent panel recommended the use of a risk-stratification tool that incorporates evidence-based risk factors for the Triad, assigning a point value in each Triad category based on risk magnitude (**Fig. 2**).[61]

This protocol is then translated into clearance and return-to-play guidelines based on the athlete's total score (**Fig. 3**).[61] Of note, a prior history of certain risk factors (eg, ED, oligomenorrhea/amenorrhea, or BSI) still confers risk points, even if the condition is not currently present. In addition to risk stratification, the team physician should use clinical judgment and take into account the athlete's unique situation in making a decision for clearance and/or return to play.[61] **Table 5** shows the assessment of risk using this tool in 2 sample runners.

Athlete A, who is determined to be at moderate risk with a score of 2, is likely to be granted provisional clearance, with routine follow-up with a dietitian and periodic risk reassessment as needed, depending on the development of any new or worsening risk factors. Special notice may be taken of the running volume/mileage at which she sustained her prior BSI. Athlete B, who is at high risk with a score of 6, may benefit from additional work-up, including laboratory assessment, DXA, and consultation with

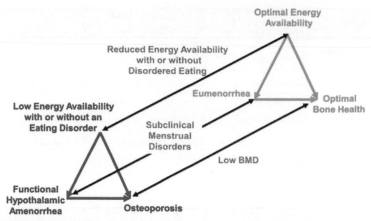

Fig. 1. Spectra of the female athlete triad. The 3 inter-related components of the Triad are energy availability, menstrual status, and bone health. Energy availability directly affects menstrual status, and, in turn, energy availability and menstrual status directly influence bone health. Optimal health is indicated by optimal energy availability, eumenorrhea, and optimal bone health, whereas, at the other end of the spectrum, the most severe presentation of the Triad is characterized by low energy availability with or without an eating disorder, functional hypothalamic amenorrhea, and osteoporosis. An athlete's condition moves along each spectrum at different rates depending on her diet and exercise behaviors. BMD, bone mineral density. (*From* Nattiv A, Loucks AB, Manore MM, et al. American College of Sports Medicine position stand. The female athlete triad. Med Sci Sports Exerc 2007;39:1867–82; Wolters Kluwer/Lippincott Williams & Wilkins; with permission.)

a sports dietitian to document adequate EA, before clearance for running. If a psychological component is detected during screening, consultation with a mental health practitioner may be prudent as well. If athlete B is able to decrease her risk, or has a satisfactorily reassuring secondary evaluation, she may be granted either limited or provisional clearance, with regular follow-up with a physician, dietitian, and any other clinical team members as needed for adequate monitoring of her health.

Treatment

Treatment of Triad conditions must address low EA, the underlying cause of the Triad. A nonpharmacologic approach involving increasing EI and/or reducing EEE, as well as normalization of BW, is the mainstay of treatment and current best practice for successful resumption of menses and improvement in bone health.[60,61] Causal evidence for the efficacy of increased EI for return of menses (ROM) has been supplied by Williams and colleagues'[165] study in primates, which showed ROM after supplemental caloric intake in the setting of ongoing training. Several case studies,[166–168] as well as a 5-year retrospective analysis,[169] have documented the association between weight gain and ROM following amenorrhea in exercising women. Studies in anorexics have documented stabilization of BMD with short-term weight gain.[170]

Treatment strategies should depend on how the athlete developed low EA (**Fig. 4**). Specific approaches are varied and depend on individual circumstances, so targets may include reversal of recent weight loss, a return to BW associated with normal menses, weight gain to achieve a BMI of greater than or equal to 18.5 kg/m^2 or greater than or equal to 90% of predicted weight, or a minimum EI of 2000 kcal/d, although higher intakes may be required.[61] These goals can be accomplished with a combination of increased EI and decreased EEE, depending on the demands of

Risk Factors	Magnitude of Risk		
	Low Risk = 0 points each	Moderate Risk = 1 point each	High Risk = 2 points each
Low EA with or without DE/ED	☐ No dietary restriction	☐ Some dietary restriction[a]; current/past history of DE;	☐ Meets DSM-V criteria for ED[b]
Low BMI	☐ BMI ≥18.5 or ≥90% EW[c] or weight stable	☐ BMI 17.5 <18.5 or <90% EW or 5 to <10% weight loss/month	☐ BMI ≤17.5 or <85% EW or ≥10% weight loss/month
Delayed Menarche	☐ Menarche <15 years	☐ Menarche 15 to <16 years	☐ Menarche ≥16 years
Oligomenorrhea and/or Amenorrhea	☐ >9 menses in 12 months[b]	☐ 6-9 menses in 12 months[b]	☐ <6 menses in 12 months[b]
Low BMD	☐ Z-score ≥−1.0	☐ Z-score −1.0[d] <−2.0	☐ Z-score ≤−2.0
Stress Reaction/Fracture	☐ None	☐ 1	☐ ≥2; ≥1 high risk or of trabecular bone sites[e]
Cumulative Risk (total each column, then add for total score)	___ points +	___ points +	___ points = ___ Total Score

Fig. 2. Female athlete triad: cumulative risk assessment. [a] Some dietary restriction as shown by self-report or low/inadequate energy intake on diet logs. [b] Current or past history. [c] Absolute BMI cutoffs should not be used for adolescents. [d] Weight-bearing sport. [e] High-risk skeletal sites associated with low BMD and delay in return to play in athletes with 1 or more components of the Triad include stress reaction/fracture of trabecular sites (femoral neck, sacrum, pelvis). BMD, bone mineral density; BMI, body mass index; DE, disordered eating; DSM-V, Diagnostic and Statistical Manual of Mental Disorders, Fifth Edition; EA, energy availability; ED, eating disorder; EW, expected weight. (*From* De Souza MJ, Nattiv A, Joy E, et al. 2014 female athlete triad coalition consensus statement on treatment and return to play of the female athlete triad: 1st International Conference held in San Francisco, California, May 2012 and 2nd International Conference held in Indianapolis, Indiana, May 2013. Br J Sports Med 2014;48:289; BMJ Publishing Group Ltd; with permission.)

the competitive schedule. If EA can be accurately estimated, a goal of greater than or equal to 45 kcal/kg FFM/d should be targeted. Changes should be gradual, with the goal of increasing weight by about 0.5 kg every 7 to 10 days. **Fig. 5** shows changes that can be made to bring a 55-kg runner with a baseline intake of 2000 kcal/d into optimal EA. Calcium-rich foods should also be encouraged, targeting an intake of 1000 to 1300 mg/d, as well as a vitamin D intake of 600 IU/d.[61,76] Time to ROM may vary considerably among amenorrheic athletes,[168–170] and may take more than a year.[169] Improvements in EA can effect positive metabolic changes within days to weeks, whereas changes in BW may take weeks to months. Improvements in BMD occur more slowly, typically trailing ROM.[171] Note that although improvements in BMD can occur with ROM, improved nutrition, and weight gain, BMD may not be restored to normal levels.[172–174]

Consideration of Pharmacologic Treatment of Triad-related Medical Conditions

Pharmacologic treatment may be warranted for the psychological treatment of ED/DE, especially if there are comorbid conditions.[61] For Triad-related health consequences of amenorrhea and osteoporosis, nonpharmacologic management is the mainstay of treatment. Pharmacologic strategies for treatment of menstrual dysfunction and osteoporosis, and/or athletes with multiple fractures related to the Triad, are largely experimental and should only be considered after a suboptimal response to at least 1 year of nonpharmacologic management or if new fractures occur.[61] For female athletes with FHA or prolonged oligomenorrhea, hormone replacement therapy (HRT) in the form of

	Cumulative Risk Score[a]	Low Risk	Moderate Risk	High Risk
Full Clearance	0 – 1 point	☐		
Provisional/Limited Clearance	2 – 5 points		☐ Provisional Clearance ☐ Limited Clearance	
Restricted from Training and Competition	≥6 points			☐ Restricted from Training/ Competition-Provisional ☐ Disqualified

Fig. 3. Female athlete triad: clearance and return-to-play (RTP) guidelines by medical risk stratification. [a] Clearance/RTP status for athletes at moderate to high risk for the triad: provisional clearance/RTP, clearance determined from risk stratification at time of evaluation (with possibility for status to change over time depending on athlete's clinical progress); limited clearance/RTP, clearance/RTP granted but with modification in training as specified by physician (with possibility for status to change depending on clinical progress and new information gathered); restricted from training/competition (provisional), athlete not cleared or able to RTP at present time, with clearance status reevaluated by physician and multidisciplinary team with clinical progress; disqualified, not safe to participate at present time and clearance status to be determined at a future date depending on clinical progress, if appropriate. (*From* De Souza MJ, Nattiv A, Joy E, et al. 2014 female athlete triad coalition consensus statement on treatment and return to play of the female athlete triad: 1st International Conference held in San Francisco, California, May 2012 and 2nd International Conference held in Indianapolis, Indiana, May 2013. Br J Sports Med 2014;48:289; BMJ Publishing Group Ltd; with permission.)

exogenous estrogen and cyclic progesterone may be indicated if there is failure of at least 1 year of nonpharmacologic management. Transdermal estrogen at a dose of 100 μg twice weekly, along with cyclic progesterone (2.5 mg daily for 10 days of every month), has been shown to improve BMD in adolescent girls with anorexia nervosa

Table 5
Sample Triad risk assessment in 2 female athletes

Risk Factor	Athlete A		Athlete B	
	Comment	Score	Comment	Score
Low EA with or without ED/DE	No dietary restriction	0	Mild restriction (vegetarian)	1
Low BMI	BMI 21	0	BMI 18.1	1
Delayed menarche	Menarche age 15 y	1	Menarche age 15 y	1
Oligomenorrhea/ amenorrhea	At present eumenorrheic; no past history of menstrual dysfunction	0	6 menses in the past 12 mo	1
Low BMD	No prior DXA	0	No prior DXA	0
BSI	History of second metatarsal shaft BSI	1	History of bilateral tibial BSI in high school	2
Total score	Moderate risk	2	High risk	6

Abbreviations: BMD, bone mineral density; BMI, body mass index; BSI, bone stress injury; EA, energy availability; ED, eating disorder; DE, disordered eating, DXA, dual-energy X-ray absorptiometry.

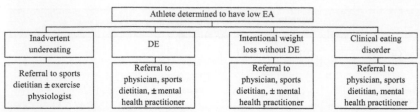

Fig. 4. Pathways to low EA and treatment recommendations. DE, disordered eating; EA, energy availability. (*Modified from* De Souza MJ, Nattiv A, Joy E, et al. 2014 Female Athlete Triad Coalition consensus statement on treatment and return to play of the female athlete triad: 1st International Conference held in San Francisco, California, May 2012 and 2nd International Conference held in Indianapolis, Indiana, May 2013. Br J Sports Med 2014;48:289; BMJ Publishing Group Ltd; with permission.)

and is an option for HRT, although studies are currently ongoing in the female athlete population.[61,175] It should be emphasized that combined hormonal contraceptives do not restore spontaneous menses and are not clearly associated with improved BMD in amenorrheic athletes.[176–178]

In athletes with FHA or prolonged oligomenorrhea, and osteoporosis, who have failed nonpharmacologic therapy, pharmacologic strategies other than HRT and oral contraceptive therapy should be prescribed only after a thorough metabolic work-up by a physician experienced in treating osteoporosis and metabolic bone disease in this population.[61] In these uncommon situations, osteoporosis medications, such as bisphosphonates and teriparatide, may be considered. According to De Souza and colleagues,[61] these treatments may be used when estrogen is contraindicated, in compliant patients who have had a lack of response to greater than or equal to 18 to 24 months of HRT, in eumenorrheic athletes/exercisers (not hypoestrogenic) who meet the criteria for pharmacologic therapy, or in athletes with multiple debilitating fractures and significant morbidity. For a full discussion and literature review of nonpharmacologic and pharmacologic management of osteoporosis and fractures in young female athletes, the authors recommend the 2014 Triad Consensus article.[61]

Baseline Statistics

    BW: 55 kg   *Body fat*: 18%   *FFM*: 45.1 kg

    EI: 2000 kcal

    Daily exercise: 1 hr at 7 min/mile pace (12.3 METs)

    EEE = MET x BW x hrs of exercise = 12.3 kcal/(kg•h) x 55kg x 1h = 676.5 kcal

Baseline EA:

    EA = (EI - EEE)/FFM = (2000 – 676.5)/45.1 = **29.3 kcal/kg FFM**

Goal Intake to achieve EA of 45 kcal/kg FFM:

    EI = (EA•FFM) + EEE = (45•45.1) + 676.5 = **2706 kcal**

EI after intervention to meet recommended intake:

    8g/kg BW of CHO   = 1760 kcal

    1.7 g/kg BW of PRO   = 374 kcal

    1 g/kg BW of fat   = 495 kcal

                          = **2629 kcal**

Fig. 5. Example of increasing EA in a 55-kg female runner. BW, body weight; CHO, carbohydrate; EA, energy availability; EEE, exercise energy expenditure; EI, energy intake; FFM, fat-free mass; MET, metabolic equivalent; PRO, protein.

Clearance/Return to Running Considerations

For any runner found to be at moderate or high risk, reassessment during the season is advised, because variables related to risk, particularly EA and menstrual status, may change during a season. Ultimately, a risk-stratification tool does not supersede clinical judgment, and physicians must take into account the athlete's unique situation in the final determination for clearance and return to play. A decision-based return-to-play model (**Fig. 6**) is useful in showing the complexity of issues that need to be considered.[61] Important risk modifiers in the female running population include those listed in **Fig. 2**, as well as age, classification as a lean-build sport, training mileage, and competitive level (high school, collegiate, elite, recreational).

IRON DEFICIENCY WITH AND WITHOUT ANEMIA

Women are at increased risk of IDA compared with men because of decreased iron intake and menstrual losses. IDA is likely more prevalent in female athletes as well.[82–84] Several explanations have been proposed to account for the iron losses observed during training, including hemolysis, hematuria, sweat loss, GI bleeding, and exercise-induced inflammation through the activity of hepcidin.[80,179,180] Vegetarians and athletes with inadequate EI seem to be at increased risk.[88,181] In women, anemia is defined by a serum hemoglobin concentration less than 12 g/dL. Serum ferritin is the most commonly used marker of body iron stores, with levels less than 12 ng/mL diagnostic of ID. There is a lack of consensus on what constitutes low ferritin (or iron depletion) in the athletic population, with thresholds ranging from less than 12 ng/mL to less than 25 ng/mL, depending on the study. As an acute phase reactant, ferritin increases independently of iron status in the setting of inflammation, and day-to-day variations may be significant.[182] Soluble transferrin receptor (sTfR), especially the sTfR/log(ferritin) index, is less variable and may more accurately reflect total body iron, with levels greater than or equal to 4.5 indicating iron depletion.[182] This index has been useful in identifying athletes with IDNA who may be more likely to respond positively to iron supplementation.[183–185]

A causal link between IDA and decreased work capacity has been discussed in the literature.[186] In endurance athletes performing submaximal exercise, this decrement is likely more related to the inability to maintain prolonged activity of iron-dependent oxidases than hemoglobin concentrations.[84] Whether subclinical IDNA leads to decreased physical performance, and should therefore be treated with iron supplementation, remains controversial.[79] Several placebo-controlled studies have shown performance benefits of iron supplementation in athletes with IDNA, including improved endurance times, faster time trials, and increased energetic efficiency.[184,187–192] However, others showed no benefit despite improvements in ferritin levels.[193–195] Further research is needed to clarify optimal cutoffs used to screen athletes, with the goal of identifying and treating those at risk of ID and performance decrement. Based on current evidence, female athletes at higher risk of ID (eg, prior history of ID/IDA, vegetarian, performance decrement, and increased fatigue) should be screened using hemoglobin and ferritin cutoffs of 12 g/dL and 20 ng/mL, respectively, to identify IDA or IDNA, in order to reduce the adverse effects that ID may have on training and performance.[79,196]

PREGNANCY

Current knowledge on the benefits of physical activity during pregnancy is encouraging. Exercise during pregnancy may decrease odds for complications such as

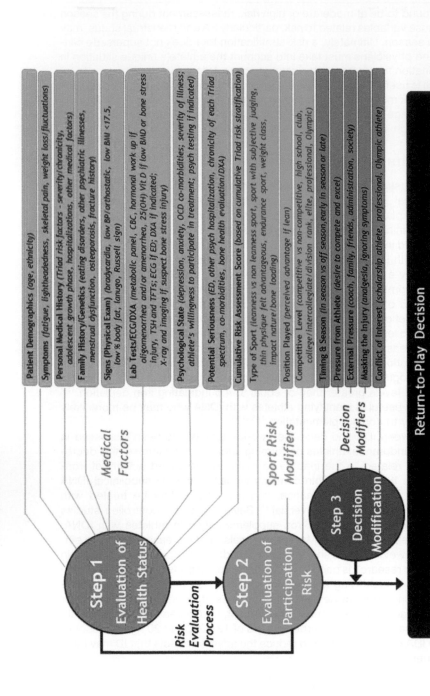

Fig. 6. Decision-based RTP model for the female athlete triad. RTP decision is determined by the primary care or team physician, and is based on a complex and comprehensive synthesis of health status, cumulative risk assessment, participation risk, sport, and decision modifiers. 25(OH) Vit D, 25-hydroxyvitamin D; BMD, bone mineral density; BMI, body mass index; BP, blood pressure; CBC, complete blood count; ECG, electrocardiogram; DXA, dual-energy X-ray absorptiometry; ED, eating disorder; OCD, obsessive-compulsive disorder; RTP, return-to-play; TFTs, thyroid function tests; TSH, thyroid-stimulating hormone. (*From* De Souza MJ, Nattiv A, Joy E, et al. 2014 Female Athlete Triad Coalition consensus statement on treatment and return to play of the female athlete triad: 1st International Conference held in San Francisco, California, May 2012 and 2nd International Conference held in Indianapolis, Indiana, May 2013. Br J Sports Med 2014;48:289; BMJ Publishing Group Ltd; with permission.)

gestational diabetes,[197–199] preeclampsia,[199–201] large for gestational age/macrosomia,[199,202–205] and preterm delivery.[206–209] Clapp[210] showed that offspring of women who exercised throughout pregnancy were significantly lighter and leaner at age 5 years compared with offspring of women who stopped exercising during pregnancy. Most guidelines recommend that healthy women with uncomplicated pregnancies accumulate at least 150 minutes of moderate intensity aerobic activity per week during pregnancy and the postpartum period,[211] although specific exercise prescriptions may vary.[212] Recommendations for calcium, vitamin D, and iron for pregnant and lactating women are listed in **Table 4**. Of note, iron requirements increase significantly during pregnancy and maternal anemia has been associated with an increased risk of preterm delivery.[213] Therefore, it is imperative that women of childbearing ages, particular those with multiple pregnancies, monitor iron status carefully.[214] The American College of Obstetricians and Gynecologists has published absolute and relative contraindications to aerobic exercise during pregnancy.[215] Further research is needed to examine the long-term effects of exercise prescription during pregnancy on both maternal and child health.

In the postpartum period, return to physical activity has been associated with decreased risk of postpartum depression.[212] The rate of return to activity varies from one woman to another, although some may be capable of engaging in an exercise within days of delivery. There are no published studies to indicate that, in the absence of medical complications, rapid resumption of activities will result in adverse effects for the mother or child.[216] No known maternal complications are associated with resumption of training,[217] and moderate weight loss while nursing is safe and does not compromise neonatal weight gain.[218] Nursing women should consider breastfeeding their infants before exercising to avoid the discomfort of engorged breasts.[219]

SUMMARY

With the continued popularity of running and steady increase of female participation in sport, the care of female runners will continue be an important topic of discussion. Advances in the understanding of the Triad and Triad-related conditions have largely informed the approach to the health of this population. An appreciation for the close relationship between EA and neuroendocrine function has equipped clinicians with the ability to promote optimal bone health and decrease risk factors for BSI and other bone consequences. The risks related to the Triad should not deter providers from encouraging participation in a sport that can be, by and large, a healthy and enjoyable endeavor for most participants. Looking forward, it is hoped that refinements in the assessment of risk factors related to the Triad, as well as advances in the treatment of Triad-related conditions, can help to ensure a vibrant and robust enjoyment of sport for all.

REFERENCES

1. 2014 Running USA Annual Marathon Report. 2015. Available at: http://www.runningusa.org/marathon-report-2015?returnTo=annual-reports. Accessed June 22, 2015.
2. Powerful Team USA roster on tap for London. 2012. Available at: http://www.usatf.org/News/Powerful-Team-USA-roster-on-tap-for-London.aspx?feed=news. Accessed June 22, 2015.
3. National Federation of State High School Associations 2013-14 High school athletics participation survey. 2014. Available at: http://www.nfhs.org/ParticipationStatics/PDF/2013-14_Participation_Survey_PDF.pdf. Accessed June 22, 2015.

4. Malina RM. Performance in the context of growth and maturation. In: Ireland ML, Nattiv A, editors. The female athlete. Philadelphia: WB Saunders; 2002. p. 49–65.

5. McDowell MA, Brody DJ, Hughes JP. Has age at menarche changed? Results from the National Health and Nutrition Examination Survey (NHANES) 1999-2004. J Adolesc Health 2007;40:227–31.

6. Anderson SE, Must A. Interpreting the continued decline in the average age at menarche: results from two nationally representative surveys of U.S. girls studied 10 years apart. J Pediatr 2005;147:753–60.

7. Herman-Giddens ME. The enigmatic pursuit of puberty in girls. Pediatrics 2013; 132:1125–6.

8. Slyper AH. The pubertal timing controversy in the USA, and a review of possible causative factors for the advance in timing of onset of puberty. Clin Endocrinol (Oxf) 2006;65:1–8.

9. Buttke DE, Sircar K, Martin C. Exposures to endocrine-disrupting chemicals and age of menarche in adolescent girls in NHANES (2003-2008). Environ Health Perspect 2012;120:1613–8.

10. Malina RM. Growth and maturation of young athletes: is training for sport a factor?. In: Chan KM, editor. Sports and children. Champagne (IL): Human Kinetics; 1998. p. 133.

11. Stager JM, Wigglesworth JK, Hatler LK. Interpreting the relationship between age of menarche and prepubertal training. Med Sci Sports Exerc 1990;22: 54–8.

12. Aksglaede L, Olsen LW, Sorensen TI, et al. Forty years trends in timing of pubertal growth spurt in 157,000 Danish school children. PLoS One 2008;3:e2728.

13. Kelly A, Winer KK, Kalkwarf H, et al. Age-based reference ranges for annual height velocity in US children. J Clin Endocrinol Metab 2014;99:2104–12.

14. Strickland SM, Metzl JD. Growth and development. In: Ireland ML, Nattiv A, editors. The female runner. Philadelphia: WB Saunders; 2002. p. 199–207.

15. Malina RM. Physical activity as a factor in growth and maturation. In: Cameron N, Bogin N, editors. Human growth and development. 2nd edition. Waltham (MA): Academic Press; 2012. p. 375–96.

16. Gomez JE. Growth and maturation. In: Anderson SJ, Harris SS, editors. Care of the young athlete. Elk Grove Village (IL): American Academy of Pediatrics; 2010. p. 17–23.

17. Christensen CL, Ruhling RO. Physical characteristics of novice and experienced women marathon runners. Br J Sports Med 1983;17:166–71.

18. van der Sluis IM, de Ridder MA, Boot AM, et al. Reference data for bone density and body composition measured with dual energy x ray absorptiometry in white children and young adults. Arch Dis Child 2002;87:341–7.

19. Malina RM, Bouchard C. Growth, maturation, and physical activity. Champaign (IL): Human Kinetics Books; 1991.

20. Malina RM. Physical growth and biological maturation of young athletes. Exerc Sport Sci Rev 1994;22:389–433.

21. Heaney RP, Abrams S, Dawson-Hughes B, et al. Peak bone mass. Osteoporos Int 2000;11:985–1009.

22. Davies JH, Evans BA, Gregory JW. Bone mass acquisition in healthy children. Arch Dis Child 2005;90:373–8.

23. Rogol AD. Sex steroids, growth hormone, leptin and the pubertal growth spurt. Endocr Dev 2010;17:77–85.

24. Theintz G, Buchs B, Rizzoli R, et al. Longitudinal monitoring of bone mass accumulation in healthy adolescents: evidence for a marked reduction after 16 years

of age at the levels of lumbar spine and femoral neck in female subjects. J Clin Endocrinol Metab 1992;75:1060–5.

25. Baxter-Jones AD, Faulkner RA, Forwood MR, et al. Bone mineral accrual from 8 to 30 years of age: an estimation of peak bone mass. J Bone Miner Res 2011;26:1729–39.

26. Ferry B, Duclos M, Burt L, et al. Bone geometry and strength adaptations to physical constraints inherent in different sports: comparison between elite female soccer players and swimmers. J Bone Miner Metab 2011;29:342–51.

27. Barrack MT, Rauh MJ, Nichols JF. Cross-sectional evidence of suppressed bone mineral accrual among female adolescent runners. J Bone Miner Res 2010;25:1850–7.

28. Fredericson M, Chew K, Ngo J, et al. Regional bone mineral density in male athletes: a comparison of soccer players, runners and controls. Br J Sports Med 2007;41:664–8.

29. Eisenmann JC, Malina RM. Age- and sex-associated variation in neuromuscular capacities of adolescent distance runners. J Sports Sci 2003;21:551–7.

30. Krahenbuhl GS, Skinner JS, Kohrt WM. Developmental aspects of maximal aerobic power in children. Exerc Sport Sci Rev 1985;13:503–38.

31. Alexander CJ. Effect of growth rate on the strength of the growth plate-shaft junction. Skeletal Radiol 1976;1:67–76.

32. Bright RW, Burstein AH, Elmore SM. Epiphyseal-plate cartilage. A biomechanical and histological analysis of failure modes. J Bone Joint Surg Am 1974;56:688–703.

33. Flachsmann R, Broom ND, Hardy AE, et al. Why is the adolescent joint particularly susceptible to osteochondral shear fracture? Clin Orthop Relat Res 2000;(381):212–21.

34. Faulkner RA, Davison KS, Bailey DA, et al. Size-corrected BMD decreases during peak linear growth: implications for fracture incidence during adolescence. J Bone Miner Res 2006;21:1864–70.

35. Maffulli N. Intensive training in young athletes. The orthopaedic surgeon's viewpoint. Sports Med 1990;9:229–43.

36. Niemeyer P, Weinberg A, Schmitt H, et al. Stress fractures in the juvenile skeletal system. Int J Sports Med 2006;27:242–9.

37. Caine D, DiFiori J, Maffulli N. Physeal injuries in children's and youth sports: reasons for concern? Br J Sports Med 2006;40:749–60.

38. Laor T, Wall EJ, Vu LP. Physeal widening in the knee due to stress injury in child athletes. AJR Am J Roentgenol 2006;186:1260–4.

39. Okamoto S, Arai Y, Hara K, et al. A displaced stress fracture of the femoral neck in an adolescent female distance runner with female athlete triad: a case report. Sports Med Arthrosc Rehabil Ther Technol 2010;2:6.

40. Goolsby MA, Barrack MT, Nattiv A. A displaced femoral neck stress fracture in an amenorrheic adolescent female runner. Sports Health 2012;4:352–6.

41. Haddad FS, Bann S, Hill RA, et al. Displaced stress fracture of the femoral neck in an active amenorrhoeic adolescent. Br J Sports Med 1997;31:70–2.

42. American Dietetic Association, Dietitians of Canada, American College of Sports Medicine, et al. American College of Sports Medicine position stand. Nutrition and athletic performance. Med Sci Sports Exerc 2009;41:709–31.

43. Burke LM, Cox GR, Culmmings NK, et al. Guidelines for daily carbohydrate intake: do athletes achieve them? Sports Med 2001;31:267–99.

44. Loucks AB. Low energy availability in the marathon and other endurance sports. Sports Med 2007;37:348–52.

45. Edwards JE, Lindeman AK, Mikesky AE, et al. Energy balance in highly trained female endurance runners. Med Sci Sports Exerc 1993;25:1398–404.

46. Zanker CL, Swaine IL. Relation between bone turnover, oestradiol, and energy balance in women distance runners. Br J Sports Med 1998;32:167–71.
47. Barrack MT, Van Loan MD, Rauh MJ, et al. Physiologic and behavioral indicators of energy deficiency in female adolescent runners with elevated bone turnover. Am J Clin Nutr 2010;92:652–9.
48. Daniels EJ. An examination of the relationship between disordered eating status and nutrient intake among NCAA cross-country runners. Northridge (CA): California State University; 2014.
49. Barrack MT, Fredericson M, Kim BY, et al. Evidence of energy deficiency and low carbohydrate intake among male and female elite collegiate endurance runners. Med Sci Sports Exerc 2015;47:S2.
50. Deuster PA, Kyle SB, Moser PB, et al. Nutritional intakes and status of highly trained amenorrheic and eumenorrheic women runners. Fertil Steril 1986;46:636–43.
51. Onywera VO, Kiplamai FK, Boit MK, et al. Food and macronutrient intake of elite Kenyan distance runners. Int J Sport Nutr Exerc Metab 2004;14:709–19.
52. De Souza MJ, Miller BE, Loucks AB, et al. High frequency of luteal phase deficiency and anovulation in recreational women runners: blunted elevation in follicle-stimulating hormone observed during luteal-follicular transition. J Clin Endocrinol Metab 1998;83:4220–32.
53. Tomten SE, Hostmark AT. Energy balance in weight stable athletes with and without menstrual disorders. Scand J Med Sci Sports 2006;16:127–33.
54. Myerson M, Gutin B, Warren MP, et al. Resting metabolic rate and energy balance in amenorrheic and eumenorrheic runners. Med Sci Sports Exerc 1991;23:15–22.
55. Mulligan K, Butterfield GE. Discrepancies between energy intake and expenditure in physically active women. Br J Nutr 1990;64:23–36.
56. Bennell KL, Malcolm SA, Thomas SA, et al. Risk factors for stress fractures in track and field athletes. A twelve-month prospective study. Am J Sports Med 1996;24:810–8.
57. Loucks AB, Thuma JR. Luteinizing hormone pulsatility is disrupted at a threshold of energy availability in regularly menstruating women. J Clin Endocrinol Metab 2003;88:297–311.
58. Loucks AB, Verdun M, Heath EM. Low energy availability, not stress of exercise, alters LH pulsatility in exercising women. J Appl Physiol 1998;84:37–46.
59. Ihle R, Loucks AB. Dose-response relationships between energy availability and bone turnover in young exercising women. J Bone Miner Res 2004;19:1231–40.
60. Nattiv A, Loucks AB, Manore MM, et al. American College of Sports Medicine position stand. The female athlete triad. Med Sci Sports Exerc 2007;39:1867–82.
61. De Souza MJ, Nattiv A, Joy E, et al. 2014 Female Athlete Triad Coalition consensus statement on treatment and return to play of the female athlete triad: 1st International Conference held in San Francisco, California, May 2012 and 2nd International Conference held in Indianapolis, Indiana, May 2013. Br J Sports Med 2014;48:289.
62. Ainsworth BE, Haskell WL, Herrmann SD, et al. 2011 compendium of physical activities: a second update of codes and MET values. Med Sci Sports Exerc 2011;43:1575–81.
63. Johnson MD. Female athletes. In: Anderson SJ, Harris SS, editors. Care of the young athlete. Elk Grove Village (IL): American Academy of Pediatrics; 2010. p. 137–52.

64. Manore MM, Kam LC, Loucks AB, et al. The female athlete triad: components, nutrition issues, and health consequences. J Sports Sci 2007;25(Suppl 1):S61–71.
65. Grandjean AC, Reimers KJ, Ruud J. Nutrition. In: Ireland ML, Nattiv A, editors. The female runner. Philadelphia: WB Saunders; 2002. p. 81–9.
66. Simonsen JC, Sherman WM, Lamb DR, et al. Dietary carbohydrate, muscle glycogen, and power output during rowing training. J Appl Physiol 1991;70: 1500–5.
67. Kirwan JP, O'Gorman D, Evans WJ. A moderate glycemic meal before endurance exercise can enhance performance. J Appl Physiol 1998;84:53–9.
68. Achten J, Jeukendrup AE. Optimizing fat oxidation through exercise and diet. Nutrition 2004;20:716–27.
69. Achten J, Halson SL, Moseley L, et al. Higher dietary carbohydrate content during intensified running training results in better maintenance of performance and mood state. J Appl Physiol 2004;96:1331–40.
70. Temesi J, Johnson NA, Raymond J, et al. Carbohydrate ingestion during endurance exercise improves performance in adults. J Nutr 2011;141:890–7.
71. Stellingwerff T, Cox GR. Systematic review: carbohydrate supplementation on exercise performance or capacity of varying durations. Appl Physiol Nutr Metab 2014;39:998–1011.
72. Jeukendrup AE. Nutrition for endurance sports: marathon, triathlon, and road cycling. J Sports Sci 2011;29(Suppl 1):S91–9.
73. Zawadzki KM, Yaspelkis BB 3rd, Ivy JL. Carbohydrate-protein complex increases the rate of muscle glycogen storage after exercise. J Appl Physiol 1992;72:1854–9.
74. Tarnopolsky MA, Bosman M, Macdonald JR, et al. Postexercise protein-carbohydrate and carbohydrate supplements increase muscle glycogen in men and women. J Appl Physiol 1997;83:1877–83.
75. Kraemer WJ, Volek JS, Bush JA, et al. Hormonal responses to consecutive days of heavy-resistance exercise with or without nutritional supplementation. J Appl Physiol 1998;85:1544–55.
76. Ross AC, Taylor CL, Yaktine AL, et al. Dietary reference intakes for calcium and vitamin D. Washington, DC: The National Academies Press; 2011.
77. Dietary reference intakes (DRIs): elements. Food and Nutrition Board, Institute of Medicine, National Academies. Available at: http://www.iom.edu/~/media/Files/ Activity Files/Nutrition/DRIs/New Material/6_ Elements Summary.pdf. Accessed June 22, 2015.
78. Dietary reference intakes for calcium and vitamin D. Washington, DC: Food and Nutrition Board, Institute of Medicine, National Academies; 2010. Available at: http://iom.nationalacademies.org/~/media/Files/Report Files/2010/Dietary-Reference-Intakes-for-Calcium-and-Vitamin-D/Vitamin D and Calcium 2010 Report Brief.pdf. Accessed July 15, 2015.
79. DellaValle DM. Iron supplementation for female athletes: effects on iron status and performance outcomes. Curr Sports Med Rep 2013;12:234–9.
80. Peeling P, Dawson B, Goodman C, et al. Athletic induced iron deficiency: new insights into the role of inflammation, cytokines and hormones. Eur J Appl Physiol 2008;103:381–91.
81. Pasricha SR, Low M, Thompson J, et al. Iron supplementation benefits physical performance in women of reproductive age: a systematic review and meta-analysis. J Nutr 2014;144:906–14.
82. Woolf K, St Thomas MM, Hahn N, et al. Iron status in highly active and sedentary young women. Int J Sport Nutr Exerc Metab 2009;19:519–35.

83. Anscheutz S, Rodgers CD, Taylor AW. Meal composition and iron status of experienced male and female distance runners. J Exerc Sci Fit 2010;8:25–33.
84. Beard J, Tobin B. Iron status and exercise. Am J Clin Nutr 2000;72:594S–7S.
85. Cook JD, Dassenko SA, Lynch SR. Assessment of the role of nonheme-iron availability in iron balance. Am J Clin Nutr 1991;54:717–22.
86. USDA national nutrient database for standard reference, release 27 (revised). Available at: http://www.ars.usda.gov/ba/bhnrc/ndl. Accessed June 22, 2015.
87. Snyder AC, Dvorak LL, Roepke JB. Influence of dietary iron source on measures of iron status among female runners. Med Sci Sports Exerc 1989;21:7–10.
88. Economos CD, Bortz SS, Nelson ME. Nutritional practices of elite athletes. Practical recommendations. Sports Med 1993;16:381–99.
89. Koehler K, Braun H, Achtzehn S, et al. Iron status in elite young athletes: gender-dependent influences of diet and exercise. Eur J Appl Physiol 2012; 112:513–23.
90. Deuster PA, Kyle SB, Moser PB, et al. Nutritional survey of highly trained women runners. Am J Clin Nutr 1986;44:954–62.
91. Hunding A, Jordal R, Paulev PE. Runner's anemia and iron deficiency. Acta Med Scand 1981;209:315–8.
92. Lampe JW, Slavin JL, Apple FS. Poor iron status of women runners training for a marathon. Int J Sports Med 1986;7:111–4.
93. Nickerson HJ, Holubets M, Tripp AD, et al. Decreased iron stores in high school female runners. Am J Dis Child 1985;139:1115–9.
94. Mettler S, Zimmermann MB. Iron excess in recreational marathon runners. Eur J Clin Nutr 2010;64:490–4.
95. NIH Consensus conference. Optimal calcium intake. NIH Consensus Development Panel on Optimal Calcium Intake. JAMA 1994;272:1942–8.
96. Benson JE, Geiger CJ, Eiserman PA, et al. Relationship between nutrient intake, body mass index, menstrual function, and ballet injury. J Am Diet Assoc 1989; 89:58–63.
97. Cohen JL, Potosnak L, Frank O, et al. A nutritional and hematologic assessment of elite ballet dancers. Phys Sportsmed 1985;13:43–54.
98. Moffatt RJ. Dietary status of elite female high school gymnasts: inadequacy of vitamin and mineral intake. J Am Diet Assoc 1984;84:1361–3.
99. Perron M, Endres J. Knowledge, attitudes, and dietary practices of female athletes. J Am Diet Assoc 1985;85:573–6.
100. Nieves JW, Melsop K, Curtis M, et al. Nutritional factors that influence change in bone density and stress fracture risk among young female cross-country runners. PM R 2010;2:740–50.
101. Kelsey JL, Bachrach LK, Procter-Gray E, et al. Risk factors for stress fracture among young female cross-country runners. Med Sci Sports Exerc 2007;39: 1457–63.
102. Bolland MJ, Barber PA, Doughty RN, et al. Vascular events in healthy older women receiving calcium supplementation: randomised controlled trial. BMJ 2008;336:262–6.
103. Bolland MJ, Grey A, Avenell A, et al. Calcium supplements with or without vitamin D and risk of cardiovascular events: reanalysis of the Women's Health Initiative limited access dataset and meta-analysis. BMJ 2011;342:d2040.
104. Holick MF. Resurrection of vitamin D deficiency and rickets. J Clin Invest 2006; 116:2062–72.
105. Holick MF. High prevalence of vitamin D inadequacy and implications for health. Mayo Clin Proc 2006;81:353–73.

106. Bischoff-Ferrari HA, Giovannucci E, Willett WC, et al. Estimation of optimal serum concentrations of 25-hydroxyvitamin D for multiple health outcomes. Am J Clin Nutr 2006;84:18–28.
107. Holick MF. Vitamin D deficiency. N Engl J Med 2007;357:266–81.
108. Dawson-Hughes B, Heaney RP, Holick MF, et al. Estimates of optimal vitamin D status. Osteoporos Int 2005;16:713–6.
109. Lehtonen-Veromaa M, Mottonen T, Irjala K, et al. Vitamin D intake is low and hypovitaminosis D common in healthy 9- to 15-year-old Finnish girls. Eur J Clin Nutr 1999;53:746–51.
110. Hamilton B, Grantham J, Racinais S, et al. Vitamin D deficiency is endemic in Middle Eastern sportsmen. Public Health Nutr 2010;13:1528–34.
111. Binkley N, Novotny R, Krueger D, et al. Low vitamin D status despite abundant sun exposure. J Clin Endocrinol Metab 2007;92:2130–5.
112. Halliday TM, Peterson NJ, Thomas JJ, et al. Vitamin D status relative to diet, lifestyle, injury, and illness in college athletes. Med Sci Sports Exerc 2011;43:335–43.
113. Constantini NW, Arieli R, Chodick G, et al. High prevalence of vitamin D insufficiency in athletes and dancers. Clin J Sport Med 2010;20:368–71.
114. Willis KS, Smith DT, Broughton KS, et al. Vitamin D status and biomarkers of inflammation in runners. Open Access J Sports Med 2012;3:35–42.
115. Ruohola JP, Laaksi I, Ylikomi T, et al. Association between serum 25(OH)D concentrations and bone stress fractures in Finnish young men. J Bone Miner Res 2006;21:1483–8.
116. Tenforde AS, Sayres LC, Sainani KL, et al. Evaluating the relationship of calcium and vitamin D in the prevention of stress fracture injuries in the young athlete: a review of the literature. PM R 2010;2:945–9.
117. Cobb KL, Bachrach LK, Greendale G, et al. Disordered eating, menstrual irregularity, and bone mineral density in female runners. Med Sci Sports Exerc 2003; 35:711–9.
118. De Souza MJ, Toombs RJ, Scheid JL, et al. High prevalence of subtle and severe menstrual disturbances in exercising women: confirmation using daily hormone measures. Hum Reprod 2010;25:491–503.
119. Tomten SE, Falch JA, Birkeland KI, et al. Bone mineral density and menstrual irregularities. A comparative study on cortical and trabecular bone structures in runners with alleged normal eating behavior. Int J Sports Med 1998;19:92–7.
120. Sowers M, Randolph JF Jr, Crutchfield M, et al. Urinary ovarian and gonadotropin hormone levels in premenopausal women with low bone mass. J Bone Miner Res 1998;13:1191–202.
121. Williams NI, Caston-Balderrama AL, Helmreich DL, et al. Longitudinal changes in reproductive hormones and menstrual cyclicity in cynomolgus monkeys during strenuous exercise training: abrupt transition to exercise-induced amenorrhea. Endocrinology 2001;142:2381–9.
122. Areta JL, Burke LM, Camera DM, et al. Reduced resting skeletal muscle protein synthesis is rescued by resistance exercise and protein ingestion following short-term energy deficit. Am J Physiol Endocrinol Metab 2014;306:E989–97.
123. Reed JL, De Souza MJ, Mallinson RJ, et al. Energy availability discriminates clinical menstrual status in exercising women. J Int Soc Sports Nutr 2015;12:11.
124. De Souza MJ, Hontscharuk R, Olmsted M, et al. Drive for thinness score is a proxy indicator of energy deficiency in exercising women. Appetite 2007;48: 359–67.
125. Reed JL, De Souza MJ, Williams NI. Changes in energy availability across the season in Division I female soccer players. J Sports Sci 2013;31:314–24.

126. Redman LM, Loucks AB. Menstrual disorders in athletes. Sports Med 2005;35: 747–55.
127. Dusek T. Influence of high intensity training on menstrual cycle disorders in athletes. Croat Med J 2001;42:79–82.
128. Bachmann GA, Kemmann E. Prevalence of oligomenorrhea and amenorrhea in a college population. Am J Obstet Gynecol 1982;144:98–102.
129. Pettersson F, Fries H, Nillius SJ. Epidemiology of secondary amenorrhea. I. Incidence and prevalence rates. Am J Obstet Gynecol 1973;117:80–6.
130. Singh KB. Menstrual disorders in college students. Am J Obstet Gynecol 1981; 140:299–302.
131. Sanborn CF, Albrecht BH, Wagner WW Jr. Athletic amenorrhea: lack of association with body fat. Med Sci Sports Exerc 1987;19:207–12.
132. Baker ER, Mathur RS, Kirk RF, et al. Female runners and secondary amenorrhea: correlation with age, parity, mileage, and plasma hormonal and sex-hormone-binding globulin concentrations. Fertil Steril 1981;36:183–7.
133. Lieberman J, De Souza MJ, Koehler K, et al. Exercise associated menstrual disturbances are less likely with increasing gynecological age. Med Sci Sports Exerc 2015;47:S3–4.
134. Schousboe JT, Shepherd JA, Bilezikian JP, et al. Executive summary of the 2013 International Society for Clinical Densitometry Position Development Conference on bone densitometry. J Clin Densitom 2013;16:455–66.
135. Gordon CM, Leonard MB, Zemel BS. International Society for Clinical Densitometry. 2013 Pediatric Position Development Conference: executive summary and reflections. J Clin Densitom 2014;17:219–24.
136. MacKelvie KJ, Khan KM, McKay HA. Is there a critical period for bone response to weight-bearing exercise in children and adolescents? A systematic review. Br J Sports Med 2002;36:250–7.
137. Weaver CM. Adolescence: the period of dramatic bone growth. Endocrine 2002; 17:43–8.
138. Bailey DA, McKay HA, Mirwald RL, et al. A six-year longitudinal study of the relationship of physical activity to bone mineral accrual in growing children: the University of Saskatchewan Bone Mineral Accrual Study. J Bone Miner Res 1999; 14:1672–9.
139. Borer KT. Physical activity in the prevention and amelioration of osteoporosis in women: interaction of mechanical, hormonal and dietary factors. Sports Med 2005;35:779–830.
140. Drinkwater BL, Nilson K, Chesnut CH 3rd, et al. Bone mineral content of amenorrheic and eumenorrheic athletes. N Engl J Med 1984;311:277–81.
141. Marcus R, Cann C, Madvig P, et al. Menstrual function and bone mass in elite women distance runners. Endocrine and metabolic features. Ann Intern Med 1985;102:158–63.
142. Myburgh KH, Bachrach LK, Lewis B, et al. Low bone mineral density at axial and appendicular sites in amenorrheic athletes. Med Sci Sports Exerc 1993;25: 1197–202.
143. Nichols DL, Sanborn CF. Female athlete and bone. In: Berning JR, Steen SN, editors. Nutrition for sport and exercise. Gaithersburg (MD): Aspen Publishers; 1998. p. 205–15.
144. Rencken ML, Chesnut CH 3rd, Drinkwater BL. Bone density at multiple skeletal sites in amenorrheic athletes. JAMA 1996;276:238–40.
145. Barrack MT, Rauh MJ, Barkai HS, et al. Dietary restraint and low bone mass in female adolescent endurance runners. Am J Clin Nutr 2008;87:36–43.

146. Vescovi JD, Scheid JL, Hontscharuk R, et al. Cognitive dietary restraint: impact on bone, menstrual and metabolic status in young women. Physiol Behav 2008; 95:48–55.

147. Khan KM, Liu-Ambrose T, Sran MM, et al. New criteria for female athlete triad syndrome? As osteoporosis is rare, should osteopenia be among the criteria for defining the female athlete triad syndrome? Br J Sports Med 2002;36:10–3.

148. Barrack MT, Rauh MJ, Nichols JF. Prevalence of and traits associated with low BMD among female adolescent runners. Med Sci Sports Exerc 2008;40: 2015–21.

149. Nichols JF, Rauh MJ, Lawson MJ, et al. Prevalence of the female athlete triad syndrome among high school athletes. Arch Pediatr Adolesc Med 2006;160: 137–42.

150. Tenforde AS, Fredericson M, Sayres LC, et al. Identifying sex-specific risk factors for low bone mineral density in adolescent runners. Am J Sports Med 2015;43:1494–504.

151. Barrack MT, Van Loan MD, Rauh MJ, et al. Body mass, training, menses, and bone in adolescent runners: a 3-yr follow-up. Med Sci Sports Exerc 2011;43: 959–66.

152. Goolsby MA, Nattiv A, Casper J. Predictors for stress fracture incidence and rate in male and female collegiate track athletes: a prospective analysis. Clin J Sport Med 2008;18:188.

153. Johnson AW, Weiss CB Jr, Wheeler DL. Stress fractures of the femoral shaft in athletes–more common than expected. A new clinical test. Am J Sports Med 1994;22:248–56.

154. Shaffer RA, Rauh MJ, Brodine SK, et al. Predictors of stress fracture susceptibility in young female recruits. Am J Sports Med 2006;34:108–15.

155. Barrow GW, Saha S. Menstrual irregularity and stress fractures in collegiate female distance runners. Am J Sports Med 1988;16:209–16.

156. Friedl KE, Nuovo JA, Patience TH, et al. Factors associated with stress fracture in young army women: indications for further research. Mil Med 1992;157: 334–8.

157. Myburgh KH, Hutchins J, Fataar AB, et al. Low bone density is an etiologic factor for stress fractures in athletes. Ann Intern Med 1990;113:754–9.

158. Rauh MJ, Macera CA, Trone DW, et al. Epidemiology of stress fracture and lower-extremity overuse injury in female recruits. Med Sci Sports Exerc 2006; 38:1571–7.

159. Nattiv A, Kennedy G, Barrack MT, et al. Correlation of MRI grading of bone stress injuries with clinical risk factors and return to play: a 5-year prospective study in collegiate track and field athletes. Am J Sports Med 2013;41: 1930–41.

160. Barrack MT, Gibbs JC, De Souza MJ, et al. Higher incidence of bone stress injuries with increasing female athlete triad-related risk factors: a prospective multisite study of exercising girls and women. Am J Sports Med 2014;42: 949–58.

161. Tenforde AS, Sayres LC, McCurdy ML, et al. Identifying sex-specific risk factors for stress fractures in adolescent runners. Med Sci Sports Exerc 2013;45:1843–51.

162. American Academy of Pediatrics. Committee on Sports Medicine and Fitness. Medical concerns in the female athlete. Pediatrics 2000;106:610–3.

163. Nattiv A, Agostini R, Drinkwater B, et al. The female athlete triad. The interrelatedness of disordered eating, amenorrhea, and osteoporosis. Clin Sports Med 1994;13:405–18.

164. Otis CL, Drinkwater B, Johnson M, et al. American College of Sports Medicine position stand. The Female Athlete Triad. Med Sci Sports Exerc 1997;29:i–ix.
165. Williams NI, Helmreich DL, Parfitt DB, et al. Evidence for a causal role of low energy availability in the induction of menstrual cycle disturbances during strenuous exercise training. J Clin Endocrinol Metab 2001;86:5184–93.
166. Kopp-Woodroffe SA, Manore MM, Dueck CA, et al. Energy and nutrient status of amenorrheic athletes participating in a diet and exercise training intervention program. Int J Sport Nutr 1999;9:70–88.
167. Dueck CA, Matt KS, Manore MM, et al. Treatment of athletic amenorrhea with a diet and training intervention program. Int J Sport Nutr 1996;6:24–40.
168. Mallinson RJ, Williams NI, Olmsted MP, et al. A case report of recovery of menstrual function following a nutritional intervention in two exercising women with amenorrhea of varying duration. J Int Soc Sports Nutr 2013;10:34.
169. Arends JC, Cheung MY, Barrack MT, et al. Restoration of menses with nonpharmacologic therapy in college athletes with menstrual disturbances: a 5-year retrospective study. Int J Sport Nutr Exerc Metab 2012;22:98–108.
170. Misra M, Prabhakaran R, Miller KK, et al. Weight gain and restoration of menses as predictors of bone mineral density change in adolescent girls with anorexia nervosa. J Clin Endocrinol Metab 2008;93:1231–7.
171. Cialdella-Kam L, Guebels CP, Maddalozzo GF, et al. Dietary intervention restored menses in female athletes with exercise-associated menstrual dysfunction with limited impact on bone and muscle health. Nutrients 2014;6:3018–39.
172. Drinkwater BL, Nilson K, Ott S, et al. Bone mineral density after resumption of menses in amenorrheic athletes. JAMA 1986;256:380–2.
173. Jonnavithula S, Warren MP, Fox RP, et al. Bone density is compromised in amenorrheic women despite return of menses: a 2-year study. Obstet Gynecol 1993; 81:669–74.
174. Keen AD, Drinkwater BL. Irreversible bone loss in former amenorrheic athletes. Osteoporos Int 1997;7:311–5.
175. Misra M, Katzman D, Miller KK, et al. Physiologic estrogen replacement increases bone density in adolescent girls with anorexia nervosa. J Bone Miner Res 2011;26:2430–8.
176. Warren MP, Brooks-Gunn J, Fox RP, et al. Persistent osteopenia in ballet dancers with amenorrhea and delayed menarche despite hormone therapy: a longitudinal study. Fertil Steril 2003;80:398–404.
177. Cobb KL, Bachrach LK, Sowers M, et al. The effect of oral contraceptives on bone mass and stress fractures in female runners. Med Sci Sports Exerc 2007;39:1464–73.
178. Gibson JH, Mitchell A, Reeve J, et al. Treatment of reduced bone mineral density in athletic amenorrhea: a pilot study. Osteoporos Int 1999;10:284–9.
179. Eichner ER. Runner's macrocytosis: a clue to footstrike hemolysis. Runner's anemia as a benefit versus runner's hemolysis as a detriment. Am J Med 1985;78: 321–5.
180. Brouns F, Beckers E. Is the gut an athletic organ? Digestion, absorption and exercise. Sports Med 1993;15:242–57.
181. Jenkinson DM, Harbert AJ. Supplements and sports. Am Fam Physician 2008; 78:1039–46.
182. Lombardi G, Lippi G, Banfi G. Iron requirements and iron status of athletes. In: Maughan RJ, editor. The encyclopaedia of sports medicine: an IOC Medical Commission publication, vol. 19. Chichester (United Kingdom): John Wiley; 2013. p. 229–41.

183. Baynes RD. Assessment of iron status. Clin Biochem 1996;29:209–15.
184. Hinton PS, Giordano C, Brownlie T, et al. Iron supplementation improves endurance after training in iron-depleted, nonanemic women. J Appl Physiol (1985) 2000;88:1103–11.
185. Brownlie T 4th, Utermohlen V, Hinton PS, et al. Tissue iron deficiency without anemia impairs adaptation in endurance capacity after aerobic training in previously untrained women. Am J Clin Nutr 2004;79:437–43.
186. Haas JD, Brownlie Tt. Iron deficiency and reduced work capacity: a critical review of the research to determine a causal relationship. J Nutr 2001;131: 676S–88S [discussion: 88S–90S].
187. Rowland TW, Deisroth MB, Green GM, et al. The effect of iron therapy on the exercise capacity of nonanemic iron-deficient adolescent runners. Am J Dis Child 1988;142:165–9.
188. Magazanik A, Weinstein Y, Abarbanel J, et al. Effect of an iron supplement on body iron status and aerobic capacity of young training women. Eur J Appl Physiol Occup Physiol 1991;62:317–23.
189. LaManca JJ, Haymes EM. Effects of iron repletion on VO2max, endurance, and blood lactate in women. Med Sci Sports Exerc 1993;25:1386–92.
190. Friedmann B, Weller E, Mairbaurl H, et al. Effects of iron repletion on blood volume and performance capacity in young athletes. Med Sci Sports Exerc 2001; 33:741–6.
191. Hinton PS, Sinclair LM. Iron supplementation maintains ventilatory threshold and improves energetic efficiency in iron-deficient nonanemic athletes. Eur J Clin Nutr 2007;61:30–9.
192. McClung JP, Karl JP, Cable SJ, et al. Randomized, double-blind, placebo-controlled trial of iron supplementation in female soldiers during military training: effects on iron status, physical performance, and mood. Am J Clin Nutr 2009;90: 124–31.
193. Fogelholm M, Jaakkola L, Lampisjarvi T. Effects of iron supplementation in female athletes with low serum ferritin concentration. Int J Sports Med 1992; 13:158–62.
194. Klingshirn LA, Pate RR, Bourque SP, et al. Effect of iron supplementation on endurance capacity in iron-depleted female runners. Med Sci Sports Exerc 1992;24:819–24.
195. Newhouse IJ, Clement DB, Taunton JE, et al. The effects of prelatent/latent iron deficiency on physical work capacity. Med Sci Sports Exerc 1989;21:263–8.
196. DellaValle DM, Haas JD. Impact of iron depletion without anemia on performance in trained endurance athletes at the beginning of a training season: a study of female collegiate rowers. Int J Sport Nutr Exerc Metab 2011;21: 501–6.
197. Dempsey JC, Sorensen TK, Williams MA, et al. Prospective study of gestational diabetes mellitus risk in relation to maternal recreational physical activity before and during pregnancy. Am J Epidemiol 2004;159:663–70.
198. Harizopoulou VC, Kritikos A, Papanikolaou Z, et al. Maternal physical activity before and during early pregnancy as a risk factor for gestational diabetes mellitus. Acta Diabetol 2010;47(Suppl 1):83–9.
199. Mudd LM, Owe KM, Mottola MF, et al. Health benefits of physical activity during pregnancy: an international perspective. Med Sci Sports Exerc 2013;45:268–77.
200. Magnus P, Trogstad L, Owe KM, et al. Recreational physical activity and the risk of preeclampsia: a prospective cohort of Norwegian women. Am J Epidemiol 2008;168:952–7.

201. Sorensen TK, Williams MA, Lee IM, et al. Recreational physical activity during pregnancy and risk of preeclampsia. Hypertension 2003;41:1273–80.
202. Alderman BW, Zhao H, Holt VL, et al. Maternal physical activity in pregnancy and infant size for gestational age. Ann Epidemiol 1998;8:513–9.
203. Mudd LM, Pivarnik J, Holzman CB, et al. Leisure-time physical activity in pregnancy and the birth weight distribution: where is the effect? J Phys Act Health 2012;9:1168–77.
204. Juhl M, Olsen J, Andersen PK, et al. Physical exercise during pregnancy and fetal growth measures: a study within the Danish National Birth Cohort. Am J Obstet Gynecol 2010;202:63.e1–8.
205. Owe KM, Nystad W, Bo K. Association between regular exercise and excessive newborn birth weight. Obstet Gynecol 2009;114:770–6.
206. Hatch M, Levin B, Shu XO, et al. Maternal leisure-time exercise and timely delivery. Am J Public Health 1998;88:1528–33.
207. Misra DP, Strobino DM, Stashinko EE, et al. Effects of physical activity on preterm birth. Am J Epidemiol 1998;147:628–35.
208. Juhl M, Andersen PK, Olsen J, et al. Physical exercise during pregnancy and the risk of preterm birth: a study within the Danish National Birth Cohort. Am J Epidemiol 2008;167:859–66.
209. Owe KM, Nystad W, Skjaerven R, et al. Exercise during pregnancy and the gestational age distribution: a cohort study. Med Sci Sports Exerc 2012;44:1067–74.
210. Clapp JF 3rd. Morphometric and neurodevelopmental outcome at age five years of the offspring of women who continued to exercise regularly throughout pregnancy. J Pediatr 1996;129:856–63.
211. US physical activity guidelines for Americans. 2008. Available at: http://www.health.gov/paguidelines. Accessed June 15, 2015.
212. Artal R, O'Toole M. Guidelines of the American College of Obstetricians and Gynecologists for exercise during pregnancy and the postpartum period. Br J Sports Med 2003;37:6–12.
213. Scholl TO. Iron status during pregnancy: setting the stage for mother and infant. Am J Clin Nutr 2005;81:1218S–22S.
214. Akabas SR, Dolins KR. Micronutrient requirements of physically active women: what can we learn from iron? Am J Clin Nutr 2005;81:1246S–51S.
215. Committee on Obstetric Practice. ACOG committee opinion. Exercise during pregnancy and the postpartum period. Number 267, January 2002. American College of Obstetricians and Gynecologists. Int J Gynaecol Obstet 2002;77:79–81.
216. Exercise during pregnancy and the postpartum period. ACOG technical bulletin number 189 – February 1994. Int J Gynaecol Obstet 1994;45:65–70.
217. Hale RW, Milne L. The elite athlete and exercise in pregnancy. Semin Perinatol 1996;20:277–84.
218. McCrory MA, Nommsen-Rivers LA, Mole PA, et al. Randomized trial of the short-term effects of dieting compared with dieting plus aerobic exercise on lactation performance. Am J Clin Nutr 1999;69:959–67.
219. Kulpa PJ, White BM, Visscher R. Aerobic exercise in pregnancy. Am J Obstet Gynecol 1987;156:1395–403.

Running Injuries During Adolescence and Childhood

Brian J. Krabak, MD, MBA[a,b,*], Brian Snitily, MD[a],
Carlo J.E. Milani, MD, MBA[a]

KEYWORDS

- Running - Injury - Youth - Pediatric

KEY POINTS

- Youth and adolescent running injuries are becoming more common as more children participate in running as a sport.
- Injuries to the youth athlete differ from those in adults because of growth-related issues.
- Early detection of injuries and correction of contributing factors can help prevent injury.

INTRODUCTION

Whether for exercise or sport, the popularity of running has greatly increased over the past few decades among all individuals, including children. In 2007, an estimated 12 million children aged 6 to 17 years participated in some form of running for exercise.[1] A 2012 study of United States youth ages 12 to 15 years showed that outside of school-based gym classes, running was the second most common activity among boys (33.5%) behind basketball and the most common activity among girls (34.9%).[2] In 2014, the National Federation of High Schools High School Participation Survey of all 51 state cross-country and track and field associations noted that a total of 1,059,206 athletes participated in track and field (580,321 boys, 478,885 girls) and 470,668 athletes participated in cross-country (252,547 boys, 218,121 girls) during the 2013/2014 season.[3] Several factors have contributed to running's increased popularity, including the development of competitive running programs at the middle and high school levels and a 2008 initiative by the United States Government to

Conflicts of Interest and Source of Funding: Nothing to disclose.
[a] Rehabilitation, Orthopedics and Sports Medicine, University of Washington, 3800 Montlake Boulevard Northeast, Box 354060, Seattle, WA 98105, USA; [b] Orthopedics and Sports Medicine, Seattle Children's Sports Medicine, 4800 Sandpoint Way NE, Seattle WA 98105, USA
* Corresponding author. University of Washington Sports Medicine, 3800 Montlake Boulevard Northeast, Box 354060, Seattle, WA 98105.
E-mail address: bkrabak@uw.edu

Phys Med Rehabil Clin N Am 27 (2016) 179–202
http://dx.doi.org/10.1016/j.pmr.2015.08.010
1047-9651/16/$ – see front matter © 2016 Elsevier Inc. All rights reserved.

increase physical activity in youths to combat obesity.[4] As the number of children who participate in running increases, however, so does the potential number of injuries. This article reviews the epidemiology of running injuries in youth and the unique physiology of the skeletally immature athlete, and discusses common injuries and treatment strategies for the youth running athlete.

EPIDEMIOLOGY

Whereas the epidemiology of running-related injuries in adults is well studied, there is limited information regarding the epidemiology of running-related injuries in children. Mehl and colleagues[5] found that between 1994 and 2007 a total of 225,344 children (boys and girls roughly equal) were treated in United States Emergency Departments for running-related injuries. Over this period, there was an annual increase in incidence of 34%, with age 12 to 14 years having the highest injury rate (45.8 per 100,000 persons).[5] Nelson and colleagues[6] reviewed Emergency Department encounters for injuries to children sustained in physical education class between 1997 and 2007. A total of 405,305 injuries were sustained in 5- to 18-year-olds during this period. Of these encounters, more than 50% could be attributed to activities involving running (running 25.1%, basketball 20.3%, football 7.8%). Similar to the Mehl study,[5] the annual rate of all injury increased over the study period.[6] Though not specific to running, younger children are more likely to have traumatic injuries and fractures in comparison with older children and adolescents, who are more likely to develop overuse injuries.[5,7]

Studies focused on high school cross-country athletes and their injuries have revealed several interesting findings. A prospective study by Rauh and colleagues[8] of 421 runners over one season found that 38.5% sustained at least one injury (defined as any reported muscle, joint, or bone problem/injury of the back or lower extremity resulting from running in a practice or meet). Girls were noted to have sustained a significantly higher overall injury rate (19.6 per 1000 athletic events [AEs]) than boys (15.0 per 1000 AEs). For girls, important predictors of injury were sustaining an injury during the summer before the season and quadriceps angle greater than 20°. Important predictors of injury for boys included a history of multiple running injuries and quadriceps angle greater than 15°. A follow-up study by Rauh[9] assessing summer training factors noted that runners who did not frequently alternate short and long mileage days ($P = .01$), ran for 8 weeks or less ($P = .31$), and ran a higher percentage predominately on hills ($P = .001$) or irregular terrains ($P = .004$) were more likely to be injured during the season. A retrospective study of high school runners (442 females and 306 males) by Tenforde and colleagues[10] noted that more than 68% of females and 59% of males reported a previous injury. Higher weekly mileage was associated with previous injuries in boys ($P = .05$) but not girls. In 2013, Tenforde and colleagues[11] reported a prospective evaluation of risk factors for stress fractures in 748 competitive high school runners (442 girls and 326 boys), and identified stress fractures in 5.4% of girls and 4.0% of boys. Tibial stress fractures were most common in girls, and the metatarsal bone was most frequently fractured in boys. These studies highlight the need to further understand the unique aspects of the child athlete and common injuries they sustain while running.

UNIQUE CONSIDERATIONS FOR THE GROWING ATHLETE

Children have varying rates of growth and development that are influenced by hormonal, genetic, and environmental factors.[12,13] Because children are skeletally immature, they are at particular risk for injury at the growth plates (physis), tendon attachment sites (apophysis), and articular cartilage at joint surfaces. The growth plate is especially vulnerable and depends on a variety of hormonal stimuli, including growth hormone (GH), insulin-like growth factor I (IGF-I), sex steroids, thyroid hormones, paracrine growth factors, and cytokines. In addition, variable rate of growth in the maturing athlete has a significant influence on biomechanics, which further puts them at risk for injury. This discussion focuses on key areas in the maturing athlete that may affect running injuries.

Bone Mineral Content

Adolescence is a period when individuals gain approximately half of their adult bone mineral content; however, the rate of bone deposition sharply declines after the age of 16 to 18 years.[14] Both men and women reach peak bone mass early in the third decade of life.[15] Of interest, some cross-sectional evidence has shown that adolescent runners have an elevated prevalence of low bone mass and decreased bone mineral accumulation with respect to expected values.[16] Although a full discussion is beyond the scope of this article, the female athlete triad, which is well described in adolescent runners, is one of the most well studied factors affecting adolescent bone development. The triad is currently understood to involve relationships between energy availability, menstrual function, and bone health.[17] In addition, new research suggests that young male athletes may exhibit processes similar to the female athlete triad, also associated with increased risk of impaired bone mineral development.[18,19] In general, low energy availability seems to be a key component of bone health during development.[20]

Endocrine

Three main endocrine axes affect growth and development during adolescence: the hypothalamic-pituitary-adrenal axis, the GH axis, and the hypothalamic-pituitary-gonadal (HPG) axis. The GH axis is largely responsible for the rapid adolescent height spurt by exerting its effect through a set of insulin-like growth factors, interaction with sex steroids, and stimulation of local IGF-I in cartilage and bone directly.[21,22] The HPG axis generally plays a larger role in skeletal maturity and bone mineralization through interactions between energy balance, sex hormones, and proper bone development.[17,23] Estrogen has been found to play a major role in skeletal maturity through effects on bone and cartilage in both girls and boys.[24] Increasing estradiol concentrations correlate with pubertal growth spurts and peak height velocity, and contribute to epiphyseal closure through multiple mechanisms, but primarily by stimulating chondrogenesis in the epiphyseal growth plate.[23,25,26] Androgen receptors are found in developing and mature osteoblasts, and are likely responsible for the greater increase in periosteal bone deposition and bone strength in men compared with women.[27,28]

Peak Height Velocity

Peak height velocity is a measure of the rate of growth speed in height. Although this can vary regionally and depends on a variety of factors, on average girls will reach their peak height velocity at 12 years of age and boys at 14 years. It has been shown that growth in children is not uniform and that maximum growth speed in the legs occurs before maximal sitting height.[29]

Peak height velocity corresponds to important physiologic changes that are important to consider. First, bone mineral density is at its lowest level just before peak height velocity.[30] Therefore, bones are at their weakest during this period of significant growth. In addition, cartilage that is growing to accommodate the increase in size of joints with growth is weaker than mature cartilage.[31] The long bones also tend to lengthen before the muscle-tendon complex, creating a tension in the muscle during periods of rapid growth.[32] Such changes put a great deal of strain on thinning growth plates and apophyses. These events highlight the importance of understanding the biological versus chronologic age of the youth runner, and the need for further research regarding appropriate training parameters for a specific athlete.[33,34]

COMMON RUNNING INJURIES
Apophyseal Injuries

Apophyseal injuries are frequently encountered in the skeletally immature runner. The apophysis represents a secondary ossification center where a tendon attaches to the bone. During period of peak growth velocity, the long bones grow in length faster than the myotendinous unit, resulting in injury to the apophysis with overtraining.[35] Apophyseal injuries can be divided into 2 categories: apophysitis (secondary to overtraining, as in distance running) or avulsion-type injuries (seen in sports requiring sudden starting and stopping, such as sprinting or soccer) (**Fig. 1**).[35,36] Although any apophysis is at risk for injury, common areas in the youth runner include the pelvis (ischial tuberosity, anterior superior and anterior inferior iliac spine), the knee (Osgood-Schlatter disease, Sinding-Larsen-Johansson lesion), the heel (Sever disease), and the fifth metatarsal (Iselin disease).[36]

Athletes will typically present with pain in the apophyseal region based on the location of the injury and an inability to continue running. Understanding the mechanism of injury and tendon attachments can help with diagnosis. Physical examination including palpation of the injured area, and passive stretch or activation of the involved muscle/tendon producing pain will confirm the diagnosis. Radiographs should be ordered to confirm a suspected avulsion fracture. Fortunately, most of these injuries will respond to a comprehensive multidisciplinary conservative treatment program.

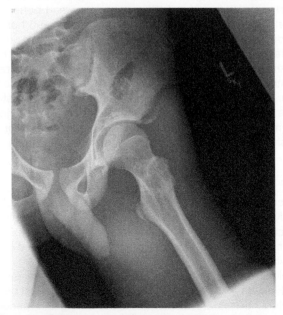

Fig. 1. Avulsion fracture of the anterior inferior iliac spine.

Rehabilitation should focus on an appropriate period of rest, use of modalities, activity modification, correction of biomechanical deficits (inflexibility or weakness), nutritional assessment, and correction of training errors that contribute to the injury. Surgery and immobilization is rarely needed and is most often used in cases of significantly displaced avulsion fractures. Further details of the most common running-associated apophyseal injuries in children are outlined in **Table 1**.

Lower Extremity Tendon Injuries

Lower extremity tendon injuries are more common than apophyseal injuries in the skeletally immature runner. Similarly to the adult runner, they are often due to over-training in the setting of biomechanics deficits involving flexibility or strength. The most common sites of injury involve the patellar tendon, Achilles tendon, or posterior tibialis tendon (**Table 2**). Similarly to apophyseal injuries, tendons can be injured during periods of peak growth velocity.[35] Early on in the clinical course, pain may occur only after athletic activities, but as the disease progresses pain may be present throughout the entirety of sporting activities or even when not participating in sports.[44] The most consistent physical examination findings are localized tenderness on the specific tendon and flexibility or strength deficits. Most tendon injuries can be treated without imaging, although ultrasonography may be used to identify any significant injury.

Aggressive nonoperative management is essential and may include a variety of modalities. Most treatment plans involve a combination of activity modifications, topical treatments including ice and analgesic creams, oral medications, bracing, and physical therapy that includes stretching and eccentric strengthening.[43] Eccentric muscle training is a mainstay in the conservative treatment of many tendinopathies, and studies have shown eccentric strength training to be effective in reducing pain associated with neovascularization.[44,49,52] Though uncommon, recalcitrant cases may require further interventions using ultrasound-guided injection of biologics or tenotomy. However, these treatments have not been studied in the child/adolescent athlete, limiting their use on the basis of evidence-based practice.

Bone

Medial tibial stress syndrome and stress fracture

Medial tibial stress syndrome (MTSS) and stress fracture are the most common causes of bone injury in runners, including skeletally immature athletes. Both MTSS and stress fractures are covered in full detail in separate reviews in this issue.[53,54] Some unique features that differ between the pediatric and adult population are noteworthy.

MTSS affects between 7.2% and 35% of all runners, including the pediatric population.[55–57] Stress fractures account for 16% of all running injuries, with high school athletes having an incidence similar to that of adults.[11,58,59] The exact etiology of MTSS is under debate, but most likely relates to a traction injury from strong leg muscles (soleus, flexor digitorum longus, flexor hallucis longus, and tibialis posterior) causing a periosteal reaction at their insertion. Continued stress will overload the bone, leading to a stress fracture. A recent systematic review by Hamstra-Wright and colleagues[60] showed that only increased body mass index (BMI), a navicular drop, and increase range of motion of ankle dorsiflexion and hip external rotation were consistently shown to increase the risk of MTSS in all age groups. A prospective study of high school cross-country runners to identify modifiable risk factors for MTSS noted that girls were 2.5 times more likely than boys to develop MTSS, and those with higher BMI were also more likely to develop MTSS.[57] Of note, age itself has not been studied as a risk factor for MTSS.

Table 1
Apophyseal injuries

Apophyseal Injury Type	Anatomy	Epidemiology Notes	Mechanism of Injury	History/ Examination Findings	Management	Other Considerations
Ischial tuberosity	Origin of long head of biceps femoris, semitendinosus, and semimembranosus muscle	Most common site of pelvic apophyseal injury[37]	Flexion of the hip with the knee extended, repetitive knee flexion, and repetitive eccentric contraction of the hamstring muscles	Posterior thigh pain and tenderness, popping sensation, and localized swelling	Apophysitis: • Rest from vigorous activity, ice, limited use of oral anti-inflammatories, and gait assessment/ correction of biomechanical issues contributing to injury Apophyseal avulsion fracture: • Displacement <2 cm: conservative management as above • Displacement >2 cm: surgical referral for consideration of ORIF[38]	May be associated with sciatic nerve injuries[39]
Anterior superior iliac spine	Origin of the sartorius and TFL	Second most common site of pelvic apophyseal injury[37]	Contraction of the sartorius, which acts to flex the hip and knee, and the TFL, which assists with abduction and lateral rotation of hip	Similar to AIIS apophyseal injury	See ischial tuberosity management above	May cause meralgia paresthetica by compression of the lateral femoral cutaneous nerve[40]

Anterior inferior iliac spine	Origin of the 2 heads of the rectus femoris muscle	Third most common site of pelvic apophyseal injury[37]	Extension of the hip and knee flexion	Findings similar to those of ischial tuberosity but at the anterior thigh	See ischial tuberosity management above	—
Osgood-Schlatter disease	Patella tendon insertion at the tibia tubercle	Most commonly seen in boys 12–15 y old and girls 8–12 y old[41]	Extension of the knee	Insidious onset of pain localized to the anterior tibial tubercle worse with running and jumping that may be associated with a palpable mass at the site	Conservative management including ice massage, oral anti-inflammatories, and protective knee padding (if kneeling regularly). Physical therapy to strengthen muscles; crossing the knee may be helpful Refractory cases with persistent symptoms may be managed surgically with drilling or excision of the tubercular mass; this is only considered after skeletal maturity	Can result in premature closure of the anterior tibial epiphysis resulting in genu recurvatum[42]
Sinding-Larsen-Johansson lesion	Patella tendon origin at the inferior pole of the patella	—	Similar to Osgood-Schlatter	Insidious onset of pain localized to the inferior pole of the patella, worse with running and jumping	A conservative approach similar to Osgood-Schlatter disease. Surgery is generally not considered even in the skeletally mature	—

(continued on next page)

Table 1
(continued)

Apophyseal Injury Type	Anatomy	Epidemiology Notes	Mechanism of Injury	History/ Examination Findings	Management	Other Considerations
Sever disease (calcaneal apophysitis)	Insertion of the Achilles tendon	Boys more commonly affected than girls. Most commonly present early in the sports season	Ankle dorsiflexion	Insidious onset of posterior heel pain. Rarely associated with swelling. Bilateral findings are common. Pain is elicited with compression of the medial and lateral heel	Conservative management including ice, relative rest, a limited trial of oral anti-inflammatories, physical therapy to stretch ankle plantarflexors and strengthen ankle dorsiflexors, and the use of heel cup orthotics. No surgical procedures are used commonly in the management of Sever disease	—
Iselin disease (fifth metatarsal head apophysitis)	Insertion of the fibularis brevis and tertius muscles	Generally thought to be rare, although true prevalence underestimated because of misdiagnosis. Most commonly seen in 10-y-old girls and 12-y-old boys	Ankle eversion, subtalar protonation, and forefoot abduction	Lateral foot pain worse with wearing shoes and weight-bearing activity. May have a tender prominence of the base of the fifth metatarsal	Conservative management including ice, relative activity restriction, appropriate footwear, and limiting running on surfaces that require foot stabilization in the coronal plane. Refractory cases may be managed with 2–3 wk in a CAM boot	—

Abbreviations: AIIS, anterior inferior iliac spine; CAM, controlled ankle movement; ORIF, open reduction and internal fixation; TFL, tensor fascia lata.

Table 2
Lower limb tendinopathies

Involved Tendon	Anatomy	Epidemiology Notes	Mechanism of Injury/ Imaging Findings	History/Examination Findings	Management
Patellar tendon	Tendon stretches from the apex of the patella, distally to the tibial tuberosity; this tissue is a continuation of the quadriceps tendon	Prevalent in jumping athletes, but also affects runners[43]	Chronic degenerative process Ultrasound imaging demonstrates abnormal tendon with localized tendon widening at the point of tenderness associated with hypoechoic areas and occasional neovascularization	May have a history positive for increased activity, but pain is typically insidious without a history of direct trauma Activity-related anterior knee pain, with focal tenderness at the inferior pole of the patella; pain is exacerbated by knee flexion and prolonged activity Early clinical course may present with pain after athletic activities only, but later pain may be present throughout entirety of sporting activities or even when not participating in sports[44] The most consistent physical examination finding is localized tenderness at the inferior pole of the patella; the most specific physical examination finding is pain with a decline squat test[43,44]	Aggressive nonoperative management is essential and may include activity modifications Treatments include ice and analgesic creams, oral medications, bracing, and physical therapy that include stretching and eccentric strengthening[43] Eccentric muscle training is a mainstay in conservative treatment Eccentric strength training shown to be effective in reducing pain associated with neovascularization[44] Some research has shown eccentric decline squat training to be superior to standard eccentric squat training[45,46] Recalcitrant cases may require further intervention using ultrasound-guided injection of biological agents, or surgical tenotomy

(continued on next page)

Table 2
(continued)

Involved Tendon	Anatomy	Epidemiology Notes	Mechanism of Injury/ Imaging Findings	History/Examination Findings	Management
Achilles tendon	Tendon stretches from the plantaris, gastrocnemius, and soleus muscles distally to the calcaneus	Strongest tendon in the body[47] Midsubstance tendinopathy (55%–65%) is more common than tendinopathy at the insertional site at the calcaneus (20%–25%)[47,48] Most commonly affects athletes in running or jumping sports[49]	Chronic degenerative process Diagnosed clinically, but ultrasound and MRI may be useful when diagnosis is unclear or when a partial tear needs to be ruled out	May complain of pain or stiffness in the Achilles 2–6 cm above the calcaneal insertion; pain is worse with activity[47] Tenderness positive in the body of the tendon or directly over the calcaneal insertion, with or without crepitus	Eccentric calf exercises have the greatest evidence and best outcomes for treatment of midsubstance Achilles tendinopathy[50–52] Recalcitrant cases may require further interventions using ultrasound-guided injection of biological agents, or surgical tenotomy
Posterior tibialis	Tendon stretches from medial border of tibia to insertion on tuberosity of the navicular	Commonly overloaded from excessive pronation, especially while running	Chronic degenerative process Diagnosed clinically, but ultrasound and MRI may be useful when diagnosis is unclear or when a partial tear needs to be ruled out	May complain of pain along the medial aspect of the ankle Tenderness positive in along the tendon near the medial malleolus	Nonoperative management is essential and may include activity modifications Treatments include ice, oral medications, physical therapy, and orthotics[43]

The presentation for children and adults for these entities is similar. Both MTSS and stress fractures of the leg present similarly, and consist of leg pain starting without obvious injury. Classically the two can be differentiated by the fact that MTSS pain may improve with activity, whereas stress-fracture pain tends to worsen with activity. Typically a child presenting with MTSS will complain of running-induced leg pain at the posteromedial aspect of the tibia in the middle or lower third of the leg. A child with a tibial stress fracture may have pain in a similar location, although it may be more focal. Both causes of leg pain can become progressively more persistent, and may even be present at rest is severe cases. Often the symptoms develop after an increase in running intensity, duration, or frequency.[61] Physical examination for both MTSS and stress fractures of the tibia may show tenderness of the tibia with or without mild swelling in the area of tenderness.[58,62,63] With this degree of similarity, these entities may be difficult to differentiate using history and examination alone.

The approach to diagnostic imaging is similar in children and adults. However, extra discretion should be exercised when obtaining imaging in children so as to limit lifetime radiation exposure. Plain radiographs are of limited value, as they inconsistently show findings in patients with MTSS and stress fractures. If radiographs are ordered, bilateral views should be considered in the skeletally immature athlete to assess subtle growth plate asymmetries.[64,65] Bone scintigraphy is of limited use, as there may be increased uptake in areas of active growth and findings are often seen in asymptomatic individuals.[64] MRI can be useful because it avoids exposure of the child to ionizing radiation and can reveal signs of a stress reaction in injured bone, particularly with stress fractures, which are not seen on plain radiographs.[66,67]

For both entities, conservative management is a mainstay of treatment. Most conservative management centers on the principles of ice, compression, and elevation in addition to progressive rehabilitation programs with a physical therapist and activity modification with reduced weight bearing, deep water running, selective bracing, correction of biomechanical deficits, and, rarely, immobilization.[68] The treatment duration and strategy for individuals with stress fractures varies depending on the location and severity of the stress fracture. The time for healing has been reported to be 6 to 8 weeks in low-risk, low-grade stress fractures, and roughly 130 days on average for high-risk stress fractures of both low and high grade.[69] Children seem to require even longer periods to heal.[70] Delayed diagnosis and mismanagement can lead to a significantly longer time to heal and delay in return to running, and may lead to avascular necrosis, osteoarthritis, and recurrence. This aspect can be particularly important for children, in whom a significant injury to the bone can cause abnormal growth and potentially lead to limb-length disparities.

Osteochondritis dissecans

Juvenile osteochondritis dissecans (JOCD) represents a unique bone injury that may present in the skeletally immature running athlete. The exact etiology of JOCD is not known, although it is widely accepted that repetitive trauma and secondary vascular effects that occur posttraumatically play a central role.[71] Other causes have been considered, including inflammation, ischemia, and heredity.[72,73] JOCD represents a separation of articular cartilage from the underlying subchondral bone, and can lead to sclerotic or fibrotic changes of the joint and the formation of a loose body.[74] Fortunately, the healing potential in the skeletally immature athlete is better than in the skeletally mature athlete.[75,76]

The knee is the most commonly affected joint in JOCD, which classically is located on the lateral aspect of the medial femoral condyle, although other areas may be affected and bilateral lesions are present 30% to 40% of the time.[77] Typically presentation is an athletic child with vague knee pain that worsens with activity or a specific traumatic event.[78] Mechanical symptoms of popping, catching, and locking are common, but may be absent before the lesion is partially or fully detached. Physical examination is often nonspecific, with tenderness of the affected condyle with the knee flexed. Knee effusions are uncommon, seen in less than 20% of children with JOCD of the knee.[77]

The talar dome is the next most commonly (though rarely) involved area of JOCD, accounting for 4% of all osteochondral lesions.[79] The medial aspect of the talar dome is more commonly affected,[80] and bilateral lesions are not uncommon (7%–25%).[81] A child presenting with JOCD of the talus will most often complain of generalized ankle pain that may localize medially or laterally depending on the location of the lesion. There may be a history of chronic instability or feeling of joint laxity before the pain.[82] Mechanical symptoms such as clicking or catching with ankle range of motion may be present, but the absence of these symptoms does not rule out JOCD. The physical examination may be notable for tenderness at the anteromedial or anterolateral aspect of the ankle, popping with passive range of motion of the ankle, and possibly an effusion. There are no special tests described in the literature for JOCD of the talus.

The diagnosis of JOCDs requires radiographs and advanced imaging. Plain radiographs of the knee (anteroposterior, lateral, tunnel, and skyline views) or ankle (anteroposterior, mortise, and lateral) should be obtained with particular focus on the common areas of involvement. Although plain radiographs may identify the lesion, MRI is considered the gold standard for evaluation of JOCD and to help determine the stability of the lesion.[74] MRI staging of the OCD (**Table 3**) will assist in determining nonoperative or operative management.[83] Bone scintigraphy and arthroscopy have been proposed as alternative diagnostic methods. Nuclear scintigraphy does not assist with staging, and arthroscopy may be normal in lesions where the articular cartilage is intact.

Management and prognosis of JOCD lesions depends on the size, location, and stability of the lesion, and the age (skeletal maturity) of the patient. In the skeletally immature patient there is a significantly increased ability to heal and a much greater role for nonoperative management.[84,85] Lesions of the lateral femoral condyle[86] and lateral talar dome[87] are the least likely to heal with conservative management alone in comparison with other locations of the knee and ankle, respectively. Most stable lesions (stages 1 and 2) are treated nonoperatively for 3 to 6 months. Conservative management including a period of non–weight bearing or immobilization followed by physical therapy is recommended depending on the location and symptoms.[31,88] Although no definitive guideline has been set regarding length of immobilization, 6 to 18 weeks has been commonly used depending on the stage and location of the JOCD, followed by continued activity modification for 3 to 6 months. Using these guidelines, more than 90% of stable JOCD lesions of the knee have good outcomes, with a return to sporting activity in 6 to 9 months.[88,89] Operative management is indicated in all skeletally mature patients with OCD or patients with unstable lesions.[90] Surgical options include arthroscopic drilling, bone grafting, reduction and fixation of the loose fragment, excision of the fragment, and osteochondral grafting. Patients managed operatively typically are able to return to their sport in 6 months. Proper management is important, as there is increased risk for the development of osteoarthritis and recurrent OCD lesions in adulthood in JOCD that is not managed appropriately.[75,91–94]

TREATMENT

Emphasis on an adolescent runner's competitive success, rather than development of running skill, especially at an early age, can lead to increased risk for overuse injuries,

Table 3
Characterization of osteochondral lesions by magnetic resonance imaging

	Arthroscopic	MRI	Radiographs (Berndt and Harty classification)
Stage I	Irregularity and softening of articular cartilage. No definable fragment	Thickening of articular cartilage and low signal change	Compression lesion. No visible fragment
Stage II	Articular cartilage breached, definable fragment, not displaced	Articular cartilage breached, low signal rim behind fragment indicating fibrous attachment	Fragment attached
Stage III	Articular cartilage breached, definable fragment, displaceable, but attached by some overlying articular cartilage	Articular cartilage breached, high signal changes behind fragment indicating synovial fluid between fragment and underlying subchondral bone	Nondisplaced fragment without attachment
Stage IV	Loose body	Loose body	Displaced fragment

From Dipaola JD, Nelson DW, Colville MR. Characterizing osteochondral lesions by magnetic resonance imaging. Arthroscopy 1991;7:102.

acute injuries, and burnout. Factors that contribute to running injuries are often organized into intrinsic and extrinsic causes. The contribution of intrinsic and extrinsic factors to the development of injury is variable depending on the runner, competition venue, and degree of participation. In addition, many injuries are the result of complex interactions between multiple risk factors in a specific setting associated with an inciting event. Owing to fundamental differences between intrinsic and extrinsic factors, treatment approaches will vary depending on the primary causes of injury. All youth runners should ideally have access to a comprehensive treatment program and treatment team including physicians, physical therapists, nutritionists, trainers, and coaches, employing each member of the team as needed to address specific injury symptoms and treatment needs.

Intrinsic factors are characterized by the individual athlete's biological and psychosocial traits. In relation to running, intrinsic factors include variations in age, gender, growth, and development. Treatment of intrinsic factors should incorporate effective pain relief and physical therapy to address neuromuscular reeducation, weakness, strength imbalance, and gait analysis to address improving biomechanics in the context of a runner's anatomic predisposition. Use of anti-inflammatory and analgesic agents such as corticosteroids, nonsteroidal anti-inflammatories, acetaminophen, and topical menthol should be used cautiously in the young athlete, as data regarding the ability of these agents to improve recovery and time to return to running are either lacking or controversial. Variations in anatomic alignment of the spine, pelvic girdle, and lower limbs should be noted. Therapeutic exercises should focus on common areas of inflexibility involving the hip flexors, iliotibial band, quadriceps, hamstrings, and gastrocsoleus complex. Strength deficits should be corrected, and treatment may focus on weakness of the hip abductors, ankle dorsiflexors, and ankle plantarflexors. Treatment should progress from muscle-specific exercises (**Figs. 2** and **3**) to functional activities (**Fig. 4**). A running-gait analysis should identify step cadence, step length, vertical displacement, trunk motion, and arm motion, with corrections made as appropriate based on the specific diagnosis.

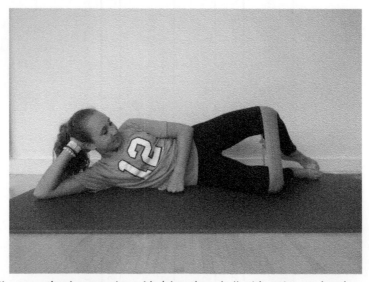

Fig. 2. Hip-strengthening exercises: side-lying clam shell with resistance band.

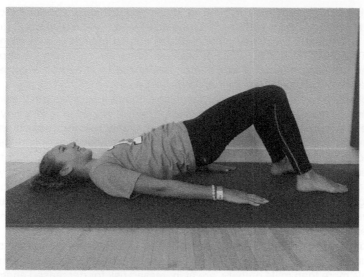

Fig. 3. Spine stabilization exercise bridging.

Extrinsic factors are associated with external forces related to training, equipment, environmental conditions of training and competition, footwear, and nutrition and energy balance. Higher training volumes have consistently been shown to increase the risk for overuse injury in multiple sports, including distance running. Therefore, managing training volumes with the goal of limiting mechanical stress at discrete sites of overuse is key to the prevention and treatment of overuse running injuries. Other factors, which have fewer data to support a role in developing running injuries, include

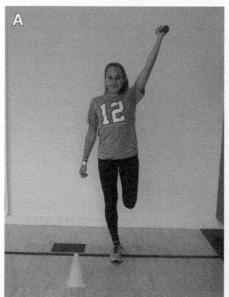
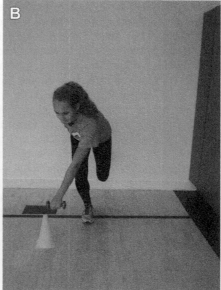

Fig. 4. (*A*) Functional exercise: single-leg stance with opposite arm reach with weight. (*B*) Functional exercise: progression to squat and diagonal reach.

poorly fitting equipment, such as running shoes and orthotics, especially when not adjusted for changes in growth rate.[95] As the adolescent runner grows and develops, coaches and parents must pay particular attention to changing equipment needs based on the child's rate of growth. For example, fitting the child with the appropriate shoes and orthoses may be a key component of the treatment and correction of biomechanics once an overuse injury has developed.

Overscheduling, that is, participation in multiple competitive events in the same day or over multiple consecutive days, creates a high ratio of workload to recovery time for the adolescent runner, and can put the athlete at higher risk for overuse and acute injury.[95] Again, coaches and parents must be aware of the amount of time the runner is allowed to recover between scheduled events, especially with respect to major competitions in which athletes attempt to push the limits of their bodies' physiologic capability. Once early signs and symptoms of overuse injuries have been identified, restricting the amount of participation in major competitive events and reduction of training volumes are integral to treating progressive overuse injuries while preserving the runner's ability to train and compete.

Nutrition, energy availability, and volume status are essential components of preparing runners for training and competition. Lean sport athletes such as runners, and female more than male runners, are at increased risk for decreased energy availability (a key component of the female athlete triad).[20] Coaches and parents of runners should identify a team of health care providers who can aid in early detection and treatment of athletes at risk for decreased energy availability. The care team should consist of medical, dietetic, mental health, and athletic training staff.[18] The main focus of treatment for athletes with low energy availability is modification of diet and exercise behaviors to increase energy availability and weight gain if needed. Given the numerous factors often driving low energy availability, treatment should use a multidisciplinary approach targeting any inappropriate training, abnormal eating behaviors, poor nutrition, body image issues, or external stressors.[18] If providers have a concern for complications associated with low bone mineral density, this multidisciplinary approach is the first-line treatment. In addition, the runner should consume calcium-rich foods with optimal calcium intake between 1000 and 1300 mg/day. The runner should have a daily intake of 600 IU of vitamin D, with higher doses possibly needed if he or she is deficient or insufficient in vitamin D. Vitamin D levels should be maintained between 32 and 50 ng/mL.[96]

Ideally the medical care team should have an established process for returning an injured runner to training or competition. There are no general evidence-based guidelines for return to running after an injured athlete is removed from participation, but the process should include evaluation of the runner's health status, participation risk, and extrinsic factors.[97] The decision regarding return to running should account for the nature of the injury, including the mechanism of injury, natural history, and known risks of participation after injury. Functional testing to evaluate readiness to return to running is essential.[97] The runner should increase training volumes gradually under the guidance of the team with the goal of running pain free. One common approach, which is not evidence-based, is to reintroduce training before competition, and to increase training distances by 10% per week. Participation in a carefully structured program should promote a safe return to running and prevent future injury.

PREVENTION

Prevention of running-related injuries should be the goal whenever possible. This principle is especially important in the pediatric population, among whom injuries can alter growth and predispose athletes to injuries and disability later in life. When considering an injury prevention program in child runners, it is important to remember the old adage that children are not small adults and have unique characteristics that put them at risk for injury; namely, children are actively growing. This growth is not a uniform process, and imbalances can develop as one system of the body matures before other areas. Other physiologic needs such as adequate caloric intake, hydration, and sleep should also be assessed. Psychological and cognitive development occurs in parallel with physical development and is an important consideration in the child runner.[98] If a prevention program for a child runner is intended to reduce harm, it is most likely to be effective if both comprehensive and personalized.

Unlike in some youth organized sports such as Little League Baseball and youth tennis, there are no widely accepted guidelines for injury prevention in the child runner. The American Academy of Pediatrics Council on Sports Medicine and Fitness (AAPCSMF) issued guidelines in 2007 on avoiding overuse injury and burnout in all youth sports.[98] AAPCSMF recommend limiting one sporting activity to a maximum of 5 days per week with at least 1 day off from any organized physical activity, and that athletes should take at least 2 to 3 months off per year from their particular sport. Similar guidelines have been made by the National Athletic Trainers' Association, who recommend that pediatric athletes should limit vigorous activity (heart rate and respiratory effort notably increased) to 16 to 20 hours per week.[99,100] Lack of healing time is thought to be one of the major factors that ultimately result in the overuse injuries seen in pediatric runners.[88,92,101,102] By encouraging regular breaks from activity, the risk of overuse injuries decreases. An additional benefit from planned breaks is the avoidance of overtraining syndrome. Overtraining syndrome may manifest as chronic muscle pain, personality changes, elevated resting heart rate, and worse sport performance.[103] Although the recommendations provided here are not specific to running, they are reasonable guidelines to offer pediatric runners, their parents, and their coaches. Limiting total running time is likely one of the most effective methods of reducing overuse injuries in pediatric runners.

All youth runners should understand the importance of proper training and an avoidance of training errors. A sudden increase in training intensity and duration has been associated with injury. To prevent injury, the 10% rule is commonly used in runners as a guide to increase training distances gradually. This rule dictates that distances run are increased 10% per week throughout the course of training. Although this approach is widely used and recommended in child runners,[98] it has not been verified to be effective in randomized trials of adults.[100,104,105] Future studies are needed to better define age-appropriate progression of training.

Both acute and overuse running injuries are attributed to relative muscle weakness or muscle imbalances.[106] Weakness of stabilizing muscles such as the gluteus medius can also predispose to injuries, such as iliotibial band syndrome and patellofemoral syndrome resulting from alterations in biomechanics.[107] It is common practice and expert opinion to include resistance training focusing on muscles such as core/spine, hip (gluteus medius), knee, and ankle stabilizers.[100] There are few large randomized controlled trials supporting the use of resistance training to prevent lower extremity injury in endurance events.[104,108,109] However, many rehabilitation programs designed to treat the injuries described in this issue involve strengthening weak muscles to correct biomechanical abnormalities. Further research may better elucidate the preventive benefit of resistance training in youth runners. Regardless of preventive effects, strengthening activities are recommended 3 times per week for all healthy children by multiple professional societies, including the American College of Sports Medicine

(ACSM) and the American Academy of Pediatrics, to support their general health and development, runners being no exception.[110,111]

The benefits of stretching to reduce injuries in adults have long been debated. A recent systematic review showed no strong evidence that stretching reduces injury in adult runners.[104] That being said, bones lengthen before muscles in children, creating a certain degree of tension that may predispose children to certain injuries such as traction apophysitis.[32,35,112] The ACSM recommends flexibility exercises 2 to 3 days per week.[113] Although these recommendations are limited to adult populations, it is common practice to incorporate stretching for young runners. Despite the benefits of this practice being unclear, there is likely little risk involved with stretching.

The use of orthoses is another method commonly considered in preventing injury in runners. Although there is little strong evidence to support the use of most orthoses for the prevention of injury, some data suggest that patellofemoral braces may help reduce anterior knee pain in runners[104] and that shock-absorbing insoles may reduce stress fractures.[104] These studies were limited to adult runners, however, and the designs of the orthoses used varied between studies. Orthotics are not strictly necessary and should be reserved for the youth runner who is recovering from an injury.

Much of the recommendations regarding injury prevention in child runners are a combination of expert opinion and extrapolation from adult studies. Given the current level of research, it seems reasonable to follow the AAPCSMF recommendations of limiting running to 5 days per week with 2 to 3 months off per year, and limiting weekly mileage to typical high school cross-country distances of 30 to 40 miles per week is reasonable for most adolescent runners.[98] However, elite high school–aged runners may train with higher mileage under appropriate supervision of a coach or trainer. Practicably more important is education for the pediatric runner, parents, and coaches regarding signs and symptoms of overuse injuries, as delayed recognition and management is thought to be a large contributor to the morbidity associated with injury.

SUMMARY

Understanding the normal growth and development of the youth athlete is essential in the development of a safe running program. Although injuries will occur, most can be treated successfully with conservative interventions and correction of training errors. Treatment should focus on athlete education, modification of training schedule, and correction of biomechanics deficits contributing to injury. Early identification and correction of these factors will allow a safe return to running sports. With proper guidance, a supportive team, and self-motivation, all youth running athletes should be able to achieve their running goals.

REFERENCES

1. The superstudy of sports participation, vol. 1: fitness activities. Hartsdale, NY: American Sports Data; 2007.
2. Fakhouri TH, Hughes JP, Burt VL, et al. Physical activity in U.S. youth aged 12-15 years, 2012. NCHS Data Brief 2014;(141):1–8.
3. National Federation of High Schools survey of participation. Available at: http://www.nfhs.org/ParticipationStatics/ParticipationStatics.aspx/. Accessed April 28, 2015.
4. Results from the School Health Policies and Practice Study 2012. Available at: http://www.cdc.gov/healthyyouth/shpps/2012/pdf/shpps-results_2012.pdf. Accessed May 5, 2015.

5. Mehl AJ, Nelson NG, McKenzie LB. Running-related injuries in school-age children and adolescents treated in emergency departments from 1994 through 2007. Clin Pediatr (Phila) 2011;50(2):126–32.

6. Nelson NG, Alhajj M, Yard E, et al. Physical education class injuries treated in emergency departments in the US in 1997-2007. Pediatrics 2009;124:918–25.

7. Stracciolini A, Casciano R, Levey Friedman H, et al. Pediatric sports injuries: an age comparison of children versus adolescents. Am J Sports Med 2013;42:965–72.

8. Rauh MJ, Koepsell TD, Rivara FP, et al. Epidemiology of musculoskeletal injuries among high school cross-country runners. Am J Epidemiol 2006;163(2):151–9.

9. Rauh MJ. Summer training factors and risk of musculoskeletal injury among high school cross-country runners. J Orthop Sports Phys Ther 2014;44(10):793–804.

10. Tenforde AS, Sayres LC, McCurdy ML, et al. Overuse injuries in high school runners: lifetime prevalence and prevention strategies. PM R 2011;3:125–31.

11. Tenforde AS, Sayres LC, McCurdy ML, et al. Identifying sex-specific risk factors for stress fractures in adolescent runners. Med Sci Sports Exerc 2013;45(10):1843–51.

12. Malina RM. Physical growth and biological maturation of young athletes. Exerc Sport Sci Rev 1994;22:389–433.

13. Jaimes C, Chauvin NA, Delgado J, et al. MR imaging of normal epiphyseal development and common epiphyseal disorders. Radiographics 2014;34(2):449–71.

14. Barrack MT, Van Loan MD, Rauh MJ, et al. Body mass, training, menses, and bone in adolescent runners: a 3-yr follow-up. Med Sci Sports Exerc 2011;43(6):959–66.

15. Baxter-Jones AD, Faulkner RA, Forwood MR, et al. Bone mineral accrual from 8 to 30 years of age: an estimation of peak bone mass. J Bone Miner Res 2011;26(8):1729–39.

16. Barrack MT, Rauh MJ, Nichols JF. Cross-sectional evidence of suppressed bone mineral accrual among female adolescent runners. J Bone Miner Res 2010;25(8):1850–7.

17. Nattiv A, Loucks AB, Manore MM, et al, American College of Sports Medicine. American College of Sports Medicine position stand. The female athlete triad. Med Sci Sports Exerc 2007;39(10):1867–82.

18. Barrack MT, Ackerman KE, Gibbs JC. Update on the female athlete triad. Curr Rev Musculoskelet Med 2013;6(2):195–204.

19. Tenforde AS, Fredericson M, Sayres LC, et al. Identifying sex-specific risk factors for low bone mineral density in adolescent runners. Am J Sports Med 2015;43(6):1494–504.

20. Loucks AB. Low energy availability in the marathon and other endurance sports. Sports Med 2007;37(4–5):348–52.

21. Rogol AD. Growth at puberty: interaction of androgens and growth hormone. Med Sci Sports Exerc 1994;26(6):767–70.

22. Van Wyk JJ, Smith EP. Insulin-like growth factors and skeletal growth: possibilities for therapeutic interventions. J Clin Endocrinol Metab 1999;84(12):4349–54.

23. Maïmoun L, Georgopoulos NA, Sultan C. Endocrine disorders in adolescent and young female athletes: impact on growth, menstrual cycles, and bone mass acquisition. J Clin Endocrinol Metab 2014;99(11):4037–50.

24. Carani C, Qin K, Simoni M, et al. Effect of testosterone and estradiol in a man with aromatase deficiency. N Engl J Med 1997;337(2):91–5.

25. Weise M, De-Levi S, Barnes KM, et al. Effects of estrogen on growth plate senescence and epiphyseal fusion. Proc Natl Acad Sci U S A 2001;98(12):6871–6.

26. Vandewalle S, Taes Y, Fiers T, et al. Sex steroids in relation to sexual and skeletal maturation in obese male adolescents. J Clin Endocrinol Metab 2014;99(8): 2977–85.

27. Bellido T, Jilka RL, Boyce BF, et al. Regulation of interleukin-6, osteoclastogenesis, and bone mass by androgens. The role of the androgen receptor. J Clin Invest 1995;95(6):2886–95.

28. Colvard DS, Eriksen EF, Keeting PE, et al. Identification of androgen receptors in normal human osteoblast-like cells. Proc Natl Acad Sci U S A 1989;86(3):854–7.

29. Beunen GP, Malina RM, Van't Hof MA, et al. Adolescent growth and motor performance, a longitudinal study of Belgian boys. Champaign (IL): Human Kinetics Books; 1989.

30. Faulkner RA, Davison KS, Bailey DA, et al. Size-corrected BMD decreases during peak linear growth: implications for fracture incidence during adolescence. J Bone Miner Res 2006;21(12):1864–70.

31. Robertson W, Kelly BT, Green DW. Osteochondritis dissecans of the knee in children. Curr Opin Pediatr 2003;15(1):38–44.

32. Philippaerts RM, Vaeyens R, Janssens M, et al. The relationship between peak height velocity and physical performance in youth soccer players. J Sports Sci 2006;24(3):221–30.

33. Lloyd RS, Oliver JL, Faigenbaum AD, et al. Chronological age vs. biological maturation: implications for exercise programming in youth. J Strength Cond Res 2014;28(5):1454–64.

34. Zwick EB, Kocher R. Growth dynamics in the context of pediatric sports injuries and overuse. Semin Musculoskelet Radiol 2014;18(5):465–8.

35. Seto CK, Statuta SM, Solari IL. Pediatric running injuries. Clin Sports Med 2010; 29(3):499–511.

36. Soprano JV, Fuchs SM. Common overuse injuries in the pediatric and adolescent athlete. Clin Pediatr Emerg Med 2007;8:7–14.

37. Rossi F, Dragoni S. Acute avulsion fractures of the pelvis in adolescent competitive athletes: prevalence, location and sports distribution of 203 cases collected. Skeletal Radiol 2001;30(3):127–31.

38. Kautzner J, Trc T, Havlas V. Comparison of conservative against surgical treatment of anterior-superior iliac spine avulsion fractures in children and adolescents. Int Orthop 2014;38(7):1495–8.

39. Dosani A, Giannoudis PV, Waseem M, et al. Unusual presentation of sciatica in a 14-year-old girl. Injury 2004;35(10):1071–2.

40. Hayashi S, Nishiyama T, Fujishiro T, et al. Avulsion-fracture of the anterior superior iliac spine with meralgia paresthetica: a case report. J Orthop Surg (Hong Kong) 2011;19(3):384–5.

41. Blankstein J, Cohen I, Heim M, et al. Ultrasonography as a diagnostic modality in Osgood–Schlatter disease: a clinical study and review of the literature. Arch Orthop Trauma Surg 2001;121:536–9.

42. Gholve PA, Scher DM, Khakharia S, et al. Osgood Schlatter syndrome. Curr Opin Pediatr 2007;19:44–50.

43. Hong E, Kraft MC. Evaluating anterior knee pain. Med Clin North Am 2014;98(4): 697–717.

44. Christian RA, Rossy WH, Sherman OH. Patellar tendinopathy—recent developments toward treatment. Bull Hosp Jt Dis (2013) 2014;72(3):217–24.

45. Purdam CR, Jonsson P, Alfredson H, et al. A pilot study of the eccentric decline squat in the management of painful chronic patellar tendinopathy. Br J Sports Med 2004;38(4):395–7.

46. Young MA, Cook JL, Purdam CR, et al. Eccentric decline squat protocol offers superior results at 12 months compared with traditional eccentric protocol for patellar tendinopathy in volleyball players. Br J Sports Med 2005;39(2):102–5.
47. Asplund CA, Best TM. Achilles tendon disorders. BMJ 2013;346:f1262.
48. Zafar MS, Mahmood A, Maffulli N. Basic science and clinical aspects of achilles tendinopathy. Sports Med Arthrosc 2009;17(3):190–7.
49. Kujala UM, Sarna S, Kaprio J. Cumulative incidence of Achilles tendon rupture and tendinopathy in male former elite athletes. Clin J Sport Med 2005;15(3):133–5.
50. Woodley BL, Newsham-West RJ, Baxter GD. Chronic tendinopathy: effectiveness of eccentric exercise. Br J Sports Med 2007;41(4):188–98.
51. Magnussen RA, Dunn WR, Thomson AB. Nonoperative treatment of midportion Achilles tendinopathy: a systematic review. Clin J Sport Med 2009;19(1): 54–64.
52. van der Plas A, de Jonge S, de Vos RJ, et al. A 5-year follow-up study of Alfredson's heel-drop exercise programme in chronic midportion Achilles tendinopathy. Br J Sports Med 2012;46(3):214–8.
53. Tenforde AS, Kraus E, Fredericson M. Bone stress injuries in runners. PM&R Clinics North America, in press.
54. Finnoff. Exertional leg pain. PM&R Clinics North America, in press.
55. Rauh MJ, Macera CA, Trone DW, et al. Selected static anatomic measures predict overuse injuries in female recruits. Mil Med 2010;175:329–35.
56. Sharma J, Golby J, Greeves J, et al. Biomechanical and lifestyle risk factors for medial tibia stress syndrome in army recruits: a prospective study. Gait Posture 2011;33:361–5.
57. Plisky MS, Rauh MJ, Heiderscheit B, et al. Medial tibial stress syndrome in high school cross-country runners: incidence and risk factors. J Orthop Sports Phys Ther 2007;37(2):40–7.
58. Chen YT, Tenforde AS, Fredericson M. Update on stress fractures in female athletes: epidemiology, treatment, and prevention. Curr Rev Musculoskelet Med 2013;6(2):173–81.
59. Changstrom BG, Brou L, Khodaee M, et al. Epidemiology of stress fracture injuries among US high school athletes, 2005-2006 through 2012-2013. Am J Sports Med 2015;43:26.
60. Hamstra-Wright KL, Bliven KC, Bay C. Risk factors for medial tibial stress syndrome in physically active individuals such as runners and military personnel: a systematic review and meta-analysis. Br J Sports Med 2015;49:362–9.
61. Taunton JE, Ryan MB, Clement DB, et al. A retrospective case-control analysis of 2002 running injuries. Br J Sports Med 2002;36(2):95–101.
62. Newman P, Adams R, Waddington G. Two simple clinical tests for predicting onset of medial tibial stress syndrome: shin palpation test and shin edema test. Br J Sports Med 2012;46:861–4.
63. Fredericson M, Jennings F, Beaulieu C, et al. Stress fracture in athletes. Top Magn Reson Imaging 2006;17(5):309–25.
64. Moran DS, Evans RK, Hadad E. Imaging of lower extremity stress fracture injuries. Sports Med 2008;38(4):345–56.
65. Bergman AG, Fredericson M, Ho C, et al. Asymptomatic tibial stress reactions: MRI detection and clinical follow-up in distance runners. Am J Roentgenol 2004; 183(3):635–8.
66. Fredericson M, Bergman AG, Hoffman KL, et al. Tibial stress reaction in runners: correlation of clinical symptoms and scintigraphy with a new magnetic resonance imaging grading system. Am J Sports Med 1995;23:472–81.

67. Spitz DJ, Newberg AH. Imaging of stress fractures in the athlete. Radiol Clin North Am 2002;40(2):313–31.
68. Robertson GA, Wood AM. Return to sports after stress fractures of the tibial diaphysis: a systematic review. Br Med Bull 2015;113(1):1–17.
69. Ardent E, Agel J, Heikes C, et al. Stress injuries to bone in college athletes: a retrospective review of experience at a single institution. Am J Sports Med 2003;31(6):959–68.
70. Niemeyer P, Weinberg A, Schmitt H, et al. Stress fractures in the juvenile skeletal system. Int J Sports Med 2006;27(3):242–9.
71. Polousky JD. Juvenile osteochondritis dissecans. Sports Med Arthrosc 2011; 19(1):56–63.
72. Yonetani Y, Nakamura N, Natsuume T, et al. Histological evaluation of juvenile osteochondritis dissecans of the knee: a case series. Knee Surg Sports Traumatol Arthrosc 2010;18:723–30.
73. Uozumi H, Sugita T, Aizawa T, et al. Histologic findings and possible causes of osteochondritis dissecans of the knee. Am J Sports Med 2009;37:2003–8.
74. Vannini F, Cavallo M, Baldassarri M, et al. Treatment of juvenile osteochondritis dissecans of the talus: current concepts review. Joints 2015;2(4):188–91.
75. Twyman RS, Desai K, Aichroth PM. Osteochondritis dissecans of the knee. A long-term study. J Bone Joint Surg Br 1991;73:461–4.
76. Kessler JI, Nikizad H, Shea KG, et al. The demographics and epidemiology of osteochondritis dissecans of the knee in children and adolescents. Am J Sports Med 2014;42:320–6.
77. Hefti F, Beguiristain J, Krauspe R, et al. Osteochondritis dissecans: a multicenter study of the European Pediatric Orthopedic Society. J Pediatr Orthop B 1999;8: 231–45.
78. Kocher MS, Tucker R, Ganley TJ, et al. Management of osteochondritis dissecans of the knee: current concepts review. Am J Sports Med 2006;34: 1181–91.
79. Thompson JP, Loomer RL. Osteochondral lesions of the talus in a sports medicine clinic. A new radiographic technique and surgical approach. Am J Sports Med 1984;12(6):460–3.
80. McCullough CJ, Venugopal V. Osteochondritis dissecans of the talus: the natural history. Clin Orthop Relat Res 1979;144:264–8.
81. Canale ST, Belding RH. Osteochondral lesions of the talus. J Bone Joint Surg Am 1980;62(1):97–102.
82. Saxena A, Eakin C. Articular talar injuries in athletes: results of microfracture and autogenous bone graft. Am J Sports Med 2007;35(10):1680–7.
83. Dipaola JD, Nelson DW, Colville MR. Characterizing osteochondral lesions by magnetic resonance imaging. Arthroscopy 1991;7:101–4.
84. Krause M, Hapfelmeier A, Möller M, et al. Healing predictors of stable juvenile osteochondritis dissecans knee lesions after 6 and 12 months of nonoperative treatment. Am J Sports Med 2013;41:2384–91.
85. Wall EJ, Vourazeris J, Myer GD, et al. The healing potential of stable juvenile osteochondritis dissecans knee lesions. J Bone Joint Surg Am 2008;90: 2655–64.
86. Samora WP, Chevillet J, Adler B, et al. Juvenile osteochondritis dissecans of the knee: predictors of lesion stability. J Pediatr Orthop 2012;32(1):1–4.
87. Gross AE, Agnidis Z, Hutchison CR. Osteochondral defects of the talus treated with fresh osteochondral allograft transplantation. Foot Ankle Int 2001;22: 385–91.

88. Jurgensen I, Bachmann G. Arthroscopic versus conservative treatment of osteochondritis dissecans of the knee: value of magnetic resonance imaging in therapy planning and follow-up. Arthroscopy 2002;18:378–86.
89. Perumal V, Wall E, Babekir N. Juvenile osteochondritis dissecans of the talus. J Pediatr Orthop 2007;27:821–5.
90. Aboussaly M, Peterson D, Salci L, et al. Surgical management of osteochondritis dissecans of the knee in the paediatric population: a systematic review addressing surgical techniques. Knee Surg Sports Traumatol Arthrosc 2014;22(6): 1216–24.
91. Linden B. Osteochondritis dissecans of the femoral condyles: a long-term follow-up study. J Bone Joint Surg Am 1977;59:769–76.
92. Din R, Annear P, Scaddan J. Internal fixation of undisplaced lesions of osteochondritis dissecans in the knee. J Bone Joint Surg Br 2006;88:900–4.
93. DiFiori JP, Benjamin HJ, Brenner JS, et al. Overuse injuries and burnout in youth sports: a position statement from the American Medical Society for Sports Medicine. Br J Sports Med 2014;48(4):287–8.
94. De Souza MJ, Nattiv A, Joy E, et al, Expert Panel. 2014 Female Athlete Triad Coalition consensus statement on treatment and return to play of the female athlete triad: 1st International Conference held in San Francisco, California, May 2012 and 2nd International Conference held in Indianapolis, Indiana, May 2013. Br J Sports Med 2014;48(4):289.
95. AMSSM overuse and burnout, 2014.
96. Female Athlete Triad Coalition, 2014.
97. Herring SA, Kibler WB, Putukian M. The team physician and the return-to-play decision: a consensus statement-2012 update. Med Sci Sports Exerc 2012; 44(12):2446–8.
98. Brenner JS, American Academy of Pediatrics Council on Sports Medicine and Fitness. Overuse injuries, overtraining, and burnout in child adolescent athletes. Pediatrics 2007;119(6):1242–5.
99. Loud KJ, Gordon CM, Micheli LJ, et al. Correlates of stress fractures among preadolescent and adolescent girls. Pediatrics 2005;115(4):e399–406.
100. McLeod TC, Decoster LC, Loud KJ, et al. National athletic trainer's association position statement: prevention of pediatric overuse injuries. J Athl Train 2011;46: 206–20.
101. Patel DS, Roth M, Kapil N. Stress fractures: diagnosis, treatment, and prevention. Am Fam Physician 2011;83(1):39–46.
102. Pihlajamaki HK, Ruohola JP, Weckstrom M, et al. Long-term outcome of undisplaced fatigue fractures of the femoral neck in young male adults. J Bone Joint Surg Br 2006;88:1574–9.
103. Small E. Chronic musculoskeletal pain in young athletes. Pediatr Clin North Am 2002;49:655–62.
104. Yeung EW, Yeung SS. Interventions for preventing lower limb soft tissue injuries in runners. Cochrane Database Syst Rev 2001;(3):CD001256.
105. Shanmugam C, Maffulli N. Sports injuries in children. Br Med Bull 2008;86: 33–57.
106. Soprano, 2005.
107. Powers CM. The influence of abnormal hip mechanics on knee injury: a biomechanical perspective. J Orthop Sports Phys Ther 2010;40(2):42–51.
108. Brushoj C, Larsen K, Albrecht-Beste E, et al. Prevention of overuse injuries by a concurrent exercise program in subjects exposed to an increase in training load: a randomized controlled trial of 1020 army recruits. Am J Sports Med 2008;36(4):663–70.

109. Rice SG, Waniewski S, American Academy of Pediatrics (AAP) Committee on Sports Medicine and Fitness, International Marathon Medical Directors Association (IMMDA). Children and marathoning: how young is too young? Clin J Sport Med 2003;13(6):369–73.
110. American College of Sports Medicine. ACSM's guidelines for exercise testing and prescription. 8th edition. Philadelphia: Lippincott Williams & Wilkins; 2010.
111. Council of Sports Medicine and Fitness. Strength by children and adolescent. Pediatrics April 2008;121(4):835–40.
112. Adirim TA, Cheng TL. Overview of injuries in the young athlete. Sports Med 2003;33(1):75–81.
113. Garber CE, Blissmer B, Deschenes MR, et al, American College of Sports Medicine. American College of Sports Medicine position stand. Quantity and quality of exercise for developing and maintaining cardiorespiratory, musculoskeletal, and neuromotor fitness in apparently healthy adults: guidance for prescribing exercise. Med Sci Sports Exerc 2011;43:1334–59.

Injuries and Health Considerations in Ultramarathon Runners

Martin D. Hoffman, MD*

KEYWORDS

- Endurance • Exercise • Injury • Medical coverage • Running • Ultramarathon

KEY POINTS

- Participation in ultramarathons has grown exponentially in recent years, but those running ultramarathons represent a small subset of runners. Ultramarathon runners can range widely in age but most are between 30 and 49 years, most are men, and as a group, ultramarathon runners tend to be well-educated.
- Injury rates appear similar for ultramarathon runners compared with other distance runners, and the types of injuries are also similar across groups. However, ultramarathon runners are observed to have fewer stress fractures and, when they occur, are more common in the foot as opposed to the lower leg, thigh, or pelvis.
- Because ultramarathons often take place in remote locations, preparticipation screening for these events is particularly important.
- Compared with shorter distance races, medical issues more unique to ultramarathon races include blisters, gastrointestinal distress, exercise-associated hyponatremia, dehydration, and transient vision impairment.
- The long-term health implications from ultramarathon running and training are not clear.

INTRODUCTION

Ultramarathons are foot races longer than the 42.195-km marathon distance, and may be continuous or staged (discontinuous) over several days. These events may take place on tracks or roads, but most are on trails, often in wilderness environments. As a result, the physiologic stress of running extended distances may be compounded by challenging terrain and environmental factors. These geographic barriers reduce the level of aid and medical support compared with urban events.

Department of Physical Medicine & Rehabilitation, Department of Veterans Affairs, Northern California Health Care System, and University of California Davis Medical Center, Sacramento, CA, USA
* Department of Physical Medicine & Rehabilitation (117), Sacramento VA Medical Center, 10535 Hospital Way, Sacramento, CA 95655-1200.
E-mail address: mdhoffman@ucdavis.edu

Phys Med Rehabil Clin N Am 27 (2016) 203–216
http://dx.doi.org/10.1016/j.pmr.2015.08.004
1047-9651/16/$ – see front matter Published by Elsevier Inc.

The most typical distances for ultramarathons are 50 km, 80 km (50 miles), 100 km, and 161 km (100 miles). More than half of ultramarathons in North America are 50 km in distance, and the second most common distance is 80 km.[1] Additionally, events longer than 161 km exist, including fixed time events and events of nonstandard distances.

Although marathon participation has shown continued steady growth for the past 3 decades,[2] participation in ultramarathons has grown exponentially in recent years.[3,4] There were more than 76,000 ultramarathon finishes in North America in 2014, which is approximately twice the number of finishes 5 years ago.[4] Despite the growth in ultra-marathon participation, the number of ultramarathon finishes is currently less than 13% of the number of marathon finishes,[1,2,4] so ultramarathon runners continue to represent a relatively small subset of runners. The present work focuses on the unique characteristics and medical issues in this running population.

CHARACTERISTICS OF ULTRAMARATHON RUNNERS

Ultramarathon runners vary widely in characteristics. This may be especially true with regard to their reasons for running ultramarathons. Many run and train for these events largely for health and social reasons, as well as for personal discovery and growth.[5,6] Although most may have personal goals driving them to run their best during a race, many are not focused on winning or age group placing. Because prize money in these events is rare, only a very few make a profession of ultramarathon running, and even those runners must rely on sponsorship support.[5]

Because competition is not the focus for many ultramarathon participants, the age of participants crosses a wide spectrum. For instance, in analyzing 161-km ultramar-athon participation from 1997 through 2008, we found finishers ranged in age from 15 to 75 years.[3] The largest proportion of ultramarathon participants are in the 30 to 39-year and 40 to 49-year age groups, with each group accounting for approximately one-third of total participants, and median age has been at 41 to 42 years for the past couple of years.[1] In general, shorter distance runners tend to be younger than ul-tramarathon runners. For perspective, the median age of recent American marathon participants has been 36 to 37 years.[2]

The fastest ultramarathon runners also tend to be slightly older than the fastest run-ners at shorter distances. The fastest marathon performances have typically been achieved by runners who are 25 to 35 years of age.[7–11] In contrast, previous cross-sectional and longitudinal analyses have shown that top ultramarathon performances can be achieved at age 40 years and beyond.[3,12–19]

Ultramarathon participation among women has been increasing,[3] although women account for only roughly 30% of ultramarathon participants in North America.[1] This compares with women accounting for more than 40% of American marathon fin-ishers[2] and approximately 60% of half-marathon finishers.[20]

Ultramarathon runners are more likely to be in a stable relationship and to have a higher education level than the general American population.[21,22] With regard to edu-cation level, we have found that more than 80% have at least a bachelor's degree, and 38% to 46% have a graduate degree.[21,22] Ultramarathon runners also tend to have professional occupations.[22–24] To some, it might be surprising that people so well-educated would voluntarily choose to run such long distances. But, the predictable findings that ultramarathon runners tend to be goal oriented and internally moti-vated,[25,26] are characteristics that likely impact both professional and personal life.

An interesting trend we have observed is that a subset of ultramarathon runners are exploring the limits of human potential by running multiple 161-km ultramarathons in a given year.[3] This is partly because the opportunity to attempt such feats has increased with a constantly increasing number of available races of this distance. For instance, there are 140,161-km ultramarathons in North America in 2015,[27] up more than three-fold from the 45 races of this distance in 2007.[3] A number of individuals have accomplished what is inconceivable for most people by completing more than ten 161-km ultramarathons in a year. Reportedly, a man finished 40,161-km ultramarathons in 2014 (https://www.strava.com/athletes/309028).

Another trend of interest observed is a decrease in the number of years of regular running before the first ultramarathon is completed.[28] In other words, those individuals running their first ultramarathon tend to have less running experience now than in the past. This may have important implications on the risk of injuries and medical issues during events.

INJURIES IN ULTRAMARATHON RUNNERS

Runners preparing to run both short and long distances are at risk for various overuse musculoskeletal injuries. A number of factors affect the injury patterns and injury incidence in runners. Potential factors of particular importance to consider for ultramarathon runners include regular training distance, age and experience level, typical running surface and exercise intensity, and use of alternate activities in training. Not a lot is known about how these factors might affect injuries in this group of athletes.

The annual incidence of injuries in ultramarathon runners appears similar to that of shorter distance runners. For instance, we found that 52% of a large cohort of 161-km ultramarathon entrants had suffered an injury severe enough to interfere with training in the previous year,[29] and 65% of active ultramarathon runners participating in a longitudinal health study (the Ultrarunners Longitudinal TRAcking or ULTRA Study) reported an exercise-related injury resulting in lost training of at least 1 day in the previous year.[30] This is comparable to the annual injury incidence rate reported among long-distance runners of 50% to 60%.[31–34]

The finding that injury rate is not higher among ultramarathon runners compared with shorter distance runners is interesting given that running distance has been found to be a risk factor for injury,[35] and the ultramarathon runners we had examined[30] were generally running greater distances than the runners in the studies of other runners.[31–34] The ultramarathon runners we examined in one study reported running an average of 3347 km in the previous year, and those who did and did not sustain an injury during the study year had similar average annual running distances.[30] In other studies of runners preparing for 161-km ultramarathons, we found that the highest running distance in 1 week during the 3 months before the events averaged between 123 and approximately 160 km, although the distance varied considerably.[29,36] We also know that it is not uncommon for these runners to have training runs of 80 km or longer in preparation for long ultramarathons.[36] In general, those running longer races put in greater training distances,[28] and presumably those with limited running distances in training for ultramarathons incorporate alternate forms of exercise besides running into their training program.

It is evident there are determinants of injury besides running distance. Likely those individuals who have withstood the stress associated with ultramarathon running have better adapted for such demands and/or have favorable intrinsic characteristics that reduce their injury risk relative to the distances they run. However, ultramarathon runners also tend to have a high use of running surfaces other than concrete or asphalt.[28] Use of running surfaces softer and with greater variation than concrete or asphalt may offer some protection from certain injuries. Differences in relative intensity and running speed, along with the associated effects this might have on stride frequency, foot strike pattern, and impact forces, could also be of importance in limiting injuries among ultramarathon runners.[37]

Although running distance does not seem to be a distinguishing factor for whether ultramarathon runners sustain injuries, we have found several other important characteristics.[30] Those sustaining an injury were younger and less experienced at running, had relatively less focus on running compared with other activities, spent a greater proportion of their exercise time at high intensities, and were more likely to have performed regular resistance training. In examining the characteristics of those with exercise-related stress fractures, the results were similar except that runners sustaining stress fractures were more likely to be women, were running greater distances, and were less likely to have performed regular resistance exercise. A previous history of exercise-related stress fracture was also found to be another risk factor for a stress fracture in this group.

The types of injuries sustained by ultramarathon runners are similar to injuries occurring in shorter distance runners (**Table 1**), but the distribution of injuries varies between groups. The knee is the most common site of injury for both ultramarathon runners[29,30]

Table 1
Number, distribution, and incidence of various exercise-related injuries in the previous 12 months among 1212 active ultramarathon runners

Injury Type and/or Location	n	Distribution, %	Incidence, %
Knee issues	291	15.3	24.0
Iliotibial band issue	191	10.1	15.8
Calf strain	159	8.4	13.1
Back injuries	150	7.9	12.4
Hamstring strain	143	7.5	11.8
Achilles tendinitis or tear	131	6.9	10.8
Ankle sprain	131	6.9	10.8
Plantar fasciitis	129	6.8	10.6
Lower leg or ankle tendinitis not involving Achilles	111	5.8	9.2
Hip flexor strain	106	5.6	8.7
Other foot and ankle injuries	54	2.8	4.5
Other leg, pelvis, or hip issues	45	2.4	3.7
Stress fracture involving foot	41	2.2	3.4
Morton neuroma	38	2.0	3.1
Metatarsalgia	38	2.0	3.1
Great toe metatarsal phalangeal joint pain (bunion)	30	1.6	2.5
Stress fracture involving tibia or fibula	23	1.2	1.9
Other lower leg injuries	18	0.9	1.5
Skin wounds, blisters, and infections	18	0.9	1.5
Other not previously specified	18	0.9	1.5
Upper extremity injuries including fractures	17	0.9	1.4
Fractures not involving the extremities	12	0.6	1.0
Stress fracture involving femur/hip	6	0.3	0.5

From Hoffman MD, Krishnan E. Health and exercise-related medical issues among 1,212 ultramarathon runners: baseline findings from the Ultrarunners Longitudinal TRAcking (ULTRA) study. PLoS One 2014;9(1):e83867; with permission.

and other distance runners.[35] However, stress fractures are a relatively less common issue in ultramarathon runners compared with shorter distance runners. We found that stress fractures accounted for 3.7% of exercise-related injuries, and 5.5% of the ultramarathon runners reported having suffered a stress fracture in the previous year.[30] Previous work has reported that stress fractures account for 5% to 16% of all injuries in runners,[38–41] and annual incidence has been reported to be as high as 25.9% among a group of elite middle and long-distance runners.[42]

In addition to stress fractures appearing to be less common in ultramarathon runners than shorter distance runners, the anatomic site for stress fractures appears to differ among running groups. Although the lower leg is typically reported as the site of most stress fractures in runners,[40,42,43] we have found that ultramarathon runners sustain most of their stress fractures in the foot.[29,30] We have suggested that the lower incidence of stress fractures in ultramarathon runners relates to the fact that, in general, only approximately half of their running is on concrete or asphalt. The higher distribution of stress fractures involving the foot may be due to greater demands sustained by the foot from running on irregular terrain.[30]

PREPARTICIPATION SCREENING FOR ULTRAMARATHONS

Ultramarathons commonly take place in remote locations that may become harsh in terms of weather conditions and terrain. Such environments necessitate considerations to greater attention to preparticipation screening. For instance, certain medical issues may not cause inordinate risk for running in urban settings, but once in a remote location, that condition may create risks that could preclude safe participation. An example might be a runner with history of epilepsy, which might be considered relatively safe for an urban marathon because a swift emergency medical response could be enacted. In contrast, a seizure experienced during an ultramarathon in a remote location would preclude a swift emergency medical response. Thus, preparticipation medical screening for clinical and medical-legal risk reduction at ultramarathons is particularly important.

When event logistics allow, the medical screening process is best performed in advance of the race.[44,45] Ideally, this means performing the screening with enough time in advance to avoid a situation in which a runner has spent considerable time and money traveling to an event and is subsequently excluded from participation, yet not too far in advance that new medical issues develop in the interim between the screening and the event.

The screening is best performed when considering the relative risk of participation, and whether the event and athlete can both reasonably accept those risks. The athlete and the event organizers must recognize that it may not be only the athlete with the medical issue who is at risk, as other athletes may inadvertently be exposed to greater risk as well. Certainly, the relative risk should be considered in the context of previous training and competition, such that uneventful training and competition may lower the perceived risk. Considerations might also include whether the athlete can participate with reduced expectations (eg, participating but not competing with full effort) or using accommodations (eg, pacers).

An approach to the preparticipation screening process for remote endurance events has been provided elsewhere.[45] The reader is referred to that work, which also details considerations relative to various medical issues, including anaphylaxis and severe allergy, seizure disorder, diabetes, previous exertional heat stroke, kidney injury, coronary artery disease, arrhythmias, following ablation therapy for conduction abnormalities, use of antiplatelet agents, pregnancy, gastrointestinal bleeding, exercise-associated hyponatremia (EAH), mental illness, and altitude illness.

MEDICAL ISSUES DURING ULTRAMARATHONS

The common medical issues that present during ultramarathons and their management have been detailed elsewhere.[44,46] Although the medical issues that present during an ultramarathon also can present during shorter races, certain medical issues tend to be more pertinent to ultramarathons because of the longer exercise durations and remote environments typical of these events. Issues most unique to ultramarathons are the focus of this review and include blisters, gastrointestinal distress, EAH, severe dehydration, and transient vision impairment.

Blisters

Blisters are the most commonly encountered medical problem in ultramarathons.[29,46–49] Although blisters rarely lead to a more severe illness, such as cellulitis,[47] they can have serious adverse effects on race performance,[29] as evident from **Table 2**. For instance, blisters and "hot spots" on the feet were reported the most (40.1%) as a factor adversely affecting race performance among finishers of a 161-km ultramarathon.[29] However, skin issues were reported as the main reason for dropping out by only 5.8% of nonfinishers.[29] In general, painful nonbloody blisters that present during a competition are best drained, while taking care to preserve the overlying skin, taped, and then lubricated. In the case of blood blisters, draining should be with caution because of the theoretic risk of infection to the exposed dermal vasculature. Prevention is best achieved by proper training, regular filing of calloused areas, avoiding changes in footwear for races, and use of lubricants.

Gastrointestinal Distress

Unlike shorter distance runs in which the primary fuel can come from stored energy sources, ultramarathon runners generally meet increased energy demands through

Table 2
Comparison of problems that impacted race performance between finishers and nonfinishers reported as percentages within each group

	Finishers	Nonfinishers	P
Blisters or "hot spots" on feet	40.1	17.3	<.0001
Nausea and/or vomiting	36.8	39.6	.60
Muscle pain	36.5	20.1	.0005
Exhaustion	23.1	13.7	.024
Inadequately heat acclimatized	21.0	28.1	.12
Inadequately trained	13.5	15.1	.66
Muscle cramping	11.4	15.8	.22
Injury during the race	9.0	10.1	.73
Ongoing injury	7.5	15.8	.010
Illness before the race	6.0	5.0	.83
Started out too fast	5.1	6.5	.52
Vision problems	2.1	3.6	.35
Difficulty making cutoff times	1.8	27.3	<.0001
Other, not categorized	11.7	26.6	.0001

From Hoffman MD, Fogard K. Factors related to successful completion of a 161-km ultramarathon. Int J Sports Physiol Perform 2011;6:32; with permission.

caloric intake during the event. Fluid intake is also essential in these longer events. These factors partly account for why gastrointestinal distress (including nausea, vomiting, abdominal cramping, and diarrhea) is commonly experienced by participants in ultramarathons (see **Table 2**).[29,50–54] One study of a 161-km ultramarathon found that 96% of the participants experienced gastrointestinal symptoms during the race.[53] In another study of 161-km ultramarathon runners, nausea and/or vomiting was found to be the most common reason self-reported for not finishing (23.0%) and the second most common problem negatively impacting race performance among finishers (36.8%).[29] Although potentially having a significant impact on race performance, nausea is typically benign, but it should be recognized that it can be an early symptom of EAH, altitude illness, and heat illness.[55]

The underlying cause of nausea and vomiting is often multifactorial, but can result from a combination of overdrinking causing an excess of unabsorbed fluids in the upper gastrointestinal tract, dehydration, and race diets with a lower percentage of calories from fat.[54,56] Therefore, ultramarathon runners should be educated to experiment during training to identify a successful strategy for meeting hydration and caloric demands during competition. When gastrointestinal distress presents during events, medical staff should recognize that these issues tend to improve with reduced exercise intensity. Antiemetic medications (eg, ondansetron or metoclopramide) also have been used successfully to help with nausea and vomiting.

Exercise-Associated Hyponatremia

EAH is defined by a serum sodium concentration below the usual normal lower limit of 135 mEq/L during or up to 24 hours after physical activity.[55,57] Confirmed deaths of public record are known to be directly attributed to complications from EAH associated with marathons, hiking, military activities, canoeing, and American football,[58–64] but to my knowledge there have been no EAH-related deaths associated with ultramarathons. Nevertheless, the incidence of EAH can be quite high in ultramarathons; incidences of 31% to 51% have been reported.[65–68] Fortunately, most cases of EAH are asymptomatic and are only detected from blood samples taken from athletes participating in research studies. As demonstrated in **Fig. 1**, the cases most likely to be symptomatic are those in which there is weight gain or inadequate weight loss due to overhydration.[69,70]

Because overhydration is a primary risk factor for EAH, current recommendations are for athletes to follow a "drink to thirst" strategy and strive to lose at least 3% to 4% of body weight during extended periods of exercise.[55,57,65] Yet, it is common that ultramarathon runners do not use this hydration strategy[36,71,72] even though it can effectively maintain adequate hydration.[36,71] Use of sodium supplements during ultramarathons is also common.[36,71,72] Yet, sodium supplementation is not effective at preventing EAH and may even worsen matters by stimulating thirst and increasing the chance of overhydration,[69] which is compounded by hormonal influences in EAH typically involving arginine vasopressin, which acts to retain water, and brain natriuretic factor, which enhances urinary sodium loss.[55] Therefore, ultramarathon runners generally should be advised to avoid excessive sodium supplementation during their runs.

Field recognition and management of EAH requires clinical suspicion for this condition. Early symptoms may include headache, mental status changes, and oliguria.[46,55,57] Unfortunately, these signs and symptoms are common with severe dehydration, heat illness, and altitude illness and can make the diagnosis of EAH challenging without point-of-care sodium analysis. However, history of high-volume fluid intake, inadequate weight loss during exercise, and/or a seizure following exercise

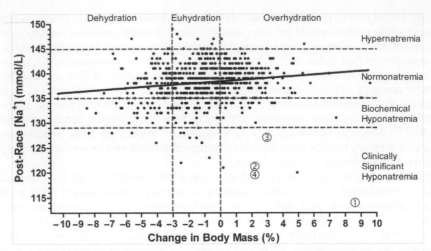

Fig. 1. Relationship of postrace serum sodium with change in body mass from registration weight for 669 observations from 5 years of data collection at 161-km ultramarathons in Northern California. Numbered open circles identify 4 confirmed cases of symptomatic EAH encephalopathy. (*From* Hoffman MD, Stuempfle KJ, Sullivan K, et al. Exercise-associated hyponatremia with exertional rhabdomyolysis: importance of proper treatment. Clin Nephrol 2014;83(4):238; with permission; and *Adapted from* Hoffman MD, Hew-Butler T, Stuempfle KJ. Exercise-associated hyponatremia and hydration status in 161-km ultramarathoners. Med Sci Sports Exerc 2013;45:784–91.)

in an individual without a known seizure disorder should raise suspicion for EAH as the underlying problem.[46,55]

Treatment for EAH is with fluid restriction and bolused hypertonic saline provided orally, if possible, or intravenously.[46,55,57] An appropriate oral solution can be prepared with 3 to 4 bouillon cubes in 125 mL of water,[73] but a solution of approximately 3 g sodium chloride (table salt) in 125 mL of water that is flavored (eg, Crystal Light, Kool Aid) may be more palatable. The typical recommendation for intravenous treatment has been up to three 100-mL boluses of 3% saline (51 mEq of sodium each),[55,57] although the need for larger volumes of hypertonic saline has been reported.[74] We also have suggested that a 50-mL ampule of sodium bicarbonate (50 mEq of sodium) might provide a reasonable alternative source of sodium if available.[46] When EAH cannot be confirmed with point-of-care testing but is considered as a likely diagnosis, the potential benefit from a 100-mL bolus of 3% hypertonic saline is thought to outweigh potential risk.[55] Alternate diagnoses should be considered when athletes do not improve with intervention, and they should be evacuated if neurologic deficits remain.

Dehydration

Dehydration results when weight loss exceeds the amount associated with released water during mobilization of glycogen stores and from fat utilization.[65,70] This typically means that body weight may decrease 3% to 4% to maintain euhydration during long periods of exercise. Although dehydration is a fairly common phenomenon in ultramarathons (see **Fig. 1**),[65] it has been well demonstrated that endurance athletes can lose 8% or greater body mass during competitions without significant clinical symptomatology or adverse consequences.[65,70] Thus, the levels of dehydration suggested by a few percent weight loss beyond 3% to 4% are generally not hazardous[75] and rarely require intravenous rehydration when oral fluids can be tolerated. Because intravenous hydration with isotonic or hypotonic fluids can have adverse consequences in an athlete with EAH,[55,65,76] and the clinical assessment of dehydration in athletes is challenging,[77,78] a cautious approach to the field management of presumed dehydration is recommended.[46]

Intravenous fluid replacement is best reserved for the severely dehydrated athlete (persistent tachycardia, poor skin turgor, and lightheadedness with standing) who is not recovering with oral fluid replacement or is having ongoing fluid losses with vomiting or diarrhea.[44,46] When point-of-care analysis of serum sodium is unavailable to confirm that the athlete is not hyponatremic, caution with intravenous hydration is warranted and the athlete should be closely observed, with hypertonic saline readily available to use if neurologic deterioration suggestive of EAH occurs.[46] Because significant symptoms related to EAH may be delayed for an hour or more after exercise while water continues to be absorbed from the gastrointestinal tract,[58,69,79] it is important to closely observe any individual with possible EAH until urination begins.

Vision Impairment

Vision impairment occurs in a small percentage of runners while participating in ultramarathons. In fact, vision problems may be severe enough to impact race performance in a small percentage of finishers and nonfinishers during 161-km ultramarathons (see **Table 2**)[29] and may become so severe that a runner is unable to continue running. The typical symptoms are a painless clouding of vision.[80] The underlying pathology is thought to be corneal edema evidenced by the observed corneal opacity.[80] The issue may recur in a subset of runners, and those with a history of refractive eye surgery seem to be at higher risk.[80] Some runners have been able to prevent recurrence by using protective eye wear and hydration lubricant eye drops. Fortunately, symptoms typically resolve without intervention within a few hours. However, it is important to recognize that the vision impairment can increase trip and fall risk or may lead to way-finding errors. When vision impairment compromises safety, it is cause for the athlete to discontinue the competition until adequate vision returns.

POTENTIAL LONG-TERM HEALTH ISSUES

It is well known that regular moderate exercise has considerable health and functional benefits. However, little is known about the potential health influences resulting from more extreme levels of exercise, including ultramarathon running. Concerns have risen that such activities may have adverse effects. Indeed, completion of a 161-km ultramarathon has been found to result in transient right ventricular dilation and dysfunction.[81,82] At present, it is not clear if repeated exposure and insufficient recovery time may lead to pathologic right ventricular adaptations, but the development of malignant ventricular arrhythmias does not appear to be associated with intense endurance exercise training.[83] Furthermore, coronary arteries of middle-aged ultramarathon runners have been found to be healthy,[84] so concerns about adverse cardiovascular effects from ultramarathon running seem premature. Other adverse health consequences, such as an increased risk of arthritis or cancer, also have been proposed, but evidence to support such concerns is lacking at present.

The ULTRA Study is a longitudinal health study of ultramarathon runners that was initiated in 2011 with primary intent to assess potential health consequences related to the high levels of exercise performed by these individuals. Thus far, only baseline findings are available, but they offer some insight into the health of this group.

Body weight and body mass index (BMI) are health-related measures affected by lifestyle. Previous cross-sectional analyses of BMI in 161-km ultramarathon runners have demonstrated that this group tends to have a healthy body weight and BMI, which is maintained with advancing age unlike what is seen in the general population.[21,85,86] Although the ULTRA Study found a negligible, but statistically significant, direct relationship between age and BMI, the strongest predictor of current BMI was BMI at age 25 years.[22] More importantly, we found strong inverse relationships between percent change in body weight since age 25 years and BMI at age 25 for both men and women. In other words, body weight shifted toward a more healthy weight in association with ultramarathon running.

As would be anticipated, individuals who are capable of running ultramarathons are healthier and have fewer medical needs than a comparable general population. Compared with self-reported data from the general population, the prevalence of virtually all chronic diseases and mental health disorders were found to be lower in the ultramarathon runners.[30] Asthma and allergies/hay fever are exceptions that appear to be higher in prevalence among ultramarathon runners compared with the general population. This may result from the effects of regular drying of the airways during exercise[87] and greater exposure to airborne allergens.[88] Although generally healthier than the general population, it should be noted that ultramarathon runners are not necessarily free of all serious illnesses. We observed a low prevalence of serious medical issues, including cancers (4.5%), coronary artery disease (0.7%), seizure disorders (0.7%), diabetes (0.7%), and human immunodeficiency virus infection (0.2%).[30]

Because ultramarathon runners may be healthier than the general population, they also miss less work.[21,46] This is partially accounted for by ultramarathon runners tending to have higher levels of education[21,22,24] and being more likely to have occupations in which minor medical issues do not prevent performance of work duties. Nevertheless, in comparison with a population of similar education and income levels, the ultramarathon runners were found to have less work loss from injury or illness.[46] The ultramarathon runners were also found to have a lower frequency of outpatient medical visits than the general population, even though medical visits specific to an exercise-related issue accounted for more than 60% of their use of the medical care system.

SUMMARY

Ultramarathon runners are a relatively small and unique group of distance runners with somewhat different medical issues than shorter distance runners. This article outlines some of those differences so that those caring for these runners in the clinic or at competitions might be better prepared.

REFERENCES

1. Anonymous. Ultrarunning 2013—the year in review. UltraRunning 2014;30–47.
2. Running USA. Running USA annual marathon report. 2014. Available at: http://www.runningusa.org/marathon-report-2014?returnTo=annual-reports. Accessed December 11, 2014.
3. Hoffman MD, Ong JC, Wang G. Historical analysis of participation in 161 km ultramarathons in North America. Int J Hist Sport 2010;27(11):1877–91.
4. Medinger J. Year in review. UltraRunning 2015;25–42.
5. David GC, Lehecka N. The spirit of the trail: culture, popularity and prize money in ultramarathoning. Available at: http://www.uta.edu/huma/agger/fastcapitalism/10_1/david_lehecka10_1.html. Accessed January 7, 2014.

6. Simpson D, Post PG, Young G, et al. "It's not about taking the easy road": the experiences of ultramarathon runners. Sport Psychol 2014;28:176–85.
7. Hunter SK, Stevens AA. Sex differences in marathon running with advanced age: physiology or participation? Med Sci Sports Exerc 2013;45(1):148–56.
8. Hunter SK, Stevens AA, Magennis K, et al. Is there a sex difference in the age of elite marathon runners? Med Sci Sports Exerc 2011;43(4):656–64.
9. Joyner MJ. Physiological limiting factors and distance running: influence of gender and age on record performances. Exerc Sport Sci Rev 1993;21:103–33.
10. USA Track and Field Web site. U.S All-time list—marathon, men. Available at: http://www.usatf.org/statistics/All-Time-Lists/MarathonMen.aspx. Accessed December 11, 2014.
11. USA Track and Field Web site. U.S. All-time list—marathon, women. Available at: http://www.usatf.org/statistics/All-Time-Lists/MarathonWomen.aspx. Accessed December 11, 2014.
12. Hoffman MD. Performance trends in 161-km ultramarathons. Int J Sports Med 2010;31(1):31–7.
13. Hoffman MD, Parise CA. Longitudinal assessment of age and experience on performance in 161-km ultramarathons. Int J Sports Physiol Perform 2015; 10(1):93–8.
14. Hoffman MD, Wegelin JA. The Western states 100-mile endurance run: participation and performance trends. Med Sci Sports Exerc 2009;41(12):2191–8.
15. Knechtle B, Rüst CA, Rosemann T, et al. Age-related changes in 100-km ultramarathon running performance. Age (Dordr) 2012;34(4):1033–45.
16. Rüst CA, Knechtle B, Eichenberger E, et al. Finisher and performance trends in female and male mountain ultramarathoners by age group. Int J Gen Med 2013;6:707–18.
17. Rüst CA, Knechtle B, Rosemann T, et al. Analysis of performance and age of the fastest 100-mile ultra-marathoners worldwide. Clinics (Sao Paulo) 2013;68(5):605–11.
18. Zingg M, Rüst CA, Lepers R, et al. Master runners dominate 24-h ultramarathons worldwide—a retrospective data analysis from 1998 to 2011. Extrem Physiol Med 2013;2(1):21.
19. Zingg MA, Knechtle B, Rüst CA, et al. Analysis of participation and performance in athletes by age group in ultramarathons of more than 200 km in length. Int J Gen Med 2013;6:209–20.
20. Running USA. Running USA annual half-marathon report. 2014. Available at: http://www.runningusa.org/2014-half-marathon-report?returnTo=annual-reports. Accessed December 11, 2014.
21. Hoffman MD, Fogard K. Demographic characteristics of 161-km ultramarathon runners. Res Sports Med 2012;20(1):59–69.
22. Hoffman MD, Chen L, Krishnan E. Body mass index and its correlates in 1,212 ultramarathon runners: baseline findings from the ULTRA study. J Phys Act Health 2015;11(8):1549–55.
23. Rauch TM, Tharion WJ, Strowman SR, et al. Psychological factors associated with performance in the ultramarathon. J Sports Med Phys Fitness 1988;28(3):237–46.
24. Thompson W, Nequin N. Ultrarunners—Who are they? UltraRunning 1983;3:22–3.
25. Acevedo EO, Dzewaltowski DA, Gill DL, et al. Cognitive orientations of ultramarathoners. Sport Psychol 1992;6:242–52.
26. Krouse RZ, Ransdell LB, Lucas SM, et al. Motivation, goal orientation, coaching, and training habits of women ultrarunners. J Strength Cond Res 2011;25(10):2835–42.
27. Stan Jensen. Stan Jensen's Web site. Available at: http://www.run100s.com. Accessed March 26, 2015.

28. Hoffman MD, Krishnan E. Exercise behavior of ultramarathon runners: baseline findings from the ULTRA study. J Strength Cond Res 2013;27(11):2939–45.
29. Hoffman MD, Fogard K. Factors related to successful completion of a 161-km ultramarathon. Int J Sports Physiol Perform 2011;6:25–37.
30. Hoffman MD, Krishnan E. Health and exercise-related medical issues among 1,212 ultramarathon runners: baseline findings from the Ultrarunners Longitudinal TRAcking (ULTRA) study. PLoS One 2014;9(1):e83867.
31. Bovens AM, Janssen GM, Vermeer HG, et al. Occurrence of running injuries in adults following a supervised training program. Int J Sports Med 1989; 10(Suppl 3):S186–90.
32. Lysholm J, Wiklander J. Injuries in runners. Am J Sports Med 1987;15:168–71.
33. Macera CA, Pate RR, Powell KE, et al. Predicting lower-extremity injuries among habitual runners. Arch Intern Med 1989;149:2565–8.
34. Walter SD, Hart LE, McIntosh JM, et al. The Ontario cohort study of running-related injuries. Arch Intern Med 1989;149:2561–4.
35. van Gent RN, Siem D, van Middelkoop M, et al. Incidence and determinants of lower extremity running injuries in long distance runners: a systematic review. Br J Sports Med 2007;41:469–80.
36. Hoffman MD, Stuempfle KJ. Sodium supplementation and exercise-associated hyponatremia during prolonged exercise. Med Sci Sports Exerc 2015;47(9): 1781–7.
37. Millet GY, Hoffman MD, Morin MB. Sacrificing economy to improve running performance—a reality in the ultramarathon? J Appl Physiol 2012;113:507–9.
38. Brubaker CE, James SL. Injuries to runners. J Sports Med 1974;2:189198.
39. James SL, Bates BT, Osternig LR. Injuries to runners. Am J Sports Med 1978; 6:40–50.
40. Matheson GO, Clement DB, McKenzie DC, et al. Stress fractures in athletes. A study of 320 cases. Am J Sports Med 1987;15:46–58.
41. McBryde AM Jr. Stress fractures in runners. Clin Sports Med 1985;4:737–52.
42. Bennell KL, Malcolm SA, Thomas SA, et al. The incidence and distribution of stress fractures in competitive track and field athletes. A twelve-month prospective study. Am J Sports Med 1996;24:211–7.
43. Brukner P, Bradshaw C, Khan KM, et al. Stress fractures: a review of 180 cases. Clin J Sport Med 1996;6:85–9.
44. Hoffman MD, Pasternak A, Rogers IR, et al. Medical services at ultra-endurance foot races in remote environments: medical issues and consensus guidelines. Sports Med 2014;44(8):1055–69.
45. Joslin J, Hoffman MD, Rogers I, et al. Special considerations in medical screening for participants in remote endurance events. Sports Med 2015;45(8): 1121–31.
46. Hoffman MD, Rogers IR, Joslin J, et al. Managing collapsed or seriously ill participants of ultra-endurance events in remote environments. Sports Med 2015;45(2): 201–12.
47. Krabak BJ, Waite B, Schiff MA. Study of injury and illness rates in multiday ultramarathon runners. Med Sci Sports Exerc 2011;43:2314–20.
48. Lipman GS, Ellis MA, Lewis EJ, et al. A prospective randomized blister prevention trial assessing paper tape in endurance distances (Pre-TAPED). Wilderness Environ Med 2014;25(4):457–61.
49. Scheer BV, Murray A. Al Andalus Ultra Trail: an observation of medical interventions during a 219-km, 5-day ultramarathon stage race. Clin J Sport Med 2011; 21:444–6.

50. Baska RS, Moses FM, Graeber G, et al. Gastrointestinal bleeding during an ultra-marathon. Dig Dis Sci 1990;35:276–9.
51. Glace B, Murphy C, McHugh M. Food and fluid intake and disturbances in gastrointestinal and mental function during an ultramarathon. Int J Sport Nutr Exerc Metab 2002;12:414–27.
52. McGowan V, Hoffman MD. Characterization of medical care at the 161-km Western States Endurance Run. Wilderness Environ Med 2015;26(1):29–35.
53. Stuempfle KJ, Hoffman MD. Gastrointestinal distress is common during a 161-km ultramarathon. J Sports Sci 2015;33(17):1814–21.
54. Stuempfle KJ, Hoffman MD, Hew-Butler T. Association of gastrointestinal distress in ultramarathoners with race diet. Int J Sport Nutr Exerc Metab 2013;23:103–9.
55. Bennett BL, Hew-Butler T, Hoffman MD, et al. Wilderness Medical Society practice guidelines for treatment of exercise-associated hyponatremia: 2014 update. Wilderness Environ Med 2014;25:S30–42.
56. Rehrer NJ, Brouns F, Beckers EJ, et al. Physiological changes and gastrointestinal symptoms as a result of ultra-endurance running. Eur J Appl Physiol Occup Physiol 1992;64:1–8.
57. Hew-Butler T, Rosner MH, Fowkes-Godek S, et al. Statement of the third international exercise-associated hyponatremia consensus development conference, Carlsbad, California, 2015. Clin J Sport Med 2015;25(4):303–20.
58. Ayus JC, Varon J, Arieff AI. Hyponatremia, cerebral edema, and noncardiogenic pulmonary edema in marathon runners. Ann Intern Med 2000;132(9):711–4.
59. Gardner JW. Death by water intoxication. Mil Med 2002;167(5):432–4.
60. Garigan TP, Ristedt DE. Death from hyponatremia as a result of acute water intoxication in an Army basic trainee. Mil Med 1999;164(3):234–8.
61. Kipps C, Sharma S, Tunstall Pedoe D. The incidence of exercise-associated hyponatraemia in the London marathon. Br J Sports Med 2011;45:14–9.
62. Myers TM, Hoffman MD. Hiker fatality from severe hyponatremia in Grand Canyon National Park. Wilderness Environ Med 2015;26(3):371–4.
63. Noakes T. Waterlogged: the serious problem of overhydration in endurance sports. Champaign (IL): Human Kinetics; 2012.
64. Siegel AJ, Verbalis JG, Clement S, et al. Hyponatremia in marathon runners due to inappropriate arginine vasopressin secretion. Am J Med 2007;120(5):461.e11-7.
65. Hoffman MD, Hew-Butler T, Stuempfle KJ. Exercise-associated hyponatremia and hydration status in 161-km ultramarathoners. Med Sci Sports Exerc 2013;45:784–91.
66. Stuempfle KJ, Lehmann DR, Case HS, et al. Hyponatremia in a cold weather ultraendurance race. Alaska Med 2002;44:51–5.
67. Hoffman MD, Stuempfle KJ, Rogers IR, et al. Hyponatremia in the 2009 161-km Western States Endurance Run. Int J Sports Physiol Perform 2012;7:6–10.
68. Lebus DK, Casazza GA, Hoffman MD, et al. Can changes in body mass and total body water accurately predict hyponatremia after a 161-km running race? Clin J Sport Med 2010;20:193–9.
69. Hoffman MD, Stuempfle KJ, Sullivan K, et al. Exercise-associated hyponatremia with exertional rhabdomyolysis: importance of proper treatment. Clin Nephrol 2014;83(4):235–42.
70. Noakes TD, Sharwood K, Speedy D, et al. Three independent biological mechanisms cause exercise-associated hyponatremia: evidence from 2,135 weighed competitive athletic performances. Proc Natl Acad Sci U S A 2005;102(51):18550–5.
71. Hoffman MD, Stuempfle KJ. Hydration strategies, weight change and performance in a 161-km ultramarathon. Res Sports Med 2014;22(3):213–25.

72. Winger J, Hoffman MD, Hew-Butler T, et al. The effect of physiology and hydration beliefs on race behavior and postrace sodium in 161-km ultramarathon finishers. Int J Sports Physiol Perform 2013;8:536–41.
73. Siegel AJ, d'Hemecourt P, Adner MM, et al. Exertional dysnatremia in collapsed marathon runners: a critical role for point-of-care testing to guide appropriate therapy. Am J Clin Pathol 2009;132(3):336–40.
74. Elsaesser TF, Pang PS, Malik S, et al. Large-volume hypertonic saline therapy in endurance athlete with exercise-associated hyponatremic encephalopathy. J Emerg Med 2013;44:1132–5.
75. Noakes TD. Hyponatremia in distance athletes: pulling the IV on the 'dehydration myth'. Phys Sportsmed 2000;28:71–6.
76. Bennett BL, Hew-Butler T, Hoffman MD, et al. In reply to clinical practice guidelines for treatment of exercise-associated hyponatremia. Wilderness Environ Med 2013;24:468–71.
77. McGarvey J, Thompson J, Hanna C, et al. Sensitivity and specificity of clinical signs for assessment of dehydration in endurance athletes. Br J Sports Med 2010;44:716–9.
78. Sharwood KA, Collins M, Goedecke JH, et al. Weight changes, medical complications, and performance during an Ironman triathlon. Br J Sports Med 2004;38(6):718–24.
79. Frizzell RT, Lang GH, Lowance DC, et al. Hyponatremia and ultramarathon running. JAMA 1986;255:772–4.
80. Høeg TB, Corrigan GK, Hoffman MD. An investigation of ultramarathon-associated visual impairment. Wilderness Environ Med 2015;26(2):200–4.
81. Lord R, Somauroo J, Stembridge M, et al. The right ventricle following ultra-endurance exercise: insights from novel echocardiography and 12-lead electrocardiography. Eur J Appl Physiol 2015;115(1):71–80.
82. Oxborough D, Shave R, Warburton D, et al. Dilatation and dysfunction of the right ventricle immediately after ultraendurance exercise: exploratory insights from conventional two-dimensional and speckle tracking echocardiography. Circ Cardiovasc Imaging 2011;4(3):253–63.
83. Andersen K, Farahmand B, Ahlbom A, et al. Risk of arrhythmias in 52 755 long-distance cross-country skiers: a cohort study. Eur Heart J 2013;34(47):3624–31.
84. Haskell WL, Sims C, Myll J, et al. Coronary artery size and dilating capacity in ultradistance runners. Circulation 1993;87(4):1076–82.
85. Hoffman MD. Anthropometric characteristics of ultramarathoners. Int J Sports Med 2008;29:1–4.
86. Hoffman MD, Lebus DK, Ganong AC, et al. Body composition of 161-km ultramarathoners. Int J Sports Med 2010;31:106–9.
87. Elers J, Pedersen L, Backer V. Asthma in elite athletes. Expert Rev Respir Med 2011;5:343–51.
88. Robson-Ansley P, Howatson G, Tallent J, et al. Prevalence of allergy and upper respiratory tract symptoms in runners of the London marathon. Med Sci Sports Exerc 2012;44:999–1004.

An Evidence-Based Videotaped Running Biomechanics Analysis

Richard B. Souza, PT, PhD, ATC, CSCS[a,b,c,*]

KEYWORDS

- Biomechanics • Running • Motion analysis • Form • Injuries • Observational
- Video analysis

KEY POINTS

- Running biomechanics play an important role in the development of injuries in recreationally active individuals.
- Performing a systematic video-based running biomechanics analysis rooted in the current evidence on running injuries can allow the clinician to develop a treatment strategy.
- The current literature has not risen to the level of proven injury prevention, suggesting that recommendations for modification of running form in uninjured runners would not be evidence based.
- When the patient presentation and physical examination findings are in agreement with abnormalities observed in a biomechanics running analysis, it serves as a potential for intervention.

INTRODUCTION

Running is an extremely common form of exercise, whether recreational or competitive. However, running injuries are also quite common. In particular, running injuries such as patellofemoral pain, iliotibial band syndrome, and stress fractures to the tibia and metatarsals have been identified as highly prevalent in runners.[1] Although causative factors of running injuries are undoubtedly multifactorial, most agree that running biomechanics play a key role in injury development.

Disclosure Statement: Dr R.B. Souza has a financial relationship with SportzPeak, Inc, a sports wellness company.

[a] Department of Physical Therapy and Rehabilitation Science, University of California, San Francisco, 185 Berry Street, Suite 350, San Francisco, CA 94107, USA; [b] Department of Radiology and Biomedical Imaging, University of California, San Francisco, 185 Berry Street, Suite 350, San Francisco, CA 94107, USA; [c] Department of Orthopaedic Surgery, University of California, San Francisco, 185 Berry Street, Suite 350, San Francisco, CA 94107, USA

* 185 Berry Street, Suite 350, San Francisco, CA 94107.

E-mail address: richard.souza@ucsf.edu

Numerous recent studies have identified abnormal biomechanics in persons with specific running injuries.[2–5] However, the vast majority of these studies used advanced technological methods, which are expensive and uncommon in standard clinical practice. Although some variables associated with running injuries require high-tech equipment, such as instrumented treadmills and 3-dimensional (3D) motion capture systems, many of the kinematic abnormalities identified in runners with injuries can be measured using a simple 2-dimensional (2D) video-based running analysis using readily available and fairly inexpensive tools.

The objective of this article is to provide a framework for a systematic video-based running biomechanics analysis plan based on the current evidence on running injuries. Although some of the proposed variables of interest ill have an impact on running performance, the primary focus of this analysis plan is to identify biomechanical factors related to common injuries in runners. Furthermore, there are many other factors that may be related or even causative for injuries while running, including training errors, current health status (ie, recent injury), and/or structural abnormalities (ie, leg length discrepancy, pes planus foot deformity etc).[6,7] However, the focus of this review is restricted to running kinematics, particularly those in the sagittal and frontal plane, which may be easily viewed with standard 2D video. A running biomechanics analysis should be an integral component of the evaluation, either for the injured runner or for screening for injury prevention, to complement a physical examination and thorough history.

ANALYSIS SETUP
Treadmill Setup

Although some studies have identified small differences in treadmill running when compared with overground running, these differences have mostly been associated with muscle activation patterns and joint forces.[8,9] In general, kinematic patterns during treadmill running are very similar to those observed during overground running.[10–12] As such, performing a video-based analysis of joint kinematics while running on a treadmill should provide valuable insight into running kinematics during overground running and is more practical for performing this evaluation.

Running velocity affects lower extremity kinematics.[13] Therefore, matching treadmill speed to a similar speed at which an injured runner experiences symptoms should be accommodated if possible. When evaluating a symptom-free runner, 1 strategy that can be used is to set the treadmill speed to match the running velocity of the runner when performing a "long run," which is a common term used for the longest distance run in the recent past. The rationale for selecting this speed is that if runners are demonstrating abnormal biomechanics while performing longer runs, these faults will accumulate over the longer exercise period and may contribute to running injuries.

Cameras

Many high-definition cameras are available at varying price points. Both image resolution and temporal resolution should be considered when selecting cameras for video-based movement analysis. Many video cameras have excellent image resolution, but are limited to 30 frames per second. Cameras with higher frame rates (eg, $\geq$120 Hz) can provide cleaner images that are easier to evaluate and more appropriate for the evaluation of running kinematics. More recently released smartphones and tablets can be adjusted to acquire video at high frame rates and provide adequate video for this purpose.

Views

When performing a video-based analysis it is recommended that, at a minimum, 2 orthogonal (at right angles to each other) views are included. The analysis provided in this article uses a lateral view and a posterior view. Others may include an anterior view or lateral views from both sides. Multiple views from each camera, including zoomed-in views on the foot and ankle as well as zoomed-out views of the entire body, can be helpful. Many of these preferences will need to be modified to work within the constraints of the clinical environment. Maintaining a reproducible camera location and a fixed orthogonal angle to the treadmill is important to performing a reliable analysis. Recent studies have found the reliability of a single camera analysis to vary significantly, with some metrics showing excellent reproducibility (knee flexion, rear foot kinematics) and others demonstrating poor reproducibility (heel-to-center of mass distance).[14] There is also evidence that experience can improve the reliability of measurements made on video-based kinematic evaluations, so it is important for the clinician to practice running evaluations regularly to improve reliability.[15]

Markers

Application of markers for identification of anatomic landmarks can be useful when performing a video-based running analysis. These markers need not be expensive retroreflective tape-based markers. Any bright colored tape can be used for this purpose. Whenever possible, tape should be applied directly to the runner's skin. This is imperative when performing research-level 3D motion analysis. However, adapting these methods for use in a clinical setting may require markers over clothes. In these situations, it is recommended that the runners wear tight-fitting running sportswear to minimize the movement of the markers from clothing during running. In the images presented throughout this article, the following landmarks are identified and marked: C7 spinous process, posterior superior iliac spines, anterior superior iliac spine, greater trochanter, lateral knee joint line, lateral malleolus, midpoint of the calf, superior and inferior portions of the heel shoe counter, and head of the fifth metatarsal. This is an example of a common set of anatomy landmarks that are useful to evaluate during running and can be modified to suit the needs to the evaluation.

Warmup and Analysis Plan

It is advisable to allow for a period of time for the runner to run on the treadmill at the target speed to accommodate to the environment. Studies have identified changes in kinematics deviating from normal running mechanics with treadmill running up to the initial 6 minutes.[16] Therefore, an acclimation period of 6 to 10 minutes should be used when possible before evaluation. It is also important consider the nature of symptom provocation in an injured runner. If a runner experiences symptoms after a number of minutes or miles, it may be necessary to acquire video with the runner in a fatigued state, after a period of running and consistent with their symptom history.

When performing a movement analysis of any type, it is critical to execute the analysis systematically. We present a distal-to-proximal analysis plan. The order of the evaluation is not critical. However, it is extremely important to perform the entire evaluation, including all segments, joints, and whole body variables consistently, to avoid missing subtle yet potentially important kinematic abnormalities. Although numerous freeware options exist with extremely helpful tools for measuring biomechanical variables on running video (angles, distances, etc), it is generally not necessary. Most of the metrics in this article can be easily identified visually on slow motion video, or evaluation when progressing through the video frame by frame. To date, cutoffs for kinematics to be identified as abnormal, or predictive of injury, do not exist. As such, the analyses included here does not provide the reader with specific angles or measures that are "abnormal." Each metric is described, and indicators of normal kinematics are provided. It is the responsibility of the evaluator to determine what threshold for normal and abnormal should be applied to an individual runner and associated with the biomechanical contributor to injury.

Phases

It is important to identify specific moments within the running cycle that can be used for evaluation. Many of the phases of the running cycle are clear. However, particularly for evaluating stride mechanics, it is important to differentiate between video frames of rapidly evolving events. Take, for example, the images provided in **Fig. 1**. **Fig. 1**A is the final frame of the swing phase, **Fig. 1**B displays initial contact, and **Fig. 1**C displays loading response (which is identified by the presence of shoe deformation in the image). Different kinematic variables are evaluated on images from different phases of running. It is important for the evaluator to become familiar with identifying each of these phases (and others as described elsewhere in this article). Inconsistent identification of phases of running in evaluating biomechanics of running gait will make performing a reliable analysis impossible.

SIDE VIEW
Foot Strike Pattern

Identification of foot strike pattern can be easily performed on slow motion video or by evaluating video in a frame-by-frame manner (**Fig. 2**). It is recommended to always confirm foot strike pattern in this fashion, because even after considerable practice, it is not uncommon to misidentify a foot strike type when observing running at full speed. Foot strike types can be categorized as forefoot strike (FFS), midfoot strike, and rear foot strike. Recent literature suggests that video-based identification of foot strike patterns by a single rater are highly reliable, although interrater measures was found to be less reliable.[17] At this time, there is limited evidence that any 1 foot strike pattern is more or less likely to cause a runner to sustain an injury. However, this is an area of active research and data on this issue are emerging.[18,19] One study on competitive collegiate runners suggested that runners with a rear foot strike pattern developed more repetitive overuse injuries when compared with runners with an FFS pattern.[20] And although these finding suggest possible association between foot

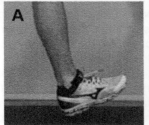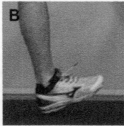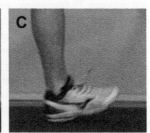

Fig. 1. Key phases of running. (*A*) The end of terminal swing is identified as to the foot remains elevated from the treadmill, just before initial contact. (*B*) Initial contact is identified as the first frame when the foot hits the ground. (*C*) Loading response is identified as the first frame in which the runner's weight is being transferred onto the lead leg and is characterized by the presence of shoe deformation.

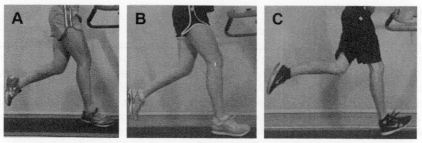

Fig. 2. Foot strike patterns. (*A*) Forefoot strike. (*B*) Midfoot strike. (*C*) Rear foot strike.

strike patterns and running injuries, more work is necessary before broad conclusions on foot strike recommendations can be made to modify injury risk.

Foot Inclination Angle at Initial Contact

The angle created by the sole of the shoe and the treadmill belt is noted as the inclination angle of the foot (relative to a global coordinate system, not the tibia) at initial contact (**Fig. 3**). This variable is not applicable for midfoot strike and FFS runners.

A recent study by Wille and colleagues[21] found inclination angle to be particularly important in estimating ground reaction forces and joint kinetics during running. Specifically, increased foot inclination angle was found to be related to higher peak knee extensor moments, increased knee energy absorbed, higher peak vertical ground reaction force, and greater braking impulse during running. Each of these variables has been implicated in injury biomechanics, suggesting that a very high foot inclination angle at initial contact may not be desirable. This may be a source for intervention in runners who experience injuries associated with high ground reaction forces or excessive joint kinetics. There are no cutoffs at which this angle is determined to be abnormal. Rather, it is likely on a sliding scale, where lower values are generally associated with lower ground reaction forces and joint kinetics, and higher values as associated with increased forces. However, it should be noted that a high foot inclination angle in isolation may be a benign finding and needs to be evaluated in the context of the entire running evaluations (see Overstriding).

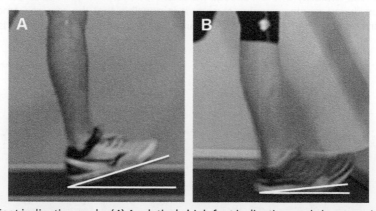

Fig. 3. Foot inclination angle. (*A*) A relatively high foot inclination angle in comparison with a horizontal line. (*B*) A relatively low foot inclination angle.

Tibia Angle at Loading Response

The vertical alignment of the lower leg during loading response can be a valuable indicator of stride mechanics. Video of the runner should be evaluated using freeze-frames at the moment of loading response (as the shoe begins to deform just after initial contact). The alignment of the lower leg relative to a vertical line in the video field of view can be evaluated easily. An extended tibia is identified when the lateral knee joint marker is posterior to the lateral malleolus marker (**Fig. 4**A). Conversely, a flexed tibia is identified when the lateral knee marker is anterior to the lateral malleolus (**Fig. 4**C), and when these 2 markers are directly vertical to one another, this would be identified as a vertical tibia (**Fig. 4**B). For a runner that suffers from impact-related running injuries, an extended tibia is not ideal. A vertical or flexed tibia allows the runner to dissipate impact more readily though knee flexion.

Similar to foot inclination angle, the tibia angle in itself may not be meaningful in isolation. It is a variable that can be grouped in a series of stride mechanics variables to better describe the characteristics of the runners stride and biomechanical risk profile.

Knee Flexion During Stance

Peak knee flexion angle during stance may occur at slightly different phases in different runners. It is recommended to scroll through stance phase frames to identify maximum knee flexion. Key aspects of knee flexion during stance include the peak amount of knee flexion and the knee joint excursion during stance (difference in angle from initial contact to peak knee flexion). In general, normal peak knee flexion approaches approximately 45° at midstance (**Fig. 5**). Although explicit cutoffs have not been developed for this variable, a runner who demonstrates considerably less than 45° of knee flexion may suggest reduced shock absorption, and intervention may be warranted. Some data exist suggesting that lower knee flexion (<40°) may be associated with certain subgroups of patients with patellofemoral pain.[22] Knee stiffness, a variable that includes both reduced knee flexion and/or increased knee flexion moment during stance phase, may be associated with tibial stress fractures.[23]

Hip Extension During Late Stance

Reduced hip extension during late stance is a common observation in the recreational runner (**Fig. 6**). It is traditionally believed that lack of hip extension may be associated with reduced flexibility of the iliopsoas muscle. However, the optimal amount of hip extension during running remains elusive. It is possible that the required amount of hip extension is not the same for each runner, but related to other characteristics of

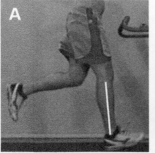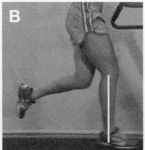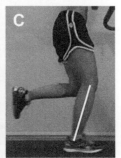

Fig. 4. Tibia angle. (*A*) Extended tibia. (*B*) Vertical tibia. (*C*) Flexed tibia.

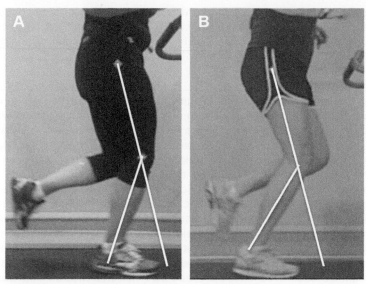

Fig. 5. Knee flexion during stance. (*A*) A runner demonstrating limited knee flexion during stance and (*B*) a normal amount of knee flexion during stance.

their running form. For example, a fairly slow runner may have a very compact stride, demonstrate approximately 10° of peak hip extension and not require any intervention. However, a different runner, with a long stride and perhaps a faster pace, may also have approximately 10° of hip extension, but also concurrently demonstrate a significant overstride pattern (landing with the foot out in front of the center of mass) with higher impact loading and braking forces. The latter runner may require stride modification or improved hip extension during running to modify these forces that could contribute to injury. Commonly observed compensations for persons with reduced hip extension include (1) increased lumbar spine extension, (2) bounding, a strategy

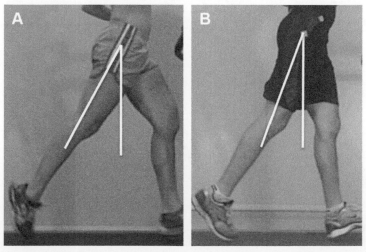

Fig. 6. Hip extension during late stance. (*A*) Runner with normal hip extension. (*B*) Runner with limited hip extension.

to increase float time to increase overall stride length in the absence of adequate hip extension, (3) increased overstriding, including excessive reaching during initial contact as a strategy to increase stride length, and (4) increased cadence to increase running speed in the presence of a limited hip extension.

Trunk Lean

Trunk lean is a variable that has received little attention in the scientific literature. However, this is not the case in the popular running non–peer-reviewed literature. Many running styles, including ChiRunning, pose running, and even barefoot running have included cues for novice runners to increase trunk lean. A focus on leaning "from the ankles," rather than increasing hip flexion to achieve the trunk lean, seems to be a priority for some styles. Many running experts suggest that trunk lean is a key component to correct running posture. However, very little has been done on the research side of this issue. A recent article by Teng and Powers[24] demonstrated that a small increase in trunk lean ($\sim 7°$) resulted in a significant lowering of the stress across the patellofemoral joint without a significant increase in ankle demand, suggesting that this strategy may be important for runners with patellofemoral pain. The overall findings were that reduced trunk flexion (more upright posture) was associated with greater knee loads. In contrast, increased trunk flexion shifted demand away from the knee joint, and to the hip and ankle (although the latter was not statistically higher).[25] However, the authors warn that this study was performed in healthy subjects and more work is necessary to understand the relationship between trunk lean and running injuries. Furthermore, the authors noted that the trunk lean in these subjects was not purely from the ankles, as is recommended by some running styles, but rather a combination of hip flexion, pelvis anterior tilt, and other small kinematic adjustments. Nonetheless, evaluating trunk lean in runners may become an important variable as additional research emerges (**Fig. 7**).

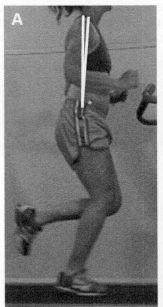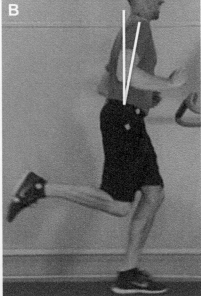

Fig. 7. Trunk lean. (*A*) A relatively upright trunk posture and (*B*) a runner a forward trunk lean.

Overstriding

Increased stride length has been found to be associated with an increased risk of tibial stress fractures in runners.[5] However, it is likely that a long stride is not the cause of high impacts associated with stress fractures and other running injuries. Rather, the presence and magnitude of overstriding may be the key risk factor. Many accomplished runners with very long strides have large amounts of hip extension without the presence of overstriding. It can be argued that these runners are not at risk for the injuries associated with high impacts.[26] It is important to differentiate stride length from overstriding in this context. Overstriding is a description of a running pattern in which the foot lands in front of the person's center of mass, and is associated with reaching, including hip flexion with knee extension, before initial contact. A recent study by Wille and colleagues[21] identified a metric that is closely related to overstriding—the distance from the heel at initial contact to the runners center of mass—is a significant predictor of knee extensor moment (the sagittal plane torque across the knee joint during stance) and braking impulse (an important contributor to shock attenuation and running energetics) during running. These data strongly suggest that overstriding is an important kinematic metric to consider when advanced technology, such as force platforms or tibia accelerometers, are not available.

As discussed, overstriding can be evaluated through a variety of metrics. Supportive measures such as the foot inclination angle at initial contact, tibial angle at loading response, and knee flexion at initial contact can inform the clinician about the tendency for overstriding. Ultimately, 1 strategy for determination of overstriding on video can be assessed by evaluating the runner at loading response.[27] By drawing a vertical line from the runner's lateral malleolus and extending upward, the relationship between the ankle position and the pelvis can be evaluated. Ideally, the vertical line will fall within the runner's pelvis, indicating that the foot is landing under the center of mass of the runner (**Fig. 8**A). If the vertical line is observed anterior to the pelvis (**Fig. 8**B), this indicates an overstride. Note that this dichotomous metric is not without limitations. In particular, it does not account for trunk flexion angle, which impacts the actual center of mass of the runner, and may be less useful for runners with a midfoot strike or FFS. Nonetheless, it is a very useful tool for identifying the presence of overstriding in runners.

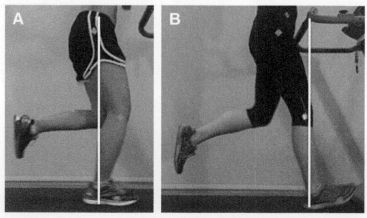

Fig. 8. Overstriding, measured at loading response. (*A*) A runner demonstrating normal stride mechanics and (*B*) a runner demonstrating an overstride, characterized by a vertical line through the lateral malleolus falling anterior to the runners pelvis.

Vertical Displacement of the Center of Mass

The vertical displacement of the center of mass is a very important metric to evaluate in runners. It is easily measured by comparing frames of video from the runner's highest point during float, to the lowest point during stance (**Fig. 9**). There are inherent errors in measuring this variable, because the actual location of the center of mass is impossible to assess on video. One strategy is to identify a location on the runner's pelvis and then to use this as a surrogate for the center of mass. Vertical displacement during running has key implications for injury mechanics as well as energetics. Increased excursion of the center of mass vertically has been found to be predictive of the peak knee extensor moment, the peak vertical ground reaction force, as well

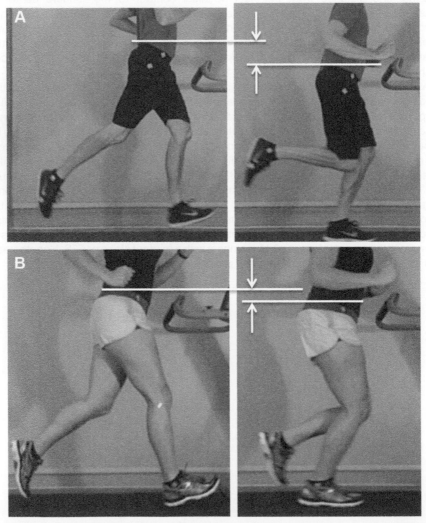

Fig. 9. Vertical displacement of the center of mass. (*A*) A bounding runner characterized by a large vertical displacement and (*B*) a relatively efficient runner with less vertical displacement.

as braking impulse during running, all very important variables in running mechanics.[21] This variable can become a problem in "bounders," runners who increase float time, often in response to other deficits (eg, reduced hip extension). The end result is increased work required by the runner to perform this type of running. It has been found that increasing cadence by 10% during running can reduce significantly the vertical displacement of the center of mass.[28]

Additional Variables

Auditory

A lot of information can be gathered from the sounds made during running. Certainly, auditory information differs between treadmills and runners of varying sizes. However, the clinician can quickly calibrate the normal or typical impact sounds of their treadmill, and this can be very useful in gathering information about impact during running. Greater noise with striking the treadmill may be associated with higher impact forces. In addition, asymmetries can quickly be identified by listening to the foot strike patterns of the runner. All of this information can be very valuable for a biomechanics running analysis.

Shaking of the treadmill

In addition to auditory information, the reaction of the treadmill at the time of impact can also provide important information. Some large, sturdy treadmills may not provide this information, but many models provide differing amounts to shaking or giving way in response to impact, and this can be very informative to the observant evaluator.

Cadence

The step rate, or cadence, should be evaluated in all runners. This variable is easily measured in a variety of ways. One strategy is to count the number of right heel strikes over a 1-minute period. This number is equivalent to the "stride rate." Multiplying this number by 2 equates to the "step rate." Several recent studies have evaluated the biomechanical consequences of manipulating cadence.[28–32] These data suggest that an increase in cadence can result in several biomechanical changes in running form, many of which may be desirable in specific runners. For example, it has been demonstrated that increasing cadence by 10% can reduce center of mass vertical excursion, braking impulse, and mechanical energy absorbed at the knee, as well as decrease peak hip adduction angle and peak hip adduction and internal rotation moments during running.[28] The optimal cadence has been an area of debate, with some suggesting that approximately 180 steps per minute being ideal. However, the majority of support for this comes from running economy studies, not studies on injury mechanics.[33,34] Although it may be too early to suggest that all runners should run at a specific cadence, it is becoming clear that cadence is an important biomechanical running variable, and one that can be easily manipulated in runners when appropriate.

POSTERIOR VIEW
Base of Support

Evaluating the base of support can be an important variable to make note of in specific runners. Running step width can vary as a function of running speed, but may also be related to common running injuries. A general rule can be followed that, when viewed from a posterior video, the left and right feet should not overlap in their ground contact location. It is not necessary that there be a large gap between the foot placement locations of the left and right feet, but there should be some space. A narrow base of support has been linked to tibial stress fractures, iliotibial band syndrome, and several kinematic patterns that have been associated with running injuries, such as excessive hip adduction and overpronation.[35–37] As such, this variable should be evaluated in all runners, and runners with a "cross-over sign" or "scissoring gait," characterized by an overly narrow base of support, may consider modification.

Heel Eversion

Foot pronation in runners is a variable that has received considerable attention over many years.[38–41] However, measuring foot pronation on 2D video presents significant challenges. One component of foot pronation that can be evaluated is heel eversion. By placing markers at the top and bottom of the shoe heel counter (**Fig. 10**), evaluation of the vertical relationship of the hindfoot can be assessed easily. It is important to evaluate not only the peak magnitude of heel eversion (ie, the relationship of the superior marker to the inferior marker), but also the rate of pronation (**Fig. 11**). The image in **Fig. 11**B occurs 5 frames after **Fig. 11**A, equating to approximately 20 milliseconds (collected at 240 frames per second). This rapid heel eversion is worthy of note as eversion velocity may play a role in specific running injuries. Several studies have linked excessive heel eversion to various running injuries, such as tibial stress fractures, patellofemoral pain, and Achilles tendonopathy.[41–43] Furthermore, it has been suggested that runners with excessive calcaneal eversion be prescribed orthotics,[44] or higher level of support shoes; however, the effectiveness of these strategies has been questioned, and current evidence is inconclusive.[45,46]

Foot Progression Angle

The foot progression angle is the transverse plane position of the foot during stance phase. As a transverse plane variable, it is not easily quantified on 2D video using our suggested setup. However, a general assessment can be made from a posterior video. A typical amount of toe-out observed during running results in the lateral aspect of the shoe being visualized from the posterior view (**Fig. 12**A). This usually equates to approximately 5° to 10° of toe-out. A mild toe-in abnormality and severe toe-in abnormality are displayed in **Fig. 12**B, C, and can be identified by the visualization of the 1st ray and medial aspect of the shoe. Abnormally toe-in foot progression angle may be associated with hip internal rotation, knee internal rotation, ankle internal rotation, or

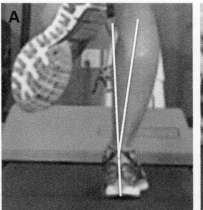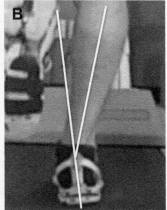

Fig. 10. Heel eversion. (A) A runner with normal alignment of the heel during running and (B) a runner with mildly excessive heel eversion during running.

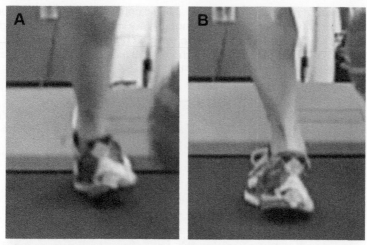

Fig. 11. Rate of heel eversion. A runner demonstrating excessive heel eversion and a high rate of heel eversion excursion. (*A*) Initial contact with the runner's heel in an inverted position and (*B*) 20 milliseconds later the heel has rotated more than 20° into eversion.

some combination of these. Several studies have identified these motions in connection with various running injuries, suggesting that this variable should be considered in a biomechanics running analysis.[47–49] Excessive toe-out is also not uncommonly seen. Although fewer studies have linked excessive toe-out or lower extremity external rotation to running injuries, it is reasonable to speculate that abnormal flexibility, including tight hip external rotators, may play a role in excessive toe-out while running. Further research is need in this area.

Heel Whips

A heel whip is another transverse plane variable that can be challenging to measure accurately on 2D video. However, a recent study has found this metric to be reliably measured from a posterior approach.[50] The whip angle is measured by comparing

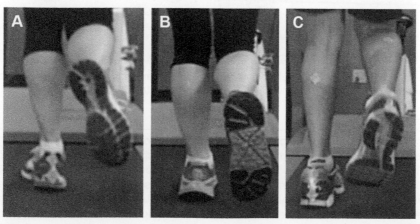

Fig. 12. Foot progression. (*A*) Normal foot progression angle. (*B*) Mild toe-in abnormality. (*C*) Severe toe-in abnormality.

the angle of the plantar surface of the shoe at initial contact with the plantar surface at the point of maximum rotation (**Fig. 13**). Although very little has been published on this variable, and the significance of this metric remains unknown, data suggest that an angular rotation of more than 5° in either the medial (see **Fig. 13**A, B) or lateral (see **Fig. 13**C, D) is observed in more than one-half of recreational runners.

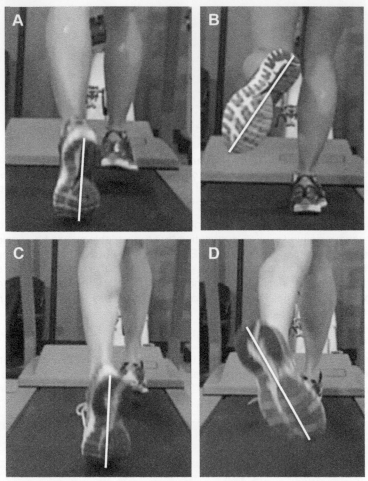

Fig. 13. Heel whips. Medial heel whip at initial swing (*A*) and maximum whip angle (*B*) and lateral heel whip at initial swing (*C*) and maximum whip (*D*).

Knee Window

Excessive hip adduction, excessive hip internal rotation, and excessive knee valgus have all been implicated in running injuries.[3,49,51,52] Each of these variables has the potential to impact the runner's "knee window." Evaluation of the knee window is a simple, dichotomous assessment of the presence or absence of a space between the knees at all times of the running cycle, and is a measure of the alignment of the hip, knee, and ankle from a posterior (or anterior) view (**Fig. 14**). The knee window does not need to be large—an excessively large knee window may suggest a varus deformity, an alignment issue that also presents with potential problems. However, the vast

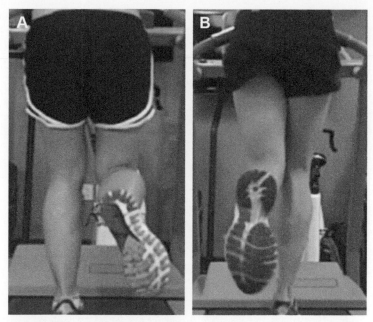

Fig. 14. Knee window. (*A*) Normal knee window and (*B*) "closed" knee window.

majority of recreational runners who fail to demonstrate a normal knee window or lose the window during the gait cycle, associated with the kinematic pattern described—namely, excessive hip adduction and internal rotation, and knee valgus. Although identification of this variable is quite simple, it should be noted that correcting an abnormally "closed" knee window is not as simple.[53] There are some limitations to this measurement. It is important for runners to wear shorts or tight-fitting pants so that this variable can be assessed. In runners with excessive soft tissue on the medial aspect of the knee, this measurement can be inaccurate. Finally, swing limb hip adduction can also create the impression of a closed knee window, even in the presence of good hip–knee–ankle alignment. Nonetheless, this measurement can be a valuable component of a biomechanics running evaluation, and several recent studies have found this variable to be modifiable through a variety of methods.[54–56]

Pelvic Drop

Assessing the amount of pelvic drop, or maximum pelvic obliquity during stance phase, can be augmented with the application of markers on the posterior superior iliac spines (**Fig. 15**). By comparing stance limb and swing limb marker positions, the amount of pelvic drop can be estimated. Excessive pelvic drop during running contributes to excessive hip adduction, a variable that has been linked to numerous running injuries.[49,51] A recent study found that a 2D quantitative assessment of this variable demonstrated excellent reliability but was poorly correlated with a 3D measurement of pelvic drop.[57] However, the clinical significance of 3D-measured pelvic drop has also been called into question.[2,58] It is possible that pelvic drop may serve as a surrogate measure for hip and/or core muscle weakness. Pelvic drop during running has been reported to be significantly related to both hip abductor strength and hip extension strength, and fatiguing of these muscles have been observed to result in excessive pelvic drop.[59,60] Looking for side to side differences can be helpful

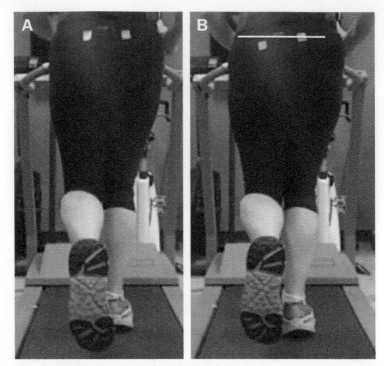

Fig. 15. Excessive pelvic drop. (*A*) At initial contact the runner's pelvis is fairly level and (*B*) during stance demonstrating excessive pelvis drop.

in detecting excessive pelvic drop and correlation with associated kinetic chain deficits should be performed to see how this contributes to injury. Although further research is necessary in this area, pelvic drop remains as a variable of interest in a biomechanics running analysis.

SUMMARY

Running biomechanics play an important role in the development of injuries in recreationally active individuals. Performing a systematic, video-based running biomechanics analysis rooted in the current evidence on running injuries can allow the clinician to develop a treatment strategy for injured runners. The majority of the current literature has not risen to the level of proven injury prevention strategies in correcting each aspect of running gait detailed in this review, suggesting that recommendations for modification of running form in uninjured runners would not be evidence based. However, when the patient presentation and physical examination findings are in agreement with abnormalities observed in a biomechanics running analysis, it serves as a potential for intervention.

The analysis plan described is not intended to be taken as a "gold standard" or a comprehensive running evaluation. Numerous other running evaluations from a biomechanics perspective are available and should be incorporated into each clinician's protocol.[61,62] It is simply a well-tested and frequently revised evaluation plan that has been successful in evaluating recreational runners. Furthermore, it is expected that this analysis plan will continue to evolve as future research emerges. Certain variables will likely materialize as critical to injury development and prevention, and others will turn out to be unrelated. Nonetheless, the components outlined in this review may serve as a template for a systematic evaluation plan to be improved upon by others, as more information about running biomechanics surfaces. Running biomechanics play a key role in injury development and prevention. Identifying simple 2D surrogates for 3D biomechanic variables of interest will allow for widespread translation of best practices, and have the best opportunity to impact this highly prevalent problem.

ACKNOWLEDGMENT

The author thanks Nicole Haas, PT, OCS, and Suzanne Souza, PT, OCS for reviewing this article, and providing invaluable clinical input.

REFERENCES

1. Taunton JE, Ryan MB, Clement DB, et al. A retrospective case-control analysis of 2002 running injuries. Br J Sports Med 2002;36(2):95–101.
2. Noehren B, Pohl MB, Sanchez Z, et al. Proximal and distal kinematics in female runners with patellofemoral pain. Clin Biomech 2012;27(4):366–71.
3. Noehren B, Schmitz A, Hempel R, et al. Assessment of strength, flexibility, and running mechanics in men with iliotibial band syndrome. J Orthop Sports Phys Ther 2014;44(3):217–22.
4. Milner CE, Hamill J, Davis I. Are knee mechanics during early stance related to tibial stress fracture in runners? Clin Biomech 2007;22(6):697–703.
5. Edwards WB, Taylor D, Rudolphi TJ, et al. Effects of stride length and running mileage on a probabilistic stress fracture model. Med Sci Sports Exerc 2009; 41(12):2177–84.
6. Johnston CA, Taunton JE, Lloyd-Smith DR, et al. Preventing running injuries. Practical approach for family doctors. Can Fam Physician 2003;49:1101–9.
7. Fields KB, Sykes JC, Walker KM, et al. Prevention of running injuries. Curr Sports Med Rep 2010;9(3):176–82.
8. Nigg BM, De Boer RW, Fisher V. A kinematic comparison of overground and treadmill running. Med Sci Sports Exerc 1995;27(1):98–105.
9. Sinclair J, Richards J, Taylor PJ, et al. Three-dimensional kinematic comparison of treadmill and overground running. Sports Biomech 2013;12(3):272–82.
10. Fellin RE, Manal K, Davis IS. Comparison of lower extremity kinematic curves during overground and treadmill running. J Appl Biomech 2010;26(4):407–14.
11. Lee SJ, Hidler J. Biomechanics of overground vs. treadmill walking in healthy individuals. J Appl Physiol 2008;104(3):747–55.
12. Riley PO, Dicharry J, Franz J, et al. A kinematics and kinetic comparison of overground and treadmill running. Med Sci Sports Exerc 2008;40(6):1093–100.
13. Brughelli M, Cronin J, Chaouachi A. Effects of running velocity on running kinetics and kinematics. J Strength Cond Res 2011;25(4):933–9.
14. Kotecki K, Rolfing J, Justman M, et al. Reliability of a standardized single-camera running gait analysis in active adults. J Orthop Sports Phys Ther 2015;43(1):A68.
15. Brunnekreef JJ, van Uden CJ, van Moorsel S, et al. Reliability of videotaped observational gait analysis in patients with orthopedic impairments. BMC Musculoskelet Disord 2005;6:17.
16. Lavcanska V, Taylor NF, Schache AG. Familiarization to treadmill running in young unimpaired adults. Hum Mov Sci 2005;24(4):544–57.
17. Damsted C, Larsen LH, Nielsen RO. Reliability of video-based identification of footstrike pattern and video time frame at initial contact in recreational runners. Gait Posture 2015;42(1):32–5.

18. Gruber AH, Umberger BR, Braun B, et al. Economy and rate of carbohydrate oxidation during running with rearfoot and forefoot strike patterns. J Appl Physiol 2013;115(2):194–201.

19. Mann R, Malisoux L, Nuhrenborger C, et al. Association of previous injury and speed with running style and stride-to-stride fluctuations. Scand J Med Sci Sports 2014. [Epub ahead of print].

20. Daoud AI, Geissler GJ, Wang F, et al. Foot strike and injury rates in endurance runners: a retrospective study. Med Sci Sports Exerc 2012;44(7):1325–34.

21. Wille CM, Lenhart RL, Wang S, et al. Ability of Sagittal kinematic variables to estimate ground reaction forces and joint kinetics in running. J Orthop Sports Phys Ther 2014;44(10):825–30.

22. Dierks TA, Manal KT, Hamill J, et al. Lower extremity kinematics in runners with patellofemoral pain during a prolonged run. Med Sci Sports Exerc 2011;43(4):693–700.

23. Milner CE, Ferber R, Pollard CD, et al. Biomechanical factors associated with tibial stress fracture in female runners. Med Sci Sports Exerc 2006;38(2):323–8.

24. Teng HL, Powers CM. Sagittal plane trunk posture influences patellofemoral joint stress during running. J Orthop Sports Phys Ther 2014;44(10):785–92.

25. Teng HL, Powers CM. Influence of trunk posture on lower extremity energetics during running. Med Sci Sports Exerc 2015;47(3):625–30.

26. Hreljac A, Marshall RN, Hume PA. Evaluation of lower extremity overuse injury potential in runners. Med Sci Sports Exerc 2000;32(9):1635–41.

27. Maschi R. How to perform a video analysis of a runner. Proceedings of the pre-conference course from the combined sections meeting of the American Physical Therapy Association; San Diego, CA, February 16, 2010.

28. Heiderscheit BC, Chumanov ES, Michalski MP, et al. Effects of step rate manipulation on joint mechanics during running. Med Sci Sports Exerc 2011;43(2):296–302.

29. Hobara H, Sato T, Sakaguchi M, et al. Step frequency and lower extremity loading during running. Int J Sports Med 2012;33(4):310–3.

30. Chumanov ES, Wille CM, Michalski MP, et al. Changes in muscle activation patterns when running step rate is increased. Gait Posture 2012;36(2):231–5.

31. Lenhart RL, Thelen DG, Wille CM, et al. Increasing running step rate reduces patellofemoral joint forces. Med Sci Sports Exerc 2014;46(3):557–64.

32. Lenhart R, Thelen D, Heiderscheit B. Hip muscle loads during running at various step rates. J Orthop Sports Phys Ther 2014;44(10):766–74. A1–4.

33. Hunter I, Smith GA. Preferred and optimal stride frequency, stiffness and economy: changes with fatigue during a 1-h high-intensity run. Eur J Appl Physiol 2007;100(6):653–61.

34. de Ruiter CJ, Verdijk PW, Werker W, et al. Stride frequency in relation to oxygen consumption in experienced and novice runners. Eur J Sport Sci 2014;14(3):251–8.

35. Meardon SA, Campbell S, Derrick TR. Step width alters iliotibial band strain during running. Sports Biomech 2012;11(4):464–72.

36. Brindle RA, Milner CE, Zhang S, et al. Changing step width alters lower extremity biomechanics during running. Gait Posture 2014;39(1):124–8.

37. Meardon SA, Derrick TR. Effect of step width manipulation on tibial stress during running. J Biomech 2014;47(11):2738–44.

38. Buchbinder MR, Napora NJ, Biggs EW. The relationship of abnormal pronation to chondromalacia of the patella in distance runners. J Am Podiatry Assoc 1979;69(2):159–62.

39. Tiberio D. The effect of excessive subtalar joint pronation on patellofemoral mechanics: a theoretical model. J Orthop Sports Phys Ther 1987;9(4):160–5.
40. Boling MC, Padua DA, Marshall SW, et al. A prospective investigation of biomechanical risk factors for patellofemoral pain syndrome: the Joint Undertaking to Monitor and Prevent ACL Injury (JUMP-ACL) cohort. Am J Sports Med 2009; 37(11):2108–16.
41. Barton CJ, Bonanno D, Levinger P, et al. Foot and ankle characteristics in patellofemoral pain syndrome: a case control and reliability study. J Orthop Sports Phys Ther 2010;40(5):286–96.
42. Milner CE, Hamill J, Davis IS. Distinct hip and rearfoot kinematics in female runners with a history of tibial stress fracture. J Orthop Sports Phys Ther 2010;40(2): 59–66.
43. Silbernagel KG, Willy R, Davis I. Preinjury and postinjury running analysis along with measurements of strength and tendon length in a patient with a surgically repaired Achilles tendon rupture. J Orthop Sports Phys Ther 2012;42(6):521–9.
44. Kannus VP. Evaluation of abnormal biomechanics of the foot and ankle in athletes. Br J Sports Med 1992;26(2):83–9.
45. Yeung SS, Yeung EW, Gillespie LD. Interventions for preventing lower limb soft-tissue running injuries. Cochrane Database Syst Rev 2011;(7):CD001256.
46. Ferber R, Hreljac A, Kendall KD. Suspected mechanisms in the cause of overuse running injuries: a clinical review. Sports Health 2009;1(3):242–6.
47. Souza RB, Powers CM. Predictors of hip internal rotation during running: an evaluation of hip strength and femoral structure in women with and without patellofemoral pain. Am J Sports Med 2009;37(3):579–87.
48. Souza RB, Powers CM. Differences in hip kinematics, muscle strength, and muscle activation between subjects with and without patellofemoral pain. J Orthop Sports Phys Ther 2009;39(1):12–9.
49. Noehren B, Davis I, Hamill J. ASB clinical biomechanics award winner 2006 prospective study of the biomechanical factors associated with iliotibial band syndrome. Clin Biomech 2007;22(9):951–6.
50. Souza RB, Hatamiya N, Martin C, et al. Medial and lateral heel whips: prevalence and characteristics in recreational runners. PM R 2015;7(8):823–30.
51. Willson JD, Davis IS. Lower extremity mechanics of females with and without patellofemoral pain across activities with progressively greater task demands. Clin Biomech 2008;23(2):203–11.
52. Herrington L. Knee valgus angle during single leg squat and landing in patellofemoral pain patients and controls. Knee 2014;21(2):514–7.
53. Willy RW, Davis IS. The effect of a hip-strengthening program on mechanics during running and during a single-leg squat. J Orthop Sports Phys Ther 2011;41(9): 625–32.
54. Willy RW, Scholz JP, Davis IS. Mirror gait retraining for the treatment of patellofemoral pain in female runners. Clin Biomech 2012;27(10):1045–51.
55. Noehren B, Scholz J, Davis I. The effect of real-time gait retraining on hip kinematics, pain and function in subjects with patellofemoral pain syndrome. Br J Sports Med 2011;45(9):691–6.
56. Barrios JA, Crossley KM, Davis IS. Gait retraining to reduce the knee adduction moment through real-time visual feedback of dynamic knee alignment. J Biomech 2010;43(11):2208–13.
57. Maykut JN, Taylor-Haas JA, Paterno MV, et al. Concurrent validity and reliability of 2d kinematic analysis of frontal plane motion during running. Int J Sports Phys Ther 2015;10(2):136–46.

58. Foch E, Milner CE. Frontal plane running biomechanics in female runners with previous iliotibial band syndrome. J Appl Biomech 2014;30(1):58–65.
59. Ford KR, Taylor-Haas JA, Genthe K, et al. Relationship between hip strength and trunk motion in college cross-country runners. Med Sci Sports Exerc 2013;45(6): 1125–30.
60. Tsatalas T, Giakas G, Spyropoulos G, et al. The effects of eccentric exercise-induced muscle damage on running kinematics at different speeds. J Sports Sci 2013;31(3):288–98.
61. Heiderscheit B. Running mechanics and clinical analysis. Sports Physical Therapy Section: American Physical Therapy Association, Independent Study Course. 2012.
62. Heiderscheit B. Biomechanics of running. Orthopaedic Physical Therapy Section, American Physical Therapy Association, Independent Study Course. 2013.

Malalignment Syndrome in Runners

Wolf Schamberger, MD, FRCPC, Dip Sports Med, Dip Electrodiagnosis*

KEYWORDS

- Pelvic malalignment • Malalignment syndrome • Back • Groin and limb pain
- Asymmetrical forces • Problems in runners • Manual therapy

KEY POINTS

- Understanding malalignment is essential for those caring for runners; approximately 80% have pelvic malalignment, which can mimic, hide, overlap with, trigger or aggravate other medical conditions.
- Malalignment syndrome includes the biomechanical changes, abnormal stresses, and resulting signs/symptoms seen with an upslip and rotational malalignment.
- A standard back examination can be misleading because it fails to assess alignment and does not look at the sites typically affected by pelvic malalignment.
- Malalignment can be corrected by following a supervised course of treatment that combines realignment, core strengthening, reestablishing movement patterns, and the timely use of appropriate complementary techniques.
- Treatment includes instruction in self-assessment and self-treatment to allow the runner to achieve and maintain realignment on a day-to-day basis and increase the chances of a full recovery and achieving his or her full potential.

INTRODUCTION

Running is an asymmetric sport in that it requires bearing weight alternately on the right and left lower extremities and absorbing the resulting unilateral forces as best as possible as these are transmitted upward through the knee, hip, pelvis, and lumbosacral region to the spine.[1] Malalignment refers to a minimal displacement from the normal alignment of any of the bones that are part of this kinetic chain and that results in abnormal biomechanical stresses that can compromise the ability to deal with these forces. This discussion focuses on the 3 most common presentations of pelvic

Disclaimer: The author denies any commercial or financial conflicts and does not have any funding sources to disclose in regard to the article on 'Malalignment syndrome in runners' that he has submitted to the *PMR Clinics of North America*.

Division of Physical Medicine and Rehabilitation, Faculty of Medicine, University of BC, Vancouver, Canada

* 73 – 101 Parkside Drive, Port Moody, British Columbia, Canada, V3H 4W6.

E-mail address: wschamberger@shaw.ca

malalignment. The term 'malalignment syndrome' refers to the biomechanical changes, signs and symptoms consistently seen in association with 2 of these presentations. Recognition of malalignment and the resulting detrimental effects should be part of the routine examination carried out by those caring for runners to avoid misdiagnosis, mistreatment, delayed recovery, and possibly failure of the runner to realize his or her full potential.

THE PELVIC RING: NORMAL AND ABNORMAL MOBILITY AND FUNCTION

The sacroiliac (SI) joint is an intricate joint that depends on its configuration and its supporting ligaments (**Figs. 1** and **2**), individual muscles (**Fig. 3**), and a system of inner and outer core muscles and myofascial slings to:

1. Allow for the smooth transfer of weight upward or downward through the lumbo–pelvic–hip complex[2] (**Fig. 4**);
2. Help ensure stability of the joint when this is functionally required; for example, on the weight-bearing side during walking and running[3–7]; and
3. Permit a minimal (2-4 mm at most) of SI joint motion: rotation around all 3 axes and movement (translation) along the corresponding planes (**Fig. 5**).[8–10]

This motion is essential for mobility and helps to absorb stress and store energy while decreasing the energy cost of running. During the gait cycle, for example, there is rotation of the pelvis as a whole, of the sacrum around one of the diagonal axes (**Fig. 6**), and of each innominate relative to the sacrum[5,9]:

a. In the coronal (or frontal) plane: upward on the weight-bearing side (see **Fig. 4B**);
b. In the sagittal plane: rotation forward (or anterior) during stance-phase, backward (or posterior) on swing-through (see **Fig. 6**); and
c. In the horizontal (or transverse) plane: outward (or outflaring) during stance phase, inward (or inflaring) with swing-through (**Fig. 7**).

Excessive rotation of an innominate relative to the sacrum around any of the 3 main axes can result in the innominate on one or both sides literally getting "stuck" in the direction of 1 or more of these 3 planes (see **Fig. 5**). Susceptibility to this occurring is attributable in part to the intricate configuration of the SI joint (**Fig. 8**):

1. It is L-shaped, with the 2 main arms of the sacral articular surface being oriented along different planes;
2. The upper and lower sacral surfaces are intimately molded to those on the innominate by way of:
   a. The concavity of 1 surface being matched by a corresponding convexity of the opposing surface[11,12];
   b. The gradual development of a crescent-shaped ridge running the length of the iliac surface, with a matching depression on the sacral side[13–15]; and
   c. Anterior widening of the sacrum, which restricts movement between the innominates by causing wedging in an anterior-to-posterior direction.

These features enhance the stability of the joint, especially on weight bearing, and also allow for some movement of 2 to 4 mm between the joint surfaces. Abnormal loading conditions that exceed this normal displacement in any direction can cause the adjoining SI joint surfaces to end up in an aberrant position so that the surfaces no longer match and stay compressed in some areas, separated in others, affecting normal movement (see **Fig. 7iii**; **Figs. 9** and **10**).[16] If the surfaces do become fixed

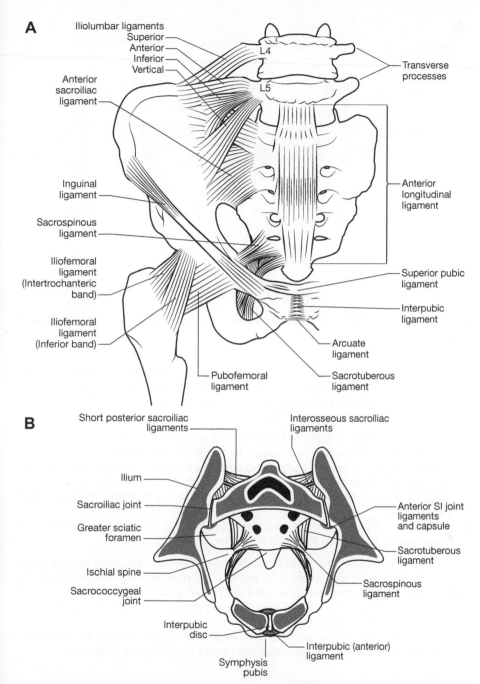

Fig. 1. Pelvic girdle: articulations and ligaments. (*A*) Anterior view. (*B*) Superior view (note the anterior widening of the sacrum).

A

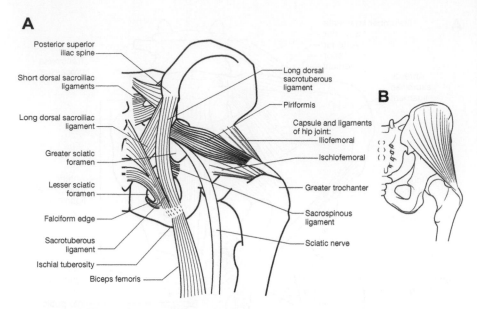

Fig. 2. (*A*) Posterior pelvic ligaments and muscles that act on the sacroiliac joint. (*B*) Gluteus maximus.

or locked in an abnormal position, major consequences include dysfunction of SI joint mobility, a disturbance of the lumbo–pelvic–hip complex and its ability to transfer weight and absorb shock, persistent malalignment of the pelvic ring and an alteration of gait.[17–19] Such a shift can be caused by:

1. Minimal excessive movement in 1 direction; for example, an awkward lift, especially with addition of a torqueing component by reaching up/downward or sideways;
2. Trauma to the pelvis itself or transmitted upward through an extremity; for example, in a motor vehicle accident or by falling onto 1 buttock (**Fig. 11**); landing hard on a straight leg, as on jumping while running cross-country, or simply missing a step (**Fig. 12**); and
3. Increased tension or spasm in muscles that attach to the pelvic ring or laxity in those needed to stabilize the joints (see **Figs. 3** and **39**).

However, in the majority of those presenting with malalignment, there is no obvious cause. One of the theories seeking to explain this phenomenon suggests that the malalignment is the outcome of a persistent asymmetry of muscle tension throughout the body caused by asymmetrical signals being generated at the segmental level (spinal cord), brain stem or cortex.[20–24]

A description of the 3 most common presentations of pelvic malalignment follows, after an outline of some basic tests that are helpful in making the diagnosis.

ASSESSING PELVIC MALALIGNMENT

The diagnosis can usually be made by:

1. Looking for the characteristic asymmetry of major landmarks specific to each of these presentations by comparing the position of one thumb to that on the other side, to detect any:

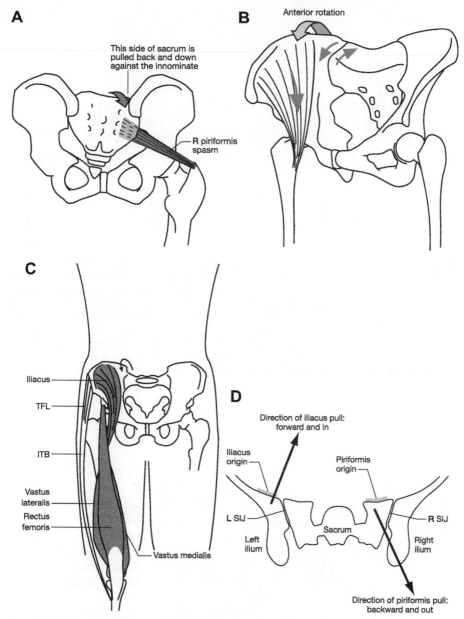

Fig. 3. Stabilization of the sacroiliac joint (SIJ) by wedging of the anteriorly widening sacrum. (*A*) Piriformis pulling the sacrum backward against the innominate. (*B*) Iliacus pulling the innominate forward against the sacrum. (*C*) Anterior innominate rotation through the action of iliacus, rectus femoris, tensor fascia lata (TFL). (*D*) Wedging effect: superior view of joints. ITB, iliotibial band.

a. Relative upward or downward displacement (**Fig. 13**):
   i. Compare the thumbs placed against the iliac crest, inferior aspect of the anterior superior iliac spine (ASIS), superior rim of the pubic bones and inferior aspect of the posterior superior iliac spine (PSIS).

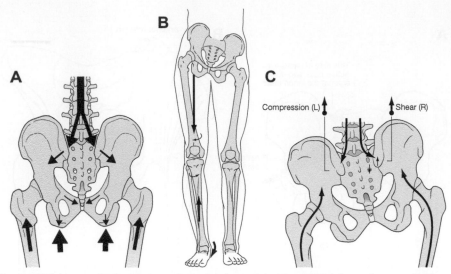

Fig. 4. Weight transfer forces through the lumbo–pelvic–hip complex from above and below. (*A*) In standing and sitting (pelvis in alignment, leg length equal). (*B*) On right 1-leg stance. (*C*) Changes in loads and forces imparted to the sacroiliac joint with a left frontal plane asymmetry. The right joint is more vertical, creating greater shear. (*From* Schamberger W. The malalignment syndrome: Diagnosing and treating a common cause of acute and chronic pelvic, limb and back pain. Edinburgh (UK): Churchill Livingstone; 2013. *Adapted from* Porterfield JA, DeRosa C. Conditions of weight bearing: asymmetrical overload syndrome (AOS). In: Vleeming A, Mooney V, Stoeckart R, editors. Movement, stability and lumbopelvic pain. Integration of research and therapy. 2nd edition. Edinburgh (United Kingdom): Churchill Livingstone; 2007. p 394; with permission.)

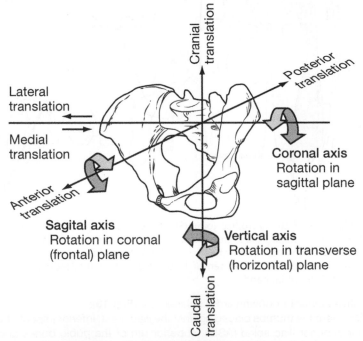

Fig. 5. Axes and planes around which sacroiliac joint movement occurs.

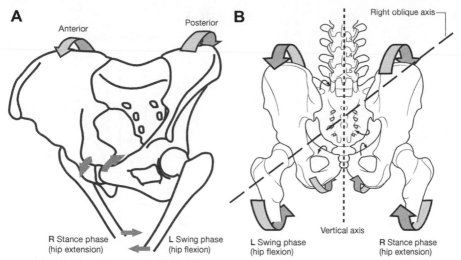

Fig. 6. Movement of the pelvic ring with normal gait. (*A*) Contrary rotation of the innominates relative to the sacrum: right anterior, left posterior. (*B*) Sacral torsion around the right oblique axis associated with the rotation of the innominates.

    b. Displacement from midline (**Fig. 14**):
       i. Compare the thumbs placed against the medial aspect of the ASIS or PSIS.
2. Doing the sitting–lying test as follows:
    a. Start with the runner lying supine on a firm surface and then assist him or her to come up into a sitting position to minimize any use of trunk or abdominal muscles in order to decrease the chance of veering off to 1 side in the process. A runner can carry out this step alone with a belt to pull up on, using the muscles in both arms.
    b. With him or her in sitting up, place a thumb lightly against the inferior aspect of the medial malleolus on each side, pointing the tip downward, so that the distal phalanx ends up positioned vertically to allow for a more accurate side-to-side comparison.
    c. Check to see if the thumbs are level with each other or if one is displaced upward relative to the other, as if the leg were shorter on that side (**Fig. 15**).
    d. While maintaining the placement of the thumbs, have the runner lie down and observe if, on doing so:
       i. The thumbs (ie, legs) move up together, or
      ii. There is a relative shift in their position, one thumb moving upward and the other downward; if that is, the case, the reverse would be evident on having him or her sit up again (**Fig. 16**).

Repeat the test once or twice to confirm your observations.

PRESENTATIONS WITH THE PELVIS ALIGNED

About 10% to 15% of the population present with the pelvis in alignment and no history of having had any adjustments (eg, manipulation, mobilization) carried out any time in the past.[25–27] Findings with 2 common variants relating to leg length are as follows.

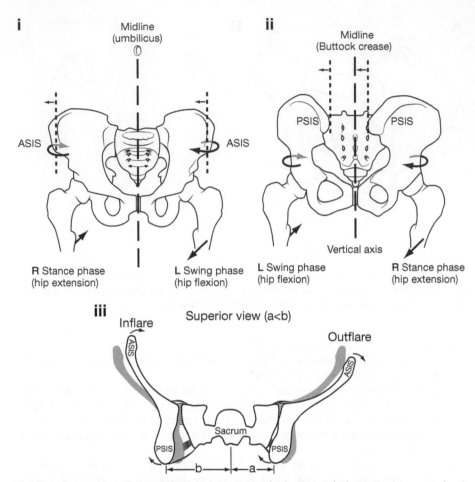

Fig. 7. Inflare and outflare of the innominates in the horizontal plane. During normal gait cycle (right stance, left swing-through phase), the right outflares, the left inflares: (i) anterior, (ii) posterior, and (iii) superior views. ASIS, anterior superior iliac spine; PSIS, posterior superior iliac spine.

Pelvis Aligned, Legs Length Equal

All the pelvic landmarks are level with their counterpart on the left in standing, sitting, and lying. The right and left ASIS and PSIS are equidistant from the midline (see **Fig. 14**Aii, Bii). The malleoli lie at the same level and move together, downward on sitting up and upward on lying down.

Pelvis Aligned, Right Anatomic (True) Leg Length Difference Present

Compared with the left side, the right iliac crest and all other right pelvic landmarks are higher in standing but are level and equidistant from midline when sitting and lying (**Fig. 17**). The right malleolus will appear to be displaced downward relative to the left one by the same amount in both sitting and lying (reflective of the true leg length difference) and the legs move together on changing from one position to the other.

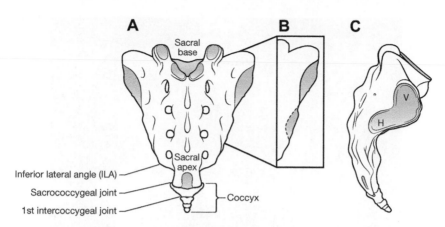

Fig. 8. Posterior aspect of the sacrum and coccyx and configuration of the adult sacroiliac (SI) joint. (*A*) Anteroposterior view: bony landmarks. (*B*) Angulated inset showing orientation of the 2 main arms of the sacral articular surface along different planes relative to the sacral axis, which creates a propellerlike shape. (*C*) Lateral view: L-shape of the SI joint (H, horizontal arm; V, vertical arm). (*Adapted from* Vleeming A, Mooney V, Stoeckart R, editors. Movement, stability and lumbopelvic pain. Integration of research and therapy. 2nd edition. Edinburgh (United Kingdom): Churchill Livingstone; 2007; with permission.)

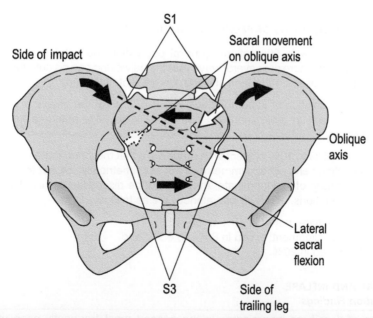

Fig. 9. Posterior rotation (*right*) and anterior rotation (*left*) demonstrating joint closure at the (level of) S1 (*right*) and S3 (*left*) to create an oblique axis. A functional destabilization occurs at S1 (*left*) and S3 (*right*), allowing the joint to move on that oblique axis. (*From* DonTigny RI. Pelvic dynamics and the S3 subluxation of the sacroiliac joint. Havre (MT): CD-ROM from DonTigny; 2004; with permission).

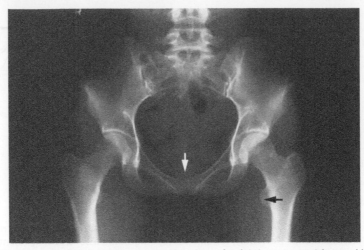

Fig. 10. Radiograph: standing anteroposterior view of pelvis in person with equal leg length and right anterior, left posterior rotational malalignment. Note the (1) femoral heads are level but the pelvic crests are oblique; (2) approximately 3 mm downward displacement of right superior pubic ramus relative to the left at symphysis pubis (*white arrow*); (3) apparent asymmetry of the (a) sacroiliac joint surfaces; for example, increased opening of the left lower joint compared with the right (see **Fig. 9**); (b) spacing between hip joint surfaces; and (c) size of lesser trochanter (LT; more of left visible - *black arrow*): with contrary rotation of the femurs (*right external, left internal*), the left LT rotates into view and seems to be larger; the right is partially hidden by overlapping with the femur.

COMMON PRESENTATIONS OF PELVIC MALALIGNMENT

As indicated, in 80% to 90% of the general population the pelvis is not in alignment.[25–27] Although there are several ways that the pelvic ring can go out of alignment, this discussion focuses on the 3 most common presentations that:

1. Can occur in isolation or in combination with 1 or both of the others; and
2. Altogether make up more than 90% of the 80% to 90% noted to have pelvic malalignment.

The remaining 5% to 10% present with other ways that the innominates and sacrum can go out of alignment, either symmetrically or asymmetrically; except for sacral torsion and a downslip of an innominate, they will not be discussed further. The 3 most common presentations, and their prevalence, are as follows:

1. Outflare and inflare: noted in 40% to 50%;
2. Rotational malalignment: noted in 80% to 85%; and
3. An upslip: noted in 20%.

OUTFLARE AND INFLARE
Examination Findings

1. Flaring of 1 or both innominates is the second most frequently seen of the 3 most common presentations of pelvic malalignment, noted in 40% to 50% altogether.[27]
2. The right or left innominate becomes fixed in excessive outward or inward rotation in the horizontal plane. The contralateral innominate, although it may be found to lie

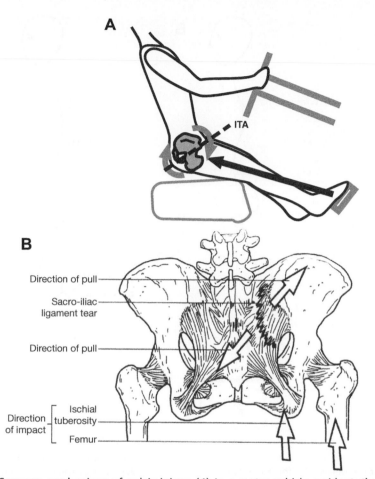

Fig. 11. Common mechanisms of pelvic injury. (*A*) In a motor vehicle accident: the force impacting on the acetabulum at an angle below the inferior transvers axis (ITA) results in anterior rotation of the innominate. (*B*) In a fall: forcing the leg upward or landing on the ischial tuberosity can stretch/disrupt the ligaments between the sacrum and ilium.

in its normal position, is usually fixed flared in the opposite direction, as if to compensate. With a right outflare and left inflare:

a. The right ASIS will have moved away from the midline of the abdomen, the left toward it (see **Fig. 14**Ai). Findings are the reverse for the PSIS: the left toward, the right away from midline, demarcated by the gluteal cleft and spinous processes (see **Fig. 14**Bi).

b. The left ASIS ends up moved forward with the inflare, the right backward with the outflare (see **Fig. 7**iii). As a result, the left one seems to be:
   i. Protruded forward in standing and sitting compared with the right and
   ii. Displaced upward (ie, h*i*gher) and the right downward (ie, l*O*wer) when observed with the runner lying supine (**Fig. 18**).

c. Barring a coexisting true leg length difference, the landmarks are level in the frontal plane in all positions and leg length is equal in sitting and lying.

d. Radiographs show the changes in the landmarks observed (**Fig. 19**).

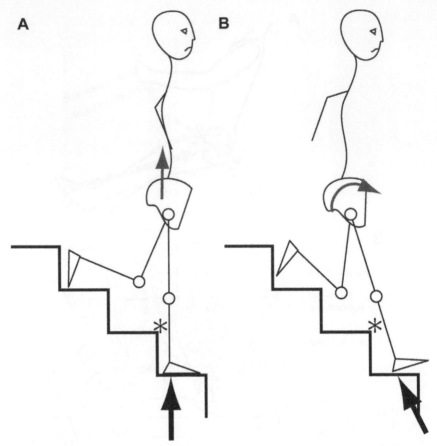

Fig. 12. Missing a step and landing with increased force on 1 extremity can cause malalignment of the pelvis. The force created can result in displacement of the innominate relative to the sacrum. At the time of impact, if the leg is positioned (*A*) vertically, this can result in upward displacement (a so-called upslip) or (*B*) at a hip-flexion angle, this can result in an anterior rotation of the innominate.

Diagnosis and Corrective Procedures: Right Outflare, Left Inflare

When a right outflare, left inflare is present, on lying supine:

1. The right ASIS is l**O**wer and displaced **O**utward, away from midline.

   Remember the mnemonic of the **4 O**s:

THE L**O**W SIDE IS THE '**O**' OR '**O**UTFLARE' SIDE.

CORRECTION IS ACHIEVED BY RESISTING **O**UTWARD MOVEMENT OF THE KNEE.

The treatment method referred to here is a form of manual therapy, known as the muscle energy technique (MET).[18,28–30] It gets the runner to harness the energy in muscles that are positioned in a way that enables them to effect the specific change. In this

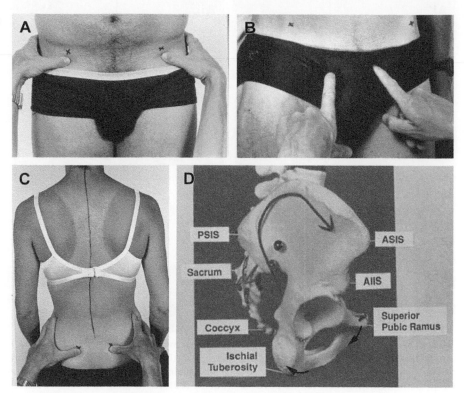

Fig. 13. Rotational malalignment: right anterior, left posterior innominate rotation. (*A*) Asymmetry of anterior superior iliac spine (ASIS; *right down, left up*). (*B*) Asymmetry of posterior superior iliac spine (PSIS) and iliac crest (*right up, left down*); obvious downward displacement of shoulder and brassiere on left secondary to compensatory scoliosis. (*C*) Right superior pubic ramus displaced downward relative to the left. (*D*) Shift of the right pelvic landmarks relative to their left counterparts: right iliac crest, PSIS, and ischial tuberosity moved upward; right ASIS, anterior inferior iliac spine (AIIS), and pubic ramus moved downward.

case, resisting abduction and external rotation of the femur by blocking outward movement of the partially flexed right knee (**Fig. 20**) reverses the origin and insertion of the right piriformis and gluteus maximus (see **Figs. 2** and **3**). These muscles can act on the innominate (which is still free to move) to rotate it forward in the horizontal plane until it again comes to lie in its normal position relative to the sacrum. The repeated contraction–relaxation of these muscles also can decrease tone and increase muscle relaxation and lengthening that, together, make it easier for the bones to slot back into their proper place.

2. The left ASIS is h*i*gher and displaced *i*nward, toward the midline.

Remember the mnemonic of the 4 *I*s:

THE H*I*GH SIDE IS THE '*I*' OR '*I*NFLARE' SIDE.

CORRECTION IS ACHIEVED BY RESISTING *I*NWARD MOVEMENT OF THE KNEE.

Blocking adduction of the left leg reverses the origin and insertion of the left gracilis and adductor longus (**Fig. 21**; see **Fig. 55**). The force generated is now directed to their

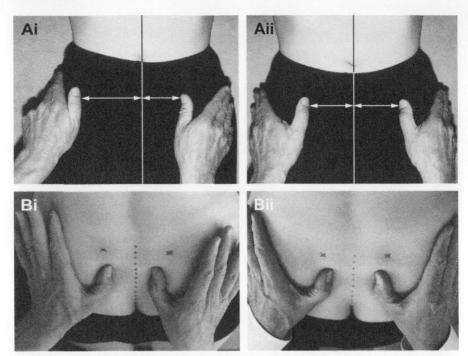

Fig. 14. (*A*) With an abnormal presentation - relative to midline, thumbs placed against inside of the anterior superior iliac spine (ASIS) show: (i) initial asymmetry, with right outflare (thumb away from midline), and left inflare (closer to midline); (ii) symmetry after correction (equidistant from midline). (*B*) Relative to midline (buttock crease, spinous processes), thumbs against inner aspect of PSIS show: (i) initial asymmetry with right outflare (thumb closer to midline), left inflare (thumb away from midline); (ii) symmetry after correction.

attachment onto the left pubic tubercle and is capable of rotating the innominate outward, back into alignment (**Fig. 22**).

Clinical Correlation for Runners

1. An outflare strains the anterior SI joint ligaments/capsule and compresses the posterior joint margins; an inflare has the opposite effect (see **Figs. 1, 2, 7**iii, and **19**B). There may be discomfort from the structures put under stress.
2. With a right inflare, left outflare, the left acetabulum faces progressively more posterolaterally as that innominate rotates outward (see **Fig. 19**A). The left superior rim comes to lie more directly anterior to the femoral head with the outward rotation of that innominate, sometimes to the point that the femoral head actually impinges against the rim as the hip joint is increasingly flexed going through swing phase. Compared with the ease with which the right leg moves through this phase:
   a. The runner may literally sense the block to this motion occurring on the left side and there may be discomfort or pain with impingement of the acetabular rim, felt in the left groin and/or hip region.[31]
   b. Left swing-through is limited. To compensate, he or she can:
      i. Bring the acetabulum facing further forward by actively increasing the extent that the pelvic ring as a whole rotates clockwise during left swing phase, partly effected by increasing active clockwise rotation of the trunk and

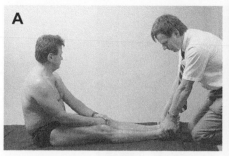
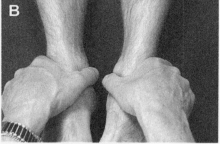

Fig. 15. Sitting part of the sitting–lying test. (*A*) Long sitting. (*B*) The left leg seems to be longer than the right.

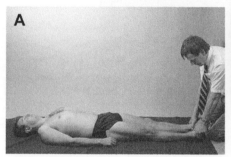
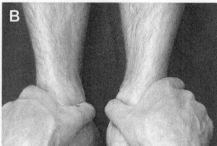

Fig. 16. Lying part of the sitting–lying test in same subject as in **Fig. 14**. (*A*) Supine lying. (*B*) There has been a shift in leg length: the right has lengthened relative to the left leg (findings are the reverse of those noted in **Fig. 14**B).

      changing the movement pattern of the arms, in an attempt to match right stride length; and

  ii. Cut back the degree of right swing-through to match that on the left and, instead, increase stride frequency to maintain the same speed.

Either compensation method leads to unwanted changes in the gait pattern that can prove costly in terms of decreased efficiency and increased energy demands.

ROTATIONAL MALALIGNMENT
Examination Findings

Innominate rotation is the most frequently seen of the 3 common presentations of pelvic malalignment, noted in 80% to 85% altogether.[26,27] An innominate can become fixed relative to the sacroiliac joint, in a position of excessive rotation in the sagittal plane, either forward (anterior) or backward (posterior). Usually, but not necessarily, the contralateral innominate is fixed in rotation in the opposite direction. Some 80% to 85% thus affected have a right anterior, left posterior and 15% to 20% a left anterior, right posterior rotation.[26,27] The SI joint may be locked on one side so that on the kinetic rotational (Gillet) test the innominate and adjoining sacrum on the locked side move as 1 unit, upward on progressive hip flexion, downward on hip extension, which is opposite to what happens normally (**Fig. 23**).

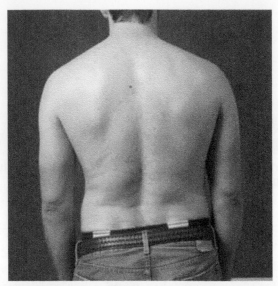

Fig. 17. Pelvic obliquity with the belt and iliac crest angled up on the right side; compensatory scoliosis and downward displacement of left shoulder and arm; head remains centered and level. Findings could be in keeping with true leg length discrepancy (right leg long), upslip or rotational malalignment.

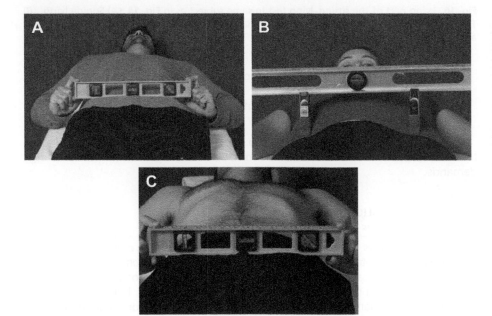

Fig. 18. Right outflare, left inflare. (*A, B*) A spirit level resting on top of the right and left anterior superior iliac spine (ASIS) shows elevation of the left side. (*B*) Feet (clamps) attached to the level rest on the ASIS; they help to raise the bubble into view (eg, for someone who is obese, pregnant). (*C*) ASIS now level, bubble in center, after correction of the outflare/inflare (same subject as in *A*).

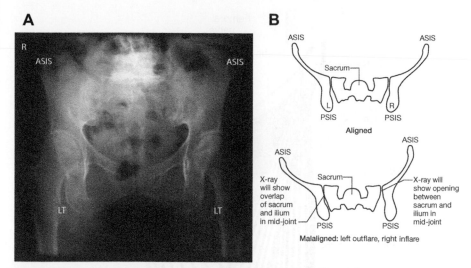

Fig. 19. Radiographic changes seen with a left outflare, right inflare. (*A*) Anteroposterior projection of pelvis and hip joints. The femoral heads remain at the same level as the left acetabulum moves outward and the right inward in the horizontal plane. Innominate width seems to be increased on the left and decreased on the right. The anterior superior iliac spine looks to be increased in overall size and broader on the outflare (*left*) side and smaller and narrower on the inflare (*right*) side. The left femoral neck lies further away from and the right one closer to the ipsilateral inferior pubic ramus. The left lesser trochanter (LT) seems to be smaller as a result of overlapping occurring with passive external rotation of the femur; on the right it seems to be larger, having been brought into view with internal rotation of that femur (see also **Fig. 10**). (*B*) Diagrammatic conceptualization of the AP beam projection onto the pelvis when aligned and with a left outflare, right inflare present; superoinferior view.

Diagnosing Rotational Malalignment

With a right anterior, left posterior rotation (see **Fig. 13**; **Fig. 24**):

1. All the anterior and posterior landmarks are displaced asymmetrically on both side-to-side and front-to-back comparison. For example:
    a. The right ASIS ends up lower compared with the ipsilateral PSIS and the left ASIS; and

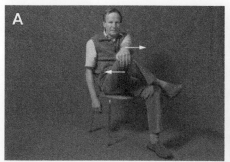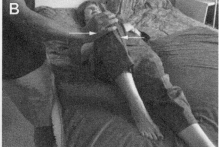

Fig. 20. Using muscle energy technique (MET) to correct a right outflare: resist active right thigh abduction and external rotation; that is, block outward movement of flexed right knee. (*A*) One-person, sitting (or lying) approach. (*B*) A 2-person approach is easy to carry out with subject lying supine, ipsilateral hip and knee flexed and foot resting on bed.

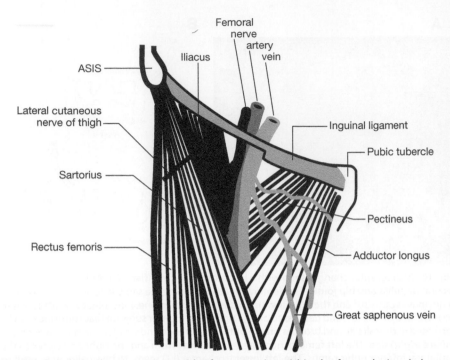

Fig. 21. Neurovascular structures at risk of compromise within the femoral triangle by any increase in tension, particularly in iliacus, psoas and pectineus. (*Note:* adductor longus origin from pubic tubercle [see **Fig. 22**], also lateral femoral cutaneous nerve traversing the canal). (*From* Schamberger W. The malalignment syndrome: Diagnosing and treating a common cause of acute and chronic pelvic, limb and back pain. Edinburgh (UK): Churchill Livingstone; 2013. *Adapted from* Anderson JE. Grant's atlas of anatomy, 7th edition. Baltimore: Williams and Wilkins, 1980.)

    b. The right pubic ramus is displaced downward and rotated forward in the sagittal plane; the left undergoes displacement in the opposite directions.

2. There is a pelvic obliquity, with the right iliac crest and ischial tuberosity ending up higher relative to left side (see **Figs. 13** and **17**).

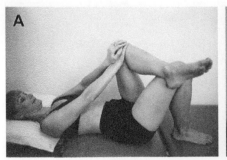
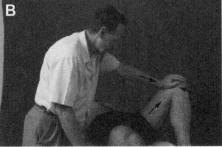

Fig. 22. To correct a left inflare, resist active left thigh adduction and internal rotation; that is, block inward movement of flexed knee. (*A*) One-person lying (or sitting) approach. (*B*) Two-person approach (*note: arrow* on left inner thigh denotes direction of adductor longus pull on right pubic tubercle attachment to rotate innominate outward).

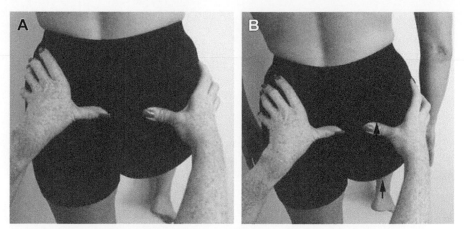

Fig. 23. Abnormal right kinetic rotational (Gillet) test, with right sacroiliac joint locked. (*A*) On initial right hip flexion to horizontal: right thumb (which marks the location of right posterior superior iliac spine [PSIS]) fails to drop down relative to the left one (marking the sacral base). (*B*) On increasing right hip flexion: the right thumb (PSIS) actually moves upward. The sacrum and PSIS are moving together as 1 locked unit, counterclockwise in the frontal plane.

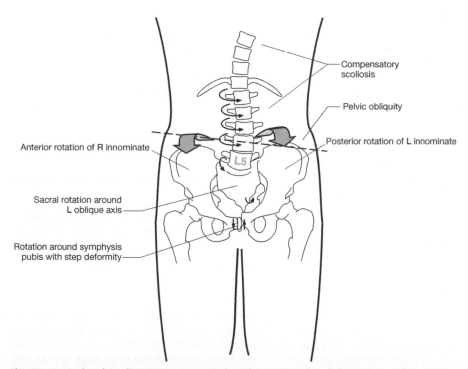

Fig. 24. Typical pelvic distortion associated with rotational malalignment: right anterior, left posterior rotation, as shown. Pubic bones are rotated and displaced relative to each other at the symphysis; sacrum in torsion around the left oblique axis. Pelvic obliquity (shown inclined to *right*) and compensatory scoliosis (thoracic segment convex to right, lumbar convex to left, with L1-4 rotated into the convexity).

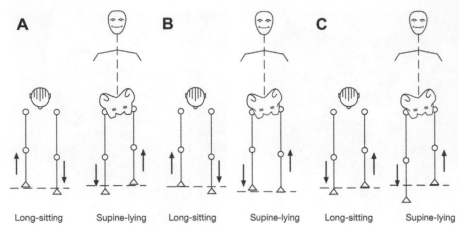

| Long-sitting | Supine-lying | Long-sitting | Supine-lying | Long-sitting | Supine-lying |

Fig. 25. Sitting–lying test: rotational malalignment presentation. All 3 subjects have right anterior, left posterior innominate rotation, with relative lengthening of the right leg compared with the left on moving from long sitting to supine lying. (*A*) The right leg is shorter sitting, longer lying; this is the most common pattern. (*B*) The right leg is shorter sitting but less so in lying. (*C*) The right leg is longer sitting and even more so in lying.

3. There is an apparent leg length difference noted in the sitting–lying test. Which leg seems to be longer or shorter is of little importance. What matters is that there is a shift in leg length on this test, with the right malleolus moving upward in sitting up and downward on lying down relative to the left (see **Figs. 15** and **16; Fig. 25**). This shift is characteristic of a right anterior, left posterior rotation; it would be in the opposite direction with a left anterior, right posterior rotation.
4. Remember the mnemonic of the **5 L**s to help determine the side of an anterior rotation:

> <u>L</u>EG <u>L</u>ENGTHENS <u>L</u>YING, <u>L</u>ANDMARKS <u>L</u>OWER.

In the case of a right anterior, left posterior rotation, the right anterior landmarks end up lower relative to those on the left and the right leg lengthens on lying down.

5. Radiographs show the changes in the landmarks observed (**Fig. 26**).

Corrective Procedures for Rotational Malalignment

There are a number of different manual therapy techniques that can be used to correct a rotational malalignment. However, MET, leverage, or a combination of the 2 techniques can be useful in that they may allow the runner to correct a recurrence between visits to the therapist or even when on the track or out on the road (**Figs. 27–34** and **37**). In the case of a:

1. Right anterior rotation:
   a. Blocking movement of the right thigh away from the trunk (ie, right hip extension) activates right gluteus maximus (**Figs. 30** and **31**). Reversal of its origin and

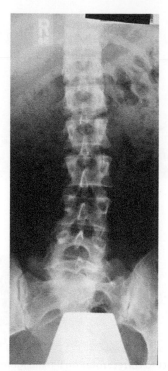

Fig. 26. Radiographic changes with malalignment: the effect on sacroiliac and facet joint orientation to the anteroposterior beam. The L1-L4 vertebral rotation into the left convexity (ie, counterclockwise) opens up the left midlumbar facet joints and accentuates the closing/compression of the right facet joints that results with the simultaneous left rotation and right side-flexion of the vertebrae. The right sacroiliac joint seems to be open along its full length, whereas only the midsection of the left one is visible as a result of overlapping and reorientation of the joint surfaces relative to the beam and to the right side (see also **Figs. 10** and **19**). L5 is sacralized on the left.

insertion allows it to rotate the right innominate in a posterior direction, by way of its attachments to the posterosuperior aspect of the ilium (see **Fig. 2**B).

b. Passively moving the right femur into increasing flexion to the point where the femoral head impinges against the anterior rim of the acetabulum creates leverage and simultaneously tightens some posterior structures, including the sacrotuberous ligament. The combined effect is a posterior rotational force on the right innominate (see **Fig. 27**A).

2. Left posterior rotation:

a. Blocking movement the left thigh toward the trunk (ie, left hip flexion) activates left iliacus (**Figs. 32** and **33**) and rectus femoris (see **Fig. 28**B); the latter also responds to blocking extension of the flexed knee (see **Fig. 28**A; **Fig. 34**). The muscles then exert an anterior rotational force by way of their attachments to the anterosuperior part of the ilium and to the pubic bone, respectively (see **Fig. 3**).

b. Passively extending the femur to the point where the femoral head impinges on the posterior acetabular rim turns the femur into a lever capable of creating an anterior rotational force on the left innominate (see **Fig. 27**B).

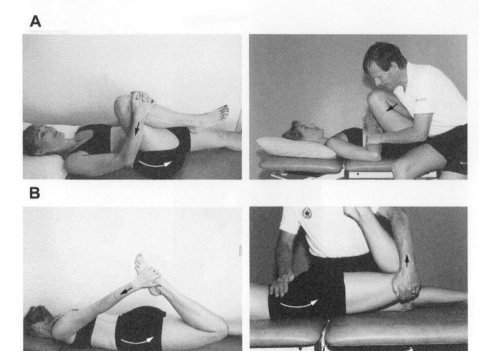

Fig. 27. Using a leverage effect to correct rotational malalignment. (*A*) Passive hip flexion to counteract a right anterior rotation: (i) 1-person and (ii) 2-person techniques. (*B*) Passive hip extension to counteract a left posterior rotation: (i) 1-person and (ii) 2-person techniques.

Clinical Correlation for Runners

1. Runners should be discouraged from routinely doing excessive unilateral stretches of iliopsoas, rectus femoris, gluteal muscles, and hamstrings, especially when the pelvis is free to move, as in standing (**Fig. 35**). For example, a right iliopsoas/quadriceps stretch tightens up right iliacus and rectus femoris; the femur may also end up far enough in extension to exert a leverage effect (see **Fig. 35**A). This maneuver is capable of:
   a. Forcing the right innominate to go out of alignment so it ends up fixed in an anterior rotated position; and
   b. Undoing any realignment that has been achieved, because it can literally force the innominate back out of alignment again.
2. To decrease this risk, stretches are best carried out simultaneously on both sides, preferably with the pelvis stabilized; for example, bilateral hamstring stretch: sitting on the floor, legs out in front; quadriceps, iliopsoas and pectineus: leaning the pelvis and trunk backward while kneeling (**Fig. 36**).
3. However, unilateral leverage maneuvers can actually be used effectively by the runner on the side of a known rotation. For example, a right anterior rotation may respond to placing the right foot on a chair and gradually leaning forward with the trunk, arms dangling downward (**Fig. 37**). The same may be accomplished by having the right foot up on a ledge and leaning forward (see **Fig. 35**B). The progressive increase in passive hip flexion turns the femur into a lever capable of correcting the rotation.

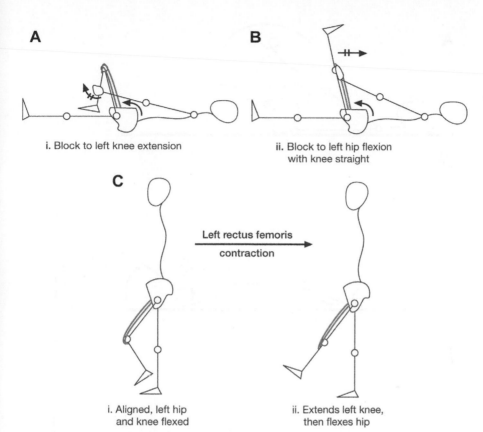

A

i. Block to left knee extension

B

ii. Block to left hip flexion
with knee straight

C

Left rectus femoris
contraction

i. Aligned, left hip
and knee flexed

ii. Extends left knee,
then flexes hip

Fig. 28. One-person muscle energy technique to correct a left posterior rotation by activating rectus femoris with the left knee (*A*) in flexion, (*B*) in extension. (*C*) Rectus femoris action in standing.

4. Unilateral stretches of a specific muscle may be indicated following realignment for:
   a. Muscles that have undergone contracture while in a shortened state during the time that malalignment was present; and
   b. Ones that fail to relax completely, show increased tone, or are actually in spasm.

UPSLIP
Examination Findings

Of the 3 most common presentations of pelvic malalignment, an upslip is the least frequently seen, appearing in isolation in 10% and in combination with a flare, rotational malalignment, or both in another 10%.[26,27] The innominate on 1 side ends up displaced straight upward relative to the adjacent sacrum and becomes fixed in that position. Again, although often no cause may be evident, some obvious ones include:

1. Having the force of an impact transmitted straight upward, either through:
   a. One extremity: for example, missing a step (see **Fig. 12**A); landing hard on 1 leg when jumping or running downhill with the knee in extension (**Fig. 38**) or
   b. The innominate itself; for example, falling directly onto an ischial tuberosity (see **Fig. 11**B).

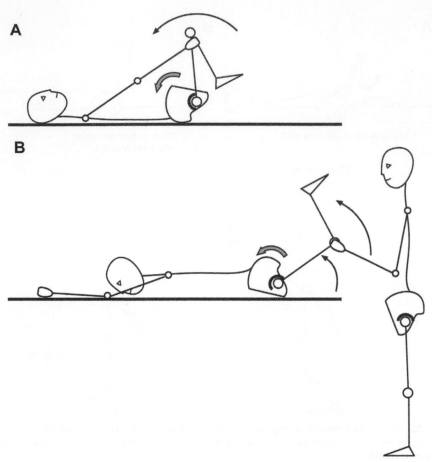

Fig. 29. Leverage effect of the femur on the innominate, by impingement against the acetabular rim (see also **Fig. 27**). Correction of (*A*) an anterior rotation; (*B*) a posterior rotation.

2. An upward traction force being applied to the innominate; for example, with a chronic increase in tension or spasm in quadratus lumborum, psoas major/minor (**Fig. 39**).

As a result, on the side of the upslip one finds:

1. The anterior and posterior pelvic landmarks are all displaced upward relative to those of the opposite innominate and to the sacrum.

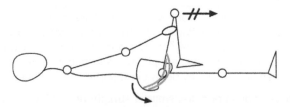

Block to right hip extension =
reversal of origin and insertion

Fig. 30. One-person muscle energy technique to correct an anterior rotation: using the gluteus maximus to create a posterior rotational force on the innominate.

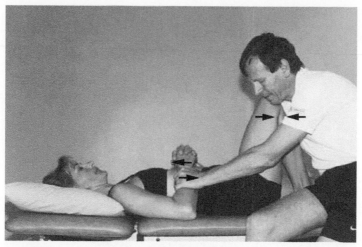

Fig. 31. Two-person muscle energy technique using the gluteus maximus to correct a right anterior rotation.

2. The ipsilateral leg is moved upward passively with the innominate, creating an apparent leg length difference. Relative to the opposite leg, it seems shortened to the same extent in both sitting and lying and the malleolus moves downward and upward, respectively, together with that on the other side (**Fig. 40**).
3. A pelvic obliquity is evident in standing, sitting, and lying.

Corrective Procedures for an Upslip

With the runner lying supine, applying gentle, repetitive traction to the leg on the upslip side usually suffices, often simply by helping to relax tense muscles around the hip/pelvic girdle that are holding the innominate in the upslip position (see **Fig. 39**; **Fig. 41**). If that fails to achieve correction, manipulation using a quick downward pull on the leg once or twice may prove successful. The runner can be instructed in self-correction (see **Fig. 41**B):

1. Starting by simply letting that leg hang down while standing on a step or stool, and

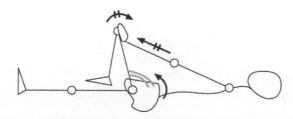

Block to left hip flexion =
anterior rotational force

Fig. 32. One-person muscle energy technique using iliacus to correct a left posterior rotation.

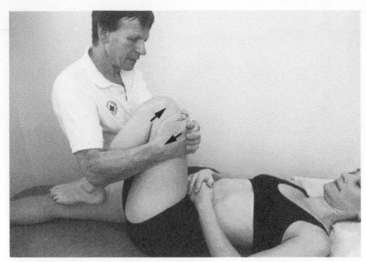

Fig. 33. Two-person muscle energy technique using iliacus to correct a left posterior rotation.

2. Progressively increasing either the time it is suspended or the amount of a weight attached, usually 20 to 30 minutes using 2.5 to 4.5 kg proves effective.

Clinical Correlation for Runners

1. The apparent leg length difference, pelvic obliquity, and compensatory scoliosis combined result in unwanted stress points, change in style, and compensatory measures; for example, leaning into the weight-bearing low side to help clear the long leg for swing-through and adjustments for side-to-side differences in stride length.[3,32]

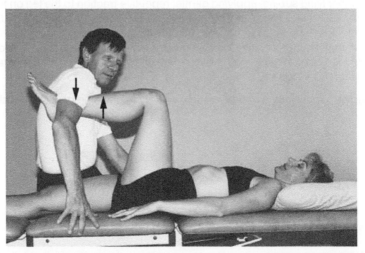

Fig. 34. Two-person muscle energy technique using the rectus femoris to correct a left posterior rotation. Having the runner's ankle/distal part of the lower leg propped up under the armpit (or lying on top of the shoulder; not shown) allows the assistant to use his body weight to advantage to generate the counterforce needed to block knee extension.

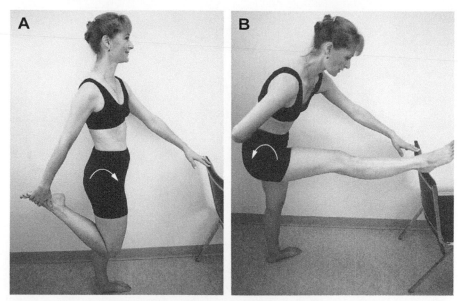

Fig. 35. (A) Popular unilateral quadriceps stretch that can cause or aggravate a preexisting right anterior rotation, by way of (1) rectus femoris pulling on its innominate origin and/or (2) the femur coming to act as a lever with increasing hip extension. (B) Unilateral hamstrings stretch (eg, straight leg propped up on a chair or table) can have a similar deleterious effect by causing/aggravating a posterior rotation. However, this same maneuver may be able to correct a preexisting right anterior rotation (see also **Fig. 37**).

2. Dysfunction of the SI joint on the side of the upslip increasing stress on the other parts of the lumbo–pelvic–hip complex bilaterally.
3. A coexisting rotational malalignment can hide an upslip; hence, it is important to recheck alignment after correction of the rotation.
4. A caution: keep the rare downslip in mind.

When dealing with a supposed upslip that fails to respond to treatment, including repeated downward traction, consider the possibility that the runner has actually sustained a downslip of the contralateral innominate. For example, a traction force on one

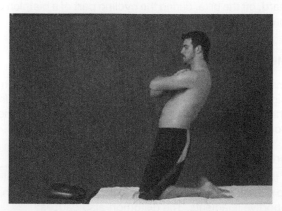

Fig. 36. Simultaneous, symmetric stretch of bilateral quadriceps, iliopsoas, and pectineus (see **Figs. 3**B, C and **19**) carried out by subject kneeling and gently leaning backward.

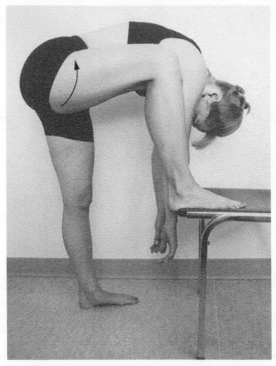

Fig. 37. A right anterior rotation may be corrected by resting the right foot on a raised surface and simply letting the trunk hang down in forward flexion as far as is comfortable. With increasing right hip flexion, the femur can eventually exert a leverage effect, with posterior rotation of the innominate (see also **Fig. 35**B). Bouncing or straining while reaching down must be avoided because it can precipitate or aggravate pain and muscle spasm.

of the lower extremities that is strong enough to pull the innominate into a downslip position can occur when the runner:

1. Has to pull upward on a straight leg, often unexpectedly and in midstride, to extract a foot that got stuck in deep mud;
2. Is thrown forward, off the bike, during the cycling part of a biathlon or triathlon while 1 foot is still caught up in the stirrup.

THE MALALIGNMENT SYNDROME

Both rotational malalignment and an upslip result in typical biomechanical changes, symptoms and signs that together constitute the malalignment syndrome.[26,27] A discussion of the characteristic findings associated with this well-defined clinical entity and the implications for runners follows.

Pelvic Ring Distortion

Displacement of the pelvic ring results in abnormal stresses on all of the joints of the lumbo–pelvic–hip complex, particularly on the adjoining surfaces of the joints and their capsule and supportive ligaments. The distortion also causes:

1. Disturbance of the normal transfer of weight through this complex (see **Fig. 4**)[3,4,8];

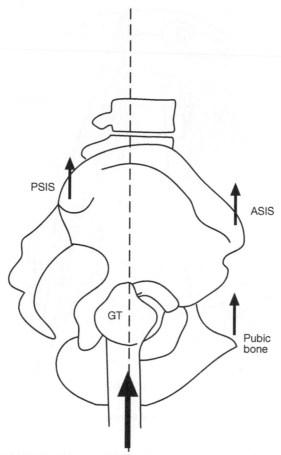

Fig. 38. Right upslip caused by a unilateral upward force on the femur transmitted through the hip joint to the innominate. ASIS, anterior superior iliac spine; PSIS, posterior superior iliac spine.

2. Irritation of neural receptors lying within any of the structures put under stress, which can result in localized and/or referred pain and paresthesias (see Case History: Runner A, below);
3. Accelerated degeneration of any sites in the lower extremities, pelvis and spine put under increased stress as a result; in particular, the discs and facet joints in the lower lumbosacral region (see **Figs. 10** and **26**; **Figs. 42** and **43**)[12,33]; and
4. Pelvic obliquity and an apparent leg length difference.

Clinical correlation for runners

Runners, who alternately bear all weight on one extremity, are likely to develop compensatory mechanisms that can affect their running biomechanics and efficiency. In an attempt to cope with any pain and/or the altered biomechanics of weight transfer, they may:

1. Actively change their pattern of weight bearing; for example:
   a. Landing more on the mid foot or forefoot to shift impact away from a painful heel area;

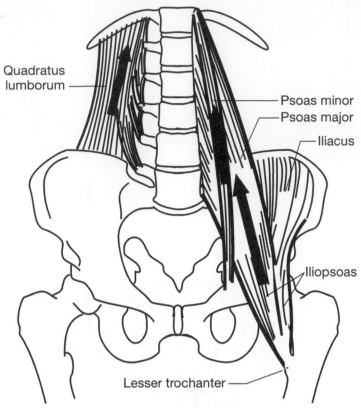

Fig. 39. Muscles capable of generating forces (*arrows*) that can result in an upslip.

    b. Tending to pronation and increasing dorsiflexion to improve shock absorption at the now more flexible foot/ankle level and decrease the forces transmitted upward; and

    c. Offload the painful site by shortening the stance phase on this side and/or shifting the center of gravity away, by leaning into the opposite direction.

2. Lean toward the side of an unstable SI joint, to approximate the surfaces and thereby increase stability (see **Fig. 4C**; **Fig. 44**).

Compensatory Curves of the Spine

The pelvic obliquity results in a compensatory scoliosis—curves in the frontal plane—to ensure the head ends up in midline as best as possible, with the eyes and ears level, to minimize any disturbance of visual function and the labyrinthine balancing mechanisms.

Clinical correlation for runners

Superimposing these compensatory lateral curves on an existing lumbar lordosis and thoracic kyphosis creates additional stresses on the spine (**Fig. 45**).

1. It can cause back pain; in particular, at the:

    a. Lumbosacral junction, where L5 interlinks with the sacrum. The lumbar convexity is formed by rotation of L1 to L4 inclusive into the convexity (see **Fig. 24**). Any

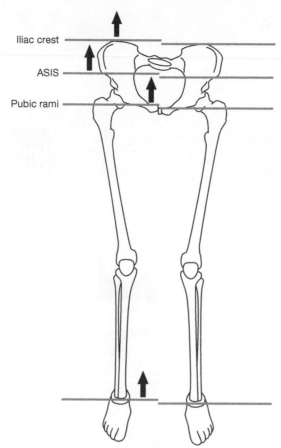

Iliac crest

ASIS

Pubic rami

Fig. 40. Sitting–lying test: right sacroiliac joint upslip. The legs move together and the right leg remains short to the same extent in sitting and lying. The right anterior and posterior pelvic landmarks are all displaced upward relative to the sacrum and left innominate. ASIS, anterior superior iliac spine.

further rotation of L4 relative to L5 puts an additional torsional stress on the L4-5 disc, results in facet joint compression on 1 side and distraction on the other, and may actually cause unwanted rotation of L5 relative to the sacrum and secondarily of the sacrum itself (**Fig. 46**).

b. Thoracolumbar junction, with transition of a lumbar lordosis to thoracic kyphosis, superimposed reversal of the compensatory curves and contrary rotation of T12 and L1, all increasing stress on the discs and facet joints in the mid back region.

c. The cervicothoracic point of reversal, often manifest as muscle tightening and/or actual pain at the base of the neck and in the shoulder/scapular regions.

2. It can aggravate any existing discomfort or actually trigger onset of back pain in a runner who already has:

a. Some degree of idiopathic scoliosis (see: "Implications for the treating physician");

b. A coexisting rotational displacement of 1 or more vertebrae (see **Fig. 46**); and

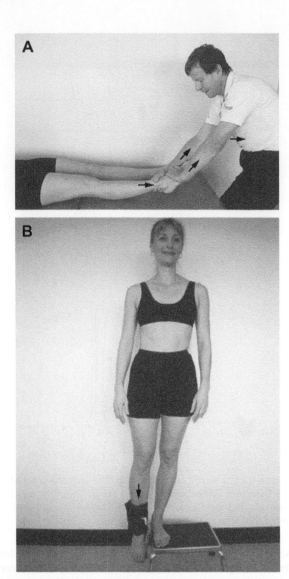

Fig. 41. Correction of a right upslip. (*A*) Two-person technique. (*B*) One-person: using the weight of the leg (with or without extra weight attached) to exert a downward traction force on the innominate and releasing tension in muscles that may be perpetuating the upslip (see **Fig. 39**).

c. A site where movement of the spine itself and between the spine and pelvis is already compromised; for example, vertebral fusion, unilateral sacralization, or lumbarization (see **Fig. 26**).

Asymmetrical Weight Bearing and Pattern of Shoe Wear

In all of those presenting with an upslip and more than 90% of those with rotational malalignment:

1. Weight-bearing shifts to the left on both sides and

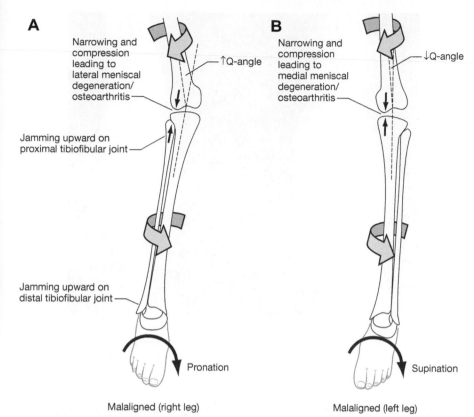

A

Narrowing and compression leading to lateral meniscal degeneration/ osteoarthritis

↑Q-angle

Jamming upward on proximal tibiofibular joint

Jamming upward on distal tibiofibular joint

Pronation

Malaligned (right leg)

B

Narrowing and compression leading to medial meniscal degeneration/ osteoarthritis

↓Q-angle

Supination

Malaligned (left leg)

Fig. 42. Effect of a malalignment-related shift toward right pronation, left supination on the knee. (*A*) Right side: the tendency toward pronation and knee valgus angulation increases the Q-angle and the pressure on the lateral compartment; excessive pronation can result in a forceful upward movement of the fibula and a jamming of the proximal tibiofibular joint (similar to what can occur with an ankle eversion sprain). (*B*) Left side: the tendency toward supination and knee varus angulation decreases the Q-angle and increases pressure on the medial compartment.

2. There is some rotation of the lower extremities and feet, outward from midline on the right side and toward it on the left (**Fig. 47**B).[26,27]

When not bearing weight, the right foot rests in increased varus angulation compared with the left (**Fig. 48**B). As a result:

1. Right heel impact is more posterolateral compared with the left, which augments forcing the right foot into valgus/pronation.
2. The right foot may quite obviously pronate whereas the left may pronate less, stay in neutral or actually supinate on weight bearing (**Figs. 49** and **50**). Although there are variations of this pattern, these all reflect a shift toward the left; for example, both feet may pronate but the right more so than the left, or both supinate but the left more so than the right.
3. The same trend is consistently reflected in the wear pattern of the shoes (**Fig. 51**):
   a. The right heel cup collapses inward, the left stays in neutral or leans outward (see **Fig. 51**A); again, any variations are consistent with this pattern (**Fig. 52**; see also **Fig. 78**A).

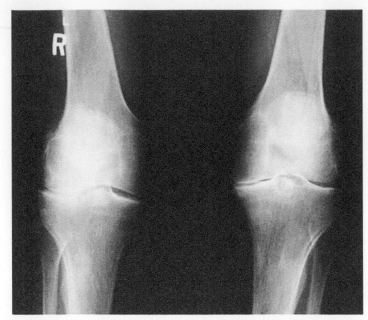

Fig. 43. Osteoarthritic changes in the knee as a result of long-term pressure redistribution similar to what can occur with a malalignment-related shift in weight bearing: accentuated wear of right lateral and left medial joint compartments (see **Figs. 49** and **50**).

b. Asymmetrical wear of the soles, especially noticeable in the forefoot region and the heel (**Fig. 53**).
c. Compaction of the midsole and often a shift of the upper: medially on the side tending to pronation (see **Fig. 51**B) and laterally on the supinating side (see **Fig. 78**A).

In some 5% to 10%, the shift is in the opposite direction: the right leg rotating inward, the left outward and the right foot tending to supination, the left to pronation (see **Fig. 47**A; **Fig. 54**). This pattern seems to be linked to anyone presenting with a left anterior, right posterior rotation and simultaneous locking of the left SI joint (or left anterior and locked, for short).[26,27]

Clinical correlation for runners

1. The increased tendency to right pronation and left supination puts contrasting stresses on specific muscles, nerves, ligaments, and joint structures from the foot upward to the hip girdle region (see **Fig. 42**; **Figs. 55–57**). Pronation stresses particularly soft tissue structures on the medial aspect of the foot and leg; supination stresses structures on the lateral aspect. Any of these can become symptomatic; typical complications are summarized here (see "Implications for the treating physician" for further discussion).
2. With increasing right pronation, the right knee progressively leans inward, tending to genu valgum with opening of the medial, compression of the lateral compartment. With left supination, the shift at the knee is toward neutral alignment or frank genu varum with opening of the lateral, compression of the medial compartment.

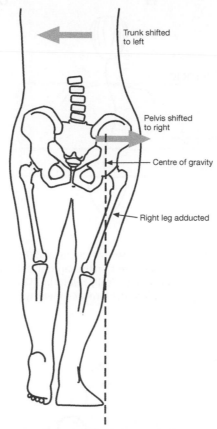

Trunk shifted
to left

Pelvis shifted
to right

Centre of gravity

Right leg adducted

Fig. 44. Compensated right Trendelenburg gait. Impaired transfer of weight through an unstable right sacroiliac joint can occur with ligament laxity, decreased muscular support, or degenerative loss of joint surface. It may be reduced or prevented by having the pelvis abduct and shift to the right to increase compression and minimize vertical shear stresses through that joint (see **Fig. 4C**).

These changes put increased stress on structures such as the right medial collateral ligament and patellofemoral compartment/patellar tendon, the left lateral collateral ligament and iliotibial (IT) band insertion, respectively. The persistent or repetitive strain can cause these structures to become tender or outright painful (eg, right patellofemoral compartment syndrome; left IT band friction syndrome). These stresses are increased by activities like running on a slope declined to the left (**Fig. 58B**). A shift in joint loading is suspected of being able to accelerate joint degeneration; in the case of the knee, of the right lateral and left medial compartment (see **Fig. 43**).[12,33]

3. The combination of right pronation and outward rotation of the leg makes it more likely for the runner to just touch or actually hit the right heel against the left ankle or inner calf. With the inwardly rotated left side, there is an increased risk of losing balance or tripping by catching the left big toe on the right heel or ankle region.

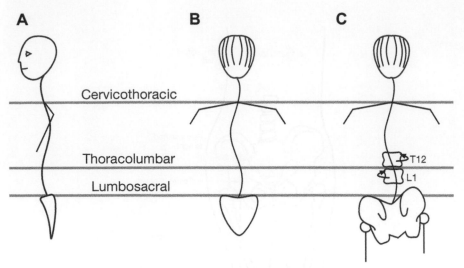

Fig. 45. Sites of spinal curve reversal and stress. (*A*) Lateral and (*B*) posterior views show overlying sites of curve reversal (and increased stress) in the sagittal and frontal plane, respectively. (*C*) Reversal at the thoracolumbar junction typically results in T12 and L1 rotating in opposite directions, with L1 still turning slightly into the lumbar convexity.

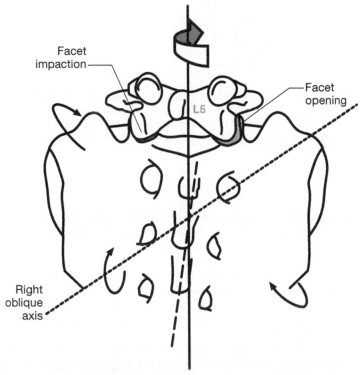

Fig. 46. Excessive clockwise rotation of the L5 complex for whatever reason results in compression or impaction of the left L5-S1 facet joint that, in turn, can cause rotation of the sacrum around the right oblique axis.

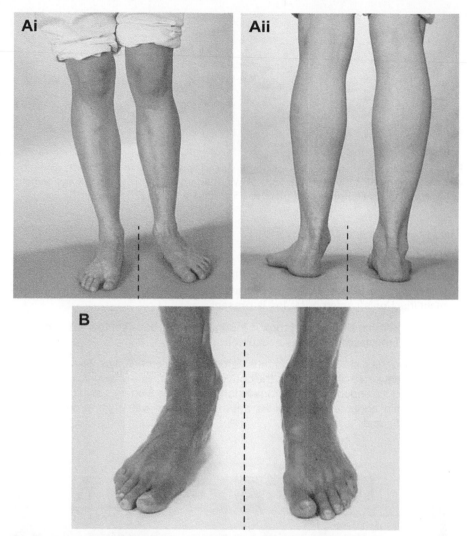

Fig. 47. Two variants of the shift in weight bearing seen with rotational malalignment. (*Ai, ii*) With the rare left anterior rotation and sacroiliac joint locking: left foot turns outward from midline and pronates, the right inward and supinates. (*Aii*) Also shows the obvious narrowing of the left Achilles tendon as it is subjected to increased tension with pronation on this side. (*B*) With one of the more common presentations: the right foot typically turns outward and pronates, the left inward and supinates.

Asymmetrical Muscle Tone

Paired muscles show tone to be increase, or "facilitated," on 1 side and decreased, or "inhibited," on the other side. The changes in tone seem to be mediated by the autonomic nervous system secondary to a mechanism, segmental or cortical, that affects the muscle spindle setting and results in either facilitation or inhibition of the resting tone.[20,26,27,34–37] The pattern of muscles affected by the pelvic malalignment is:

1. Asymmetrical: some are automatically tensed up on the right, others on the left side, whereas their partner on the opposite side seems to be relaxed; for example,

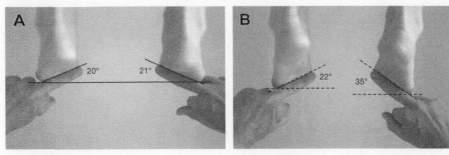

Fig. 48. Angulation of the feet at rest (same subject, sitting). (*A*) In alignment: symmetric varus angulation of the sole of the feet. (*B*) With an upslip and rotational malalignment: right varus angulation is increased (here to 35° compared with 22° on the *left*).

left quadratus lumborum, iliopsoas, hip abductors/tensor fascia lata (TFL), triceps surae; right piriformis, biceps femoris (**Figs. 59** and **60**); and

2. Consistent, regardless of what type of an upslip (right or left) or rotational malalignment (right or left anteroposterior) is present.

Malalignment can also cause a chronic increase in tone, and eventual tenderness, in muscles and myofascial slings as a result of:

1. Increasing the distance between muscle origin and insertion, typically affecting:
   a. The paravertebral muscles on the convex (ie, longer) side of a curve in the spine;
   b. The left hip abductors and peroneus longus with the tendency to left supination; right hip adductors and tibialis anterior/posterior with right pronation (see **Fig. 55**); and

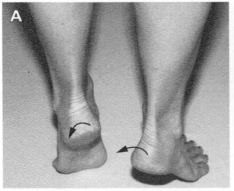
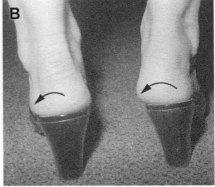

Fig. 49. (*A*) Toe-walking can bring out the asymmetry of weight bearing seen with an upslip and rotational malalignment: inward whip and collapse of the heel (calcaneal eversion) on the pronating right side, outward whip and calcaneal inversion on the supinating left side. (*B*) A similar pattern, accentuated by walking on high heels: right pronates, with heel shifting inward (partly off the medial edge); the left supinates, with heel shifting slightly over the lateral edge. *Note:* increased tension (narrowing) of Achilles tendon on right pronating side in both subjects.

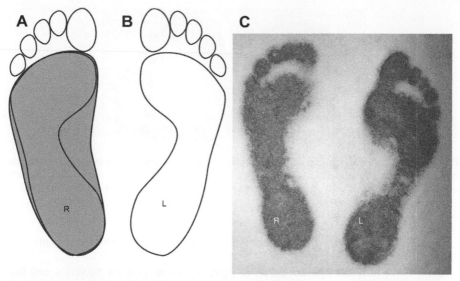

Fig. 50. Foot contact surface. (*A*) On an orthotic versus (*B*) barefoot on sand. (*C*) Barefoot weight-bearing pattern seen from below a glass surface, reflecting the typical malalignment-related shift in weight bearing: medially on the pronating right, noticeably increased foot surface contact in the midfoot region; laterally on the supinating left, decreasing contact especially along the inner longitudinal arch region.

    c. The hamstrings on the side of an anterior rotation; rectus femoris and iliopsoas on the side of a posterior rotation (**Fig. 61**).
2. The muscle being constantly in some degree of contraction in an attempt to splint a painful area, stabilize a joint, or combination of these; typical involved are:
    a. The paravertebral muscles lying alongside the thoracolumbar junction, with the contrary rotation of T12 and L1 at the site of curve reversal causing

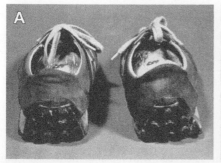 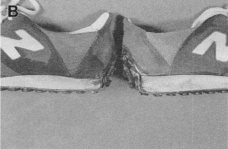

Fig. 51. Reflection of the shift in weight bearing with malalignment (see Case History: Runner A). (*A*) With the more common patterns of rotational malalignment and an upslip: the tendency to right pronation, left supination, leads to heel cup collapse toward the left. (*B*) Medial view of the same running shoes showing compression of the inside of the right heel/sole (on *left* in photo) compared with the left shoe (on *right* in photo).

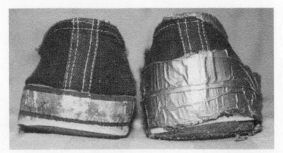

Fig. 52. The pattern of heel cup collapse in someone who pronates bilaterally still reflects the typical shift in weight bearing with malalignment: right leans in much more than the left, leading to desperation measures using duct tape to reinforce the right heel cup medially.

additional biomechanical stresses on the adjacent discs and facet joints (see **Fig. 45**).

b. The key muscles that act on an SI joint: piriformis, gluteus maximus and iliopsoas (see **Figs. 2**, **3** and **39**), especially if the joint has become:

   i. Unstable as a result of ligament laxity and/or actual joint degeneration, or

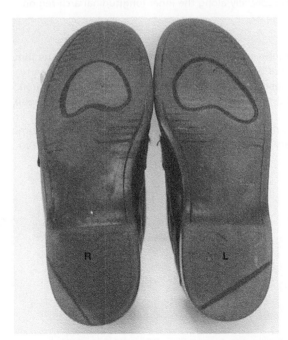

Fig. 53. Typical asymmetrical wear pattern of the soles seen with malalignment. Right (*R*) side: increased wear posterolaterally in the heel (reflecting the increased varus angulation of the right foot at impact; see **Fig. 48**) and medially in the forefoot (reflecting the tendency to pronation). Left (*L*) side: wear in the heel affects a wider area, located more posteriorly and medially (reflecting the comparatively decreased varus angulation at impact) and more laterally in the forefoot (reflecting the tendency to supination).

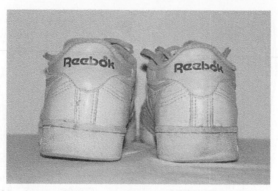

Fig. 54. Pattern of heel cup collapse typically seen with left anterior and locked rotational malalignment, reflecting the tendency to left pronation, right supination.

  ii. Painful from irritation of joint surfaces, supporting capsule and/or ligaments.
 c. The myofascial slings[6,15,17,29,32,38–40]; for example, those that help to stabilize the pelvis and spine:
  i. The anterior oblique support systems, formed in part by the anterior abdominal fascia connected to the external/internal obliques and rectus abdominis; and

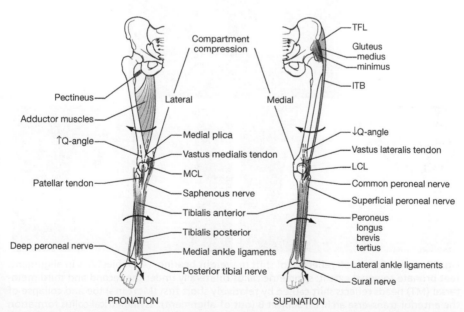

Fig. 55. Structures put under stress by the malalignment-related shift in weight-bearing, tending to right pronation and left supination. ITB, iliotibial band; LCL, lateral collateral ligament; MCL, medial collateral ligament.

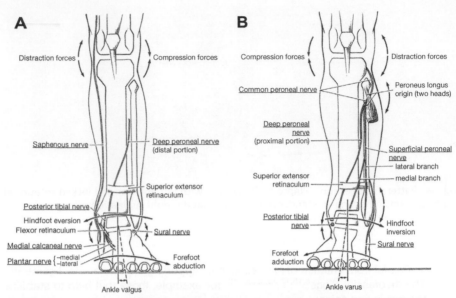

Fig. 56. Peripheral nerves in the left leg affected by a shift in weight bearing. (*A*) Nerves affected by pronation forces. (*B*) Nerves affected by supination forces. (Schamberger 1987).

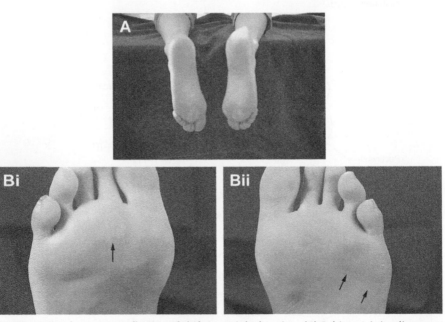

Fig. 57. Callus formation reflective of shift in weight bearing. (*A*) Subject A is in alignment, feet pronate to equal extent: symmetric callus bilaterally under the second and third metatarsal (MT) heads reflects shift caused by relatively short first (Morton's) toe and collapse of the anterior transverse arch. (*B*) Subject B (out of alignment): asymmetrical callus formation reflects malalignment-related shift in weight bearing, (*Bi*) more medially on the pronating right side, under the second MT head (indicated by single *arrow*) and (*Bii*) more laterally on the supinating left side, under the fourth and fifth MT heads (indicated by the two *arrows*).

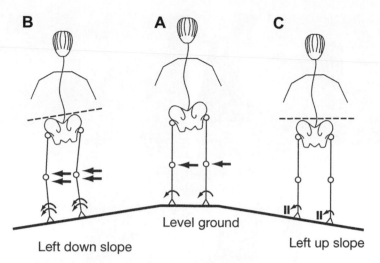

Fig. 58. The effect of slope on the malalignment-related shift toward right pronation, left supination. (A) Usual shift, with both feet leaning into left side, noted when on level ground. This tendency (B) is accentuated on a grade sloping down to the left and (C) decreased on a grade sloping up to the left.

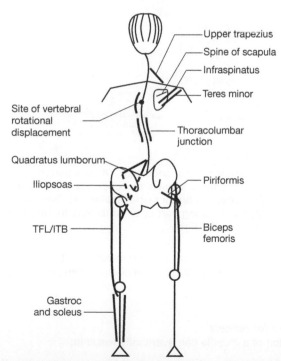

Fig. 59. Typical sites of increased muscle tension (and often tenderness) seen with pelvic malalignment and also minimal rotation of a vertebra (here shown at the interscapular level). If a muscle involved shows increased tone bilaterally, the one indicated here is usually the one affected more severely. TFL/ITB, tensor fascia lata/iliotibial band.

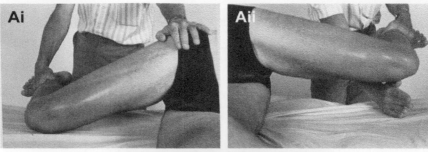

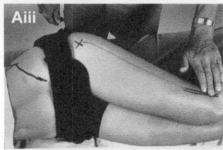

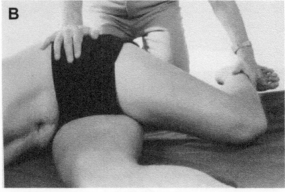

Fig. 60. Ober's test for limitation of hip adduction. (*A*) In a person with an upslip or rotational malalignment: (*Ai*) the right adducts to touch the plinth, (*Aii*) left adduction is limited, and (*Aiii*) the facilitated left tensor fascia lata/iliotibial band complex proves consistently tense (and usually tender along part or all of its length). (*B*) After realignment: left adduction now equals that on the right.

ii. The posterior oblique system, formed in part by latissimus dorsi on 1 one side connected by the thoracolumbar fascia to gluteus maximus on the opposite side.

Clinical correlation for runners
Chronic contraction of a muscle can eventually result in:

1. Tension myalgia, as well as development of trigger points within the muscle;
2. Irritation and inflammation at the myotendinous and fibro-osseous junctions; and
3. Inhibition or alteration of movement patterns that involve the tender muscle or the myofascial sling that it is part of; and

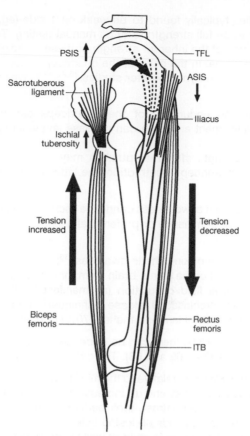

Fig. 61. Changes in tension resulting with the shift of a muscle origin toward or away from the insertion with an innominate anterior rotation: tension increased in biceps femoris, decreased in iliacus, rectus femoris and tensor fascia lata/iliotibial band (ITB) complex. The reverse changes occur with a posterior rotation.

4. Referral from the myotome itself and/or a trigger point to a distant site(s).

Asymmetry of Muscle Strength and Bulk

Muscle strength is affected in a typical asymmetrical pattern that is more readily apparent in the lower extremities. Compared with their partner on the opposite side, a functional weakness ranging from 3+ to 4+/5 is consistently seen:

1. In the right: ankle invertors (tibialis anterior/posterior); hip flexors (iliopsoas, quadriceps) and extensors (primarily gluteus maximus); hip adductors; extensor hallucis longus.
2. In the left: ankle evertors (peroneus longus/brevis); hip abductors (gluteus medius/minimus; TFL); hip external/internal rotators; hamstrings.

This asymmetrical pattern of weakness is consistently seen with either a right or left upslip and all the variations on rotational malalignment except for the left anterior, right anterior and left SI joint locked one, in which the findings are reversed.

Some of the muscles typically found to be weak on 1 side (eg, right quadriceps) may actually seem to be full strength (5/5) on manual testing. This finding is likely to be more a reflection of the inherent strength of these muscles which the examiner just cannot overcome. In the case of the quadriceps, side-to-side differences may be detectable only on dynamometer studies,[26,27,34,41] which have also shown that:

1. Both the power and endurance of the quadriceps can be reduced in the presence of malalignment and both can increase immediately following realignment; and
2. The increase in strength after manipulation may be greater for an eccentric than a concentric quadriceps contraction; the latter will frequently not improve at all.

The asymmetrical pattern of weakness cannot be ascribed to laterality; for example, handed/footedness, eye dominance or preferential hearing lateralization.[26,27] Explanations proposed include:

1. Impaired proprioceptive or kinesthetic awareness[36];
2. Dysfunction at the level of the spine, brain stem, or cortex[35];
3. Impaired cerebrospinal fluid circulation (as manifest by the ability to achieve realignment using the craniosacral release technique)[20]; and
4. Lateralization of motor dominance to the left (70%) or right (15%).

As the malalignment persists, there can be evidence of a change in muscle bulk on side-to-side comparison (**Figs. 62** and **63**). The difference may reflect:

1. Reorientation of muscle fibers relative to the midline, placing some muscles in a position of advantage so that they end up increasing in size because of increased efficiency and/or demand; in contrast, their partner on the opposite side may now work at a disadvantage and ends up losing bulk;
2. Wasting as a result of a change in style of walking or running, in an attempt to:
   a. Accommodate the biomechanical changes that have occurred;
   b. Off-load a painful structure; for example, joint, tendon, or other soft tissue; or
   c. Minimize the use of a muscle that has become painful, leading to disuse wasting.

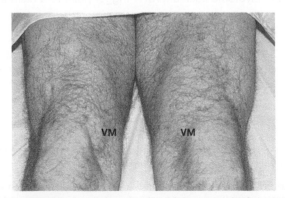

Fig. 62. Quadriceps asymmetry in a person with malalignment (right anterior, left posterior innominate rotation): wasting of right and hypertrophy of left vastus medialis (VM).

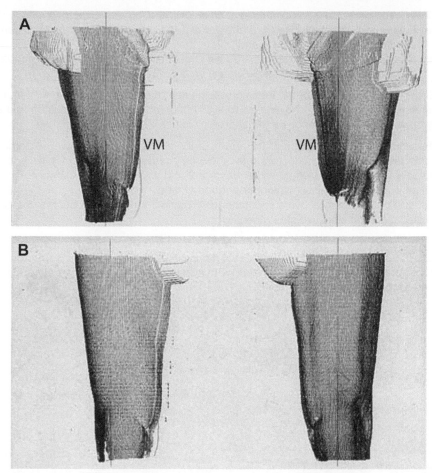

Fig. 63. Quadriceps bulk of the person in **Fig. 62**, delineated with a laser scanner. (*A*) Asymmetry of vastus medialis (VM) noted with the malalignment: right wasted, left hypertrophied. (*B*) Almost symmetric VM bulk within 4 months of maintaining alignment and return to regular activities (ie, no selective muscle strengthening). (*From* Schamberger W. The malalignment syndrome: Diagnosing and treating a common cause of acute and chronic pelvic, limb and back pain. Edinburgh (UK): Churchill Livingstone; 2013.)

c. A muscle contracting inappropriately; for example, out of sequence with other muscles in an 'inner' or 'outer' sling or failing to respond at all on attempted volitional contraction.[37,42]

Clinical correlation for runners

1. The runner may sense that 1 leg (typically the right) is weaker or somewhat unstable on weight bearing compared with the other one (see: 'Impaired balance and recovery') and may experience one leg fatiguing more readily or feeling sore as from overuse (see Case History: Runner A and B).

2. The runner participating in biathlons or triathlons, the leg on 1 side may:
   a. Feel weak on the bike in terms of the amount of power it can generate and a tendency to fatigue more easily; and
   b. Seem to move differently compared with the other side, with movement not being as spontaneous (or even awkward) on the weak side (**Fig. 64**).

Some authors have attributed these problems to a malalignment-related leg length difference, with one study showing up to a 5% decrease in power generated and a loss of pedal stroke efficiency on the short leg side.[24]

3. Realignment results in immediate return of full strength in most lower extremity muscles. The left hip abductors may show only partial improvement initially, but usually recovers full strength within days or 2 to 3 weeks at the most once alignment is being maintained for longer periods of time.
4. Muscle bulk usually recovers spontaneously within 2 to 3 months, but may be assisted by doing selective strengthening.

Asymmetrical Ligament Tension

The biomechanical changes that occur with these 2 presentations can affect ligaments secondarily by placing them:

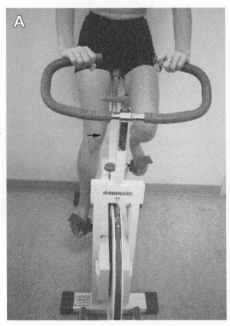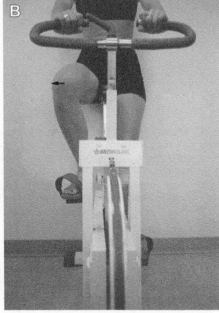

Fig. 64. Relationship of the knees to the midline (crossbar) in a cyclist with an upslip or rotational malalignment and the typical rotation of the legs (right outward, left inward; see **Figs. 42, 47**B**, 55**). (*A*) On pushing down on the pedal, the right knee moves toward midline, combining hip/knee extension, foot pronation, and a tendency to genu valgum. (*B*) On coming up, the right knee moves away from midline, with external rotation of the leg as the knee flexes. In contrast, the left knee maintains a relatively neutral position, traveling primarily in the sagittal plane throughout both phases.

1. Under increased tension; examples include: (**Figs. 65** and **66**); examples include:
    a. The medial collateral ligament of the knee on the side of excessive pronation and secondary shift toward genu valgum; the lateral collateral ligament on the neutral or supinating side, with shift toward genu varum (see **Figs. 55** and **56**);
    b. Posterior and interosseous SI joint ligaments (**Figs. 1**A and **2**A), also the sacro-tuberous and sacrospinous, on the side of a posterior rotation (see **Figs. 65**A and **66**B);
    c. Long dorsal sacroiliac ligament with an upslip or anterior rotation (see **Fig. 65**B); and
    d. The medial ankle ligaments and flexor retinaculum on the pronating side, lateral ligaments on the supinating side (**Figs. 55**, **56** and **79**).
2. In a slackened position:
    Tension would be decreased in the counterparts of the ligaments mentioned in point #1, above; for example, the sacrotuberous, sacrospinous with an anterior rotation, the long dorsal sacroiliac ligament with a posterior rotation.

Clinical correlation for runners

1. Ligaments put under tension:
    a. These gradually lengthen, decreasing their ability to support a joint. On realignment, laxity of these ligaments predisposes to recurrence of the malalignment, until they finally regain their normal length.
    b. The pain-transmitting C nerve fibers within ligaments can neither stretch as quickly nor as much as the elastic components, making them vulnerable to irritation, inflammation, and even disruption. They can become a source of localized and/or referred pain and paresthesias, long before elongation of the elastic components has reached its limit (see Case History: Runner A).[43–45]

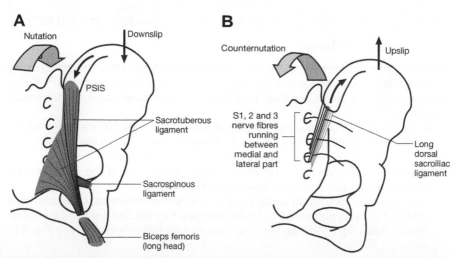

Fig. 65. Ligaments put under tension by the movement of an innominate or the sacrum relative to each other. (*A*) Posterior rotation or a downslip: sacrotuberous, sacrospinous, also interosseous ligaments (not shown; see **Fig. 1**B). (*B*) Anterior rotation or an upslip: long dorsal sacroiliac ligament. PSIS, posterior superior iliac spine.

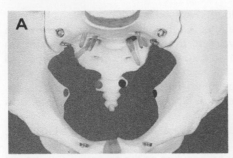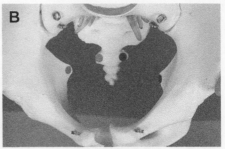

Fig. 66. Sacrospinous ligament origins and insertions on an anteroposterior view of pelvis. (*A*) The distance between the right origin and insertion (*light dots*) is equal to that on the left (*black dots*). (*B*) With rotational malalignment (right anterior, left posterior): the origin and insertion are brought closer together on the right and separated on the left.

2. Ligaments put in a slackened position:
   a. These gradually undergo shortening, or contracture, and may limit joint range of motion.
   b. They can be one cause of post-realignment pain (see "Implications for the treating physician").

Asymmetrical Lower Extremity Range of Motion

Side-by-side comparison shows asymmetry of the range of motion attainable in any joint from the neck down to the great toes (**Figs. 67–71**). Differences of 10° to 15° are not uncommon. However, adding up the total range available in a particular line of movement (eg, hip flexion and extension) on 1 side equals that available on the opposite side. Barring any abnormalities of the joints (eg, degeneration, inflammatory conditions, contracture), realignment results in immediate return of equal bilateral ranges of motion. Frequently, the total range available in a particular direction actually comes to exceed that noted before correction by 5° to 15°, as key muscles relax and allow other joints to regain their normal range of motion (see **Figs. 67**B and **68**C).

Clinical correlation for runners

1. Changes in pelvic and lower extremity ranges of motion can affect the gait cycle by causing side-to-side differences of the swing-through and stance phase.[32,38] Any compensatory measures are likely to alter style, decrease efficiency and increase energy costs.
2. The malalignment results in changes that, in combination, will make it harder for the runner to bring the straight leg upward on 1 side. For example, in the runner with a right anterior rotation, this movement can be limited in part by:
   a. Physical obstruction from the downward displacement of the right anterior acetabular rim with anterior rotation (see **Fig. 67**Ai);
   b. The increased tone noted particularly in right gluteus maximus, biceps femoris and piriformis, in part owing to facilitation (see **Fig. 59**) and the further separation of their origin and insertion that occurs with this movement (see **Fig. 61**); and
   c. Other factors, such as contracture of soft tissues that have been put into a relaxed or shortened state (e.g. right sacrotuberous and sacrospinous ligaments relaxed with right anterior rotation) (**Figs. 65**B and **66**B, respectively), may also come into play.

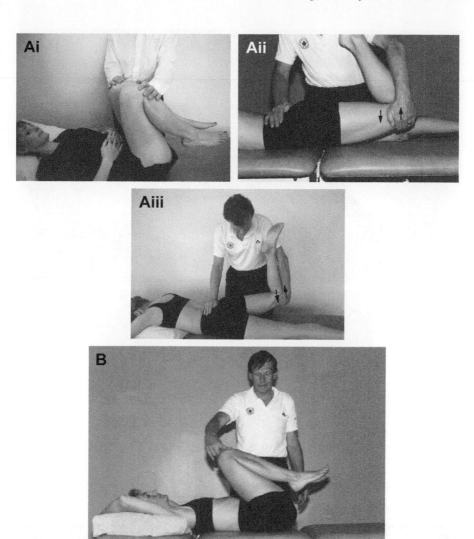

Fig. 67. Effect of alignment on passive hip flexion and extension, tested with knees in flexion. (*A*) With rotational malalignment (right anterior, left posterior): (*Ai*) limitation of right hip flexion (105°) compared with the left (115°); (*Aii*) limitation of left hip extension (10°) compared with (*Aiii*) that on the right of 25°. (*B*) In alignment: hip flexion is now equal and actually increased to 130°, with extension equal at 25°.

3. Limitations would affect particularly a sprinter, who usually depends on greater stride length, and a hurdler or steeplechaser, who has to clear a barrier; all require more of the available range of motion of certain joints than a middle or distance runner. Some runners may be able to adapt their style to take advantage of these asymmetries of available ranges. For example, the fact that 1 hurdler preferentially approaches a jump with the right leg leading may reflect an increase in right hip flexion and left internal rotation (relative to their counterparts) that makes it easier to carry out the jump this way. However, it puts that same hurdler at a disadvantage

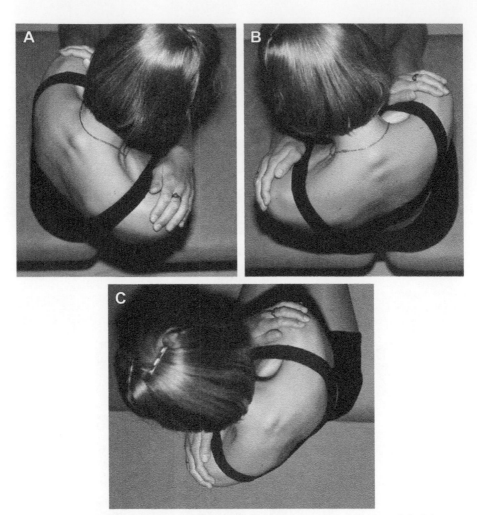

Fig. 68. Trunk rotation in sitting. (*A, B*) Malalignment of the pelvis is present. (*A*) Right rotation to 45°. (*B*) Left rotation limited to 35°. (*C*) On realignment, left came to equal right rotation, with improvement to 55° now evident bilaterally.

and increased risk of injury if for some reason he or she is thrown off stride (eg, clipping a hurdle; an awkward landing and recovery) and has to take the next jump with the left leg leading and the right one trailing. He or she is then forced into and may even exceed the relative limitation of left hip flexion and right internal rotation, with the attendant risk of injury (**Fig. 69**).

Limitations of particular concern include:

1. Left pelvic and often also trunk rotation in the horizontal plane; that is, counterclockwise (see **Fig. 68**B; **Fig. 70**). The runner can try to compensate for the effect on stride length by:
   a. Actively increasing left trunk rotation in an attempt to bring the pelvis further back on the left and lengthen stance phase on that side;

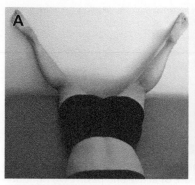
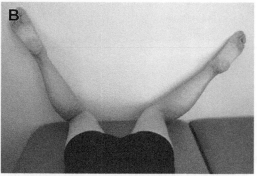

Fig. 69. Internal rotation of the hip. (*A*) In alignment: symmetric (40° bilaterally). (*B*) With malalignment present: right decreased, left increased (30° vs 50°, respectively). In both situations, total equals 80°.

      b. Voluntarily decrease left swing-through to match the limitation on the right side; or

      c. A combination of increased trunk rotation and reduction in swing-through.

  2. Hip extension or flexion (see **Fig. 67**)

      a. Any limitation of these could decrease the ability of the leg to go through full swing-through or stance phase, respectively. In an attempt to achieve equal

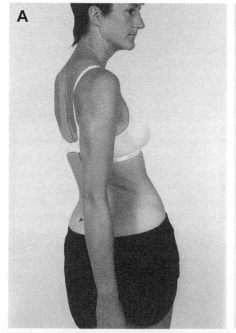
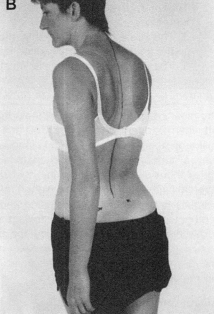

Fig. 70. Asymmetry of pelvic rotation around the vertical axis in the horizontal plane typically seen with rotational malalignment. (*A*) Active clockwise rotation to 40°. (*B*). Active counterclockwise rotation limited to 30°. Note the decreased facial, shoulder girdle, and chest profile compared with that seen in (*A*).

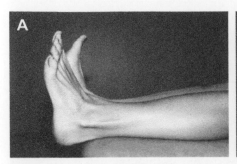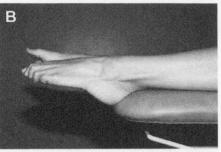

Fig. 71. Effect of an upslip and the more common patterns of rotational malalignment on ankle range of motion assessment, with relative increase of active and passive (*A*) right dorsiflexion and (*B*) left plantarflexion.

stride length, the runner can actively increase ankle plantarflexion on swing-through, go into a supination pattern of weight bearing earlier in stance phase, and/or land more on the forefoot to increase the length of the respective extremity.

3. Limitation of left ankle dorsiflexion, right plantarflexion (**Fig. 71**):
   a. Right dorsiflexion is increased, contributing to the tendency to pronation and risk of developing plantar fasciitis and Achilles tendonitis on this side (see **Figs. 47**B, **49**A, B, and **79**, also "Implications for the treating physician").[46]
   b. Left plantar flexion is increased, augmenting the tendency to supination. Together, these make for a more rigid foot, poor at shock absorption, increasing:
      i. The stress on proximal joints, muscles and soft tissue structures as more of the impact is now transmitted upward; and
      ii. The risk of sustaining an ankle strain or stress fracture on this side.

Apparent or Functional Leg Length Difference

The most common finding is that the right iliac crest ends up higher than that on the left when standing (see **Figs. 13**C, D and **17**). The pelvic obliquity persists in sitting, unlike someone with an anatomic long leg whose pelvis would now be level; however, a concomitant underlying anatomic leg length difference could not be ruled out at this point. Most likely, the right side will continue to be higher, although a reversal (with the left side now higher) may become evident on sitting. That a pelvic obliquity is present in both standing and sitting merely suggests that pelvic malalignment is likely present but knowing this, or which iliac crest is higher, is not necessarily helpful in determining the side of an anterior rotation or an upslip. Also, leg length per se can be affected by other factors, including contracture and asymmetry of tension in the muscles and ligaments of the pelvic girdle and hip region.

Clinical correlation for runners

1. Confirmation of the apparent leg length difference and the type of malalignment present depends on looking at the runner in several positions (standing, sitting and lying), checking for leg length changes on the sitting–lying test and assessment of pelvic landmarks.

2. Differences in leg length of as much as 2 to 4 cm:
   a. Can be attributable entirely to the presence of rotational malalignment, an up-slip, or a combination of these; and
   b. May reverse completely on changing from long sitting to supine lying.
3. Whereas 80% to 85% of the adult population present with pelvic malalignment, only 6% to 12% of them actually have an anatomic leg length difference of 5 mm or more.[26,27,47] Some runners may benefit from a heel lift once in alignment to avoid stresses attributable to the leg length difference and secondary changes (eg, pelvic obliquity, compensatory scoliosis).

Impaired Balance and Recovery

A problem with balance and recovery is most noticeable on kinetic testing, particularly single leg stance (see **Fig. 23**). For example, the runner may have no problem supporting weight on the left leg alone, whereas carrying out the maneuver on the right side is at best achieved with increased concentration on the effort or may result in an obvious swaying of the pelvis and/or trunk to maintain balance. At worst, the runner is unable to carry out the maneuver at all.[37,48] An obvious side-to-side difference may also become evident on toe walking and hopping on 1 foot (see **Fig. 49**).

The imbalance is likely a reflection of a combination of factors, including:

1. The asymmetry of weight bearing, with relative instability noted on the side of pronation where:
   a. The foot and ankle are unlocked and more mobile (**Fig. 72**A); and

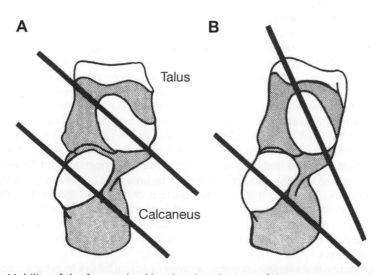

A   **B**

Talus

Calcaneus

Fig. 72. Mobility of the foot and ankle related to the axes of the transverse tarsal joint. (*A*) When the calcaneus is in eversion (eg, pronation), the conjoint axis between the talonavicular and calcaneocuboid joints are parallel to one another so that increased motion occurs in the transverse tarsal joint. (*B*) When the calcaneus is in inversion (eg, supination) the axes are no longer parallel and there is decreased motion and increased stability of the transverse tarsal joint. (*From* Mann R. Biomechanics of running. In: Mack RP, editor. American Academy of Orthopedic Surgeons: symposium on the foot and leg in running sports. St Louis (MO): CV Mosby; 1982. p. 1–29.)

b. The Q-angle increases and the knee ends up no longer positioned directly over the foot (see **Figs. 42**A, and **55**).
2. The asymmetry of muscle strength and tension.
3. Asymmetry of proprioceptive input from the pelvis, lower extremity joints and soft tissues, including the soles of the feet (see **Fig. 50**).

Clinical correlation for runners

The runner can experience a sensation of a knee or hip giving way unexpectedly, sometimes preceded by a sharp pain, yet examination may fail to show any joint instability or tenderness. One explanation proposes that subconscious or conscious pain originates from soft tissues or nerves that:

1. Are already in trouble because of the malalignment; and
2. Lie either in the vicinity of a joint or can refer pain to this joint or to a distant site; for example, the T12/L1 lateral cutaneous branch referring to the lateral hip region (**Fig. 83**A3, B3); the hip joint ligaments referring to the lateral knee joint area (see **Fig. 1**A; **Fig. 73**).

The pain can cause a reflex relaxation of muscles that support the joint and result in it giving way. For example:

1. Relaxation of the quadriceps can make the knee buckle, an impulse that temporarily shuts down piriformis and gluteus maximus can have a similar effect on the hip joint, allowing it to collapse into flexion. Both mechanisms could cause the runner to stumble or fall.
2. Episodic giving way of one leg has also been ascribed to sudden failure of one or more of the key muscles that ensure stability of the SI joint, resulting in the so-called slipping clutch phenomenon. The sensation of something giving way in the hip girdle region is more likely to occur on initial weight bearing when standing up and also on entering the stance phase while walking or running.[49]
3. Recurrent ankle sprains are often attributed to having a chronic unstable ankle with lengthening of ligaments resulting from cumulative sprains. However, in those who are out of alignment, no lengthening or obvious instability or even tenderness may be evident on examination. The shift toward right pronation and left supination, as well as the relative weakness of right ankle invertors and left evertors, predispose to a right eversion, left inversion sprain. However, some runners have obvious difficulty when trying to move the foot and ankle in a specific direction on command (eg, the right down/up and in to test invertors, the left down and out for evertors); this difficulty can usually be overcome simply by providing tactile, verbal, and/or visual feedback. The fact that, in the absence of obvious ligament laxity, this apparent deficit can sometimes resolve with realignment suggests that the runner may be experience a feeling of instability, a problem of insecure foot placement and a tendency to recurrent ankle sprains which is attributable to one or more of the following factors:
   a. The functional weakness, possibly a delay or actual failure to initiate a contraction (also referred to as a pseudoparesis[37,48]) of right ankle invertors or left evertors;
   b. Some instability of the joint secondary to the malalignment; for example, of the right transverse tarsal joint, with the increase in dorsiflexion/tendency to pronation (see **Fig. 72**); and
   c. Temporary ligament (and possibly joint) deafferentation, with impaired proprioception and kinesthetic awareness, a conjecture supported by research on

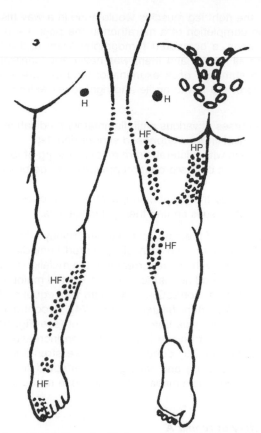

Fig. 73. Referred pain patterns from the iliofemoral and pubofemoral ligaments of the hip joint noted with hip joint instability. H, location of the hip joint; HF, referral from the femoral attachments; HP, referral from the pelvic attachments. (*Adapted from* Hackett GS. Ligament and tendon relaxation (skeletal disability) treated by prolotherapy (fibro-osseous proliferation). 3rd edition. Charles C. Thomas, Springfield, IL 1958.)

subjects who recently sustained a sprain or who had chronic unstable ankles but no evidence of ligament laxity.[50,51]

Case Histories

The following case histories illustrate some of the phenomena seen as a result of the biomechanical and other changes that are part of the malalignment syndrome.

Runner A: referred pain phenomenon presenting as heel pain

A 2:20 marathon runner first became aware of right heel pain after a 12-mile run along winding trails. There were no obvious problems during the run, no twisting or undue jarring. The pain became persistent, varied in intensity, and could be felt consistently on weight bearing but sometimes also when just resting. Pain at heel strike led to a change in gait, favoring the right side, eventually resulting in obvious wasting of the right buttock and lower extremity muscles. After a run of

10 miles or longer, the right leg muscles would ache in a way his muscles used to feel in both legs on completion of a marathon in the past. He had never had any back pain. Radiographs, a computed tomography scan, and a bone scan of the foot and ankle were all normal and there was never any localizable tenderness or pain elicited on the standard back examination and on stressing the soft tissue structures and joints of the pelvic girdle and right lower extremity. The pain failed to respond to:

1. Analgesics and courses of various antiinflammatory medications;
2. The use of a right heel lift for a supposed shorter right leg;
3. Provision of orthotics with bilateral 4 mm medial posting of forefoot and hindfoot to counter the problem of overpronation presumed to be present on both sides; and
4. Standard physiotherapy treatments, acupuncture and, once, an injection of xylocaine into all the soft tissues around the right calcaneus.

Seven years after onset of the pain, an osteopath rightly attributed the pain to the pelvis being out of alignment. The pain disappeared immediately on realignment using the MET; it returned with any recurrence of the malalignment during the initial treatment period, but stopped altogether once he started maintaining alignment for longer periods of time. After correction, leg length was equal and he was noted to supinate slightly to equal extent bilaterally (**Fig. 74**), in contrast with the obvious pronation noted on the right side before realignment (see **Fig. 51A**). Right muscle bulk recovered to equal that on the left just with an increase in his walking and running and without him having done any selective strengthening (see **Figs. 62** and **63**). However, his training and racing were affected from the onset of the heel pain so that he never again managed to run close to the times he had posted previously.

Analysis of case history of runner A

1. This runner's heel pain was erroneously attributed to a number of problems, leading to inappropriate treatment measures that could easily have resulted in further harm. The shift in weight bearing was missed because of failure to examine the wear of his

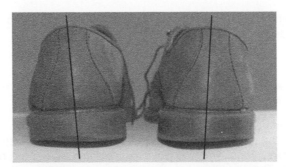

Fig. 74. This runner had a pattern of right foot pronation, left supination evident when malalignment was present (see **Figs. 47**B and **51**). On realignment, the true weight-bearing pattern became evident: bilateral, symmetric supination, with both heel cups now leaning out 5° (see Case History: Runner A; also Runner B, see **Fig. 78**B).

shoes and assess the gait pattern under stress; for example, toe walking and hopping. In reality, excessive pronation was occurring only on the right side (see
Fig. 51A). Provision of orthotics posted medially on both sides merely reinforced
the malalignment-related biomechanical forces on the left side that were already
causing the left foot to supinate (see **Fig. 55**; **Fig. 75**). It also failed to counter the
right pronation, because this was in part owing to outward rotation of the lower ex-
tremity/foot and increased ankle dorsiflexion possible on this side (see **Fig. 47**B
and **71**). The diagnosis of supposed leg length difference had been based on examination of leg length in only 1 position: supine lying.

2. The heel pain resulted from irritation of S1 root fibers supplying the sacrospinous
   and sacrotuberous ligaments, because these were subjected to increased stress
   by the malalignment (**Figs. 76** and **77**). On the basis of referral, the brain had
   mistakenly attributed them to originating from the calcaneal bone and possibly
   the skin overlying the heel, which are part of the S1 sclerotome and dermatome,
   respectively.

3. The combination of failure to come up with the correct diagnosis and the ensuing
   pursuit of misguided treatment measures over the 7-year period effectively ended
   his running career at the national and international level.

***Runner B: biomechanical stresses on the left tensor fascia lata/iliotibial band
complex***
A 26-year-old long distance runner was seen within days of having failed in his third
attempt at finishing a marathon. On each occasion, he had become aware of
increasing pain over the lateral aspect of the left hip and upper thigh from around
the 15-mile mark and had to withdraw from the race within the next 5 miles because
the pain became unbearable. The pain would settle quickly with rest, allowing him to
return to training within days. The 2 previous episodes had been attributed to a left

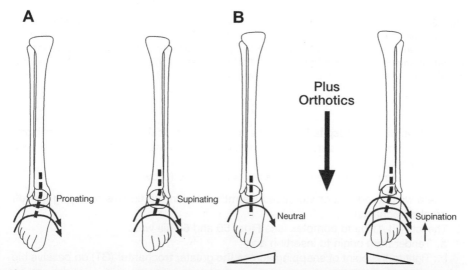

Fig. 75. A person with right anterior, left posterior innominate rotation. (*A*) Tendency to
right pronation, left supination. (*B*) The effect of providing bilateral orthotics with a medial
raise (posting): a decrease of right pronation, worsening of left supination.

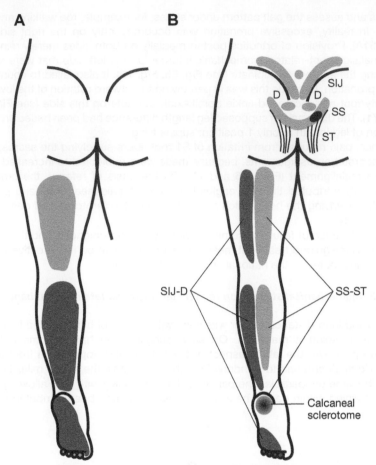

Fig. 76. Nerve root versus referred pattern of dysesthesias. (*A*) S1 radiculopathy pattern. (*B*) Referred pattern from lower posterior sacroiliac (SIJ-D), sacrotuberous (ST), and sacrospinous (SS) ligaments associated with sacroiliac joint instability. (*Adapted from* Hackett GS. Ligament and tendon relaxation (skeletal disability) treated by prolotherapy (fibro-osseous proliferation). 3rd ed. Charles C. Thomas, Springfield, IL 1958).

trochanteric bursitis, despite the fact that injections of local anesthetic and cortisone into and around the bursa shortly after each of these attempts had failed to bring even temporary relief.

The examination after the third attempt showed the following:

1. There was no edema or increased warmth noted in the tissues overlying the left greater trochanter.
2. The left TFL/IT band complex (see **Figs. 55** and **60**Aiii) was:
   a. Tender from origin to insertion and
   b. Tight to the point of snapping across the greater trochanter (GT) on passive hip extension/flexion.
3. Muscles in the lower extremities showed asymmetrical weakness; specifically, strength in left hip abductors was 4/5 compared with full (5/5) in the right ones.

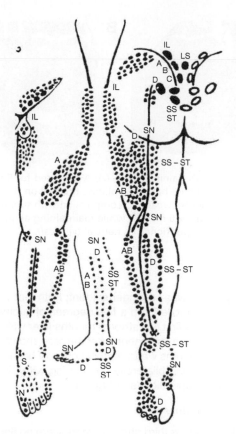

Fig. 77. Referral patterns from the posterior sacroiliac ligaments. From the superior segments: Relaxation (laxity) of the lumbosacral (LS) and upper portion of the sacroiliac articulations (A and B) occur together so frequently that their referred pain area from the iliolumbar ligament and AB are combined in one dermatome. From the inferior segments (C and D): Relaxation occurs together so frequently that their referred pain areas from D and sacrospinous and sacrotuberous (SS-ST) are combined in one dermatome. SN, sciatic nerve. (*Adapted from* Hackett GS. Ligament and tendon relaxation (skeletal disability) treated by prolotherapy (fibro-osseous proliferation). 3rd ed. Charles C. Thomas, Springfield, IL 1958.)

4. Left hip adduction was restricted compared with the right side (see **Fig. 60**Aii).
5. Rotational malalignment (right anterior, left posterior) had resulted in a shift of weight bearing: the right foot rolled inward, the left outward, a pattern that was confirmed by the collapse of the heel cups of his runners to the left (see **Fig. 78**A).

After realignment:

1. The left TFL/IT band complex showed no tenderness and tone now equaled that on the right, allowing the left to adduct to the same extent as the right one (see **Fig. 60**B).
2. Left hip abductor strength normalized at 5/5, on par with that on the right side.

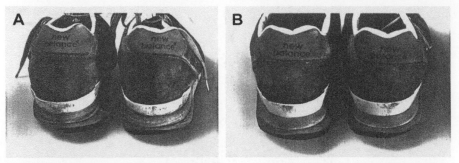

Fig. 78. Case history: runner B's training shoes. (*A*) A pair used for 6 months before correction of the malalignment. Note the heel cup collapse (inward on the right, outward on the left) and increased left lateral heel wear and compression with supination. (*B*) A pair (identical make to those in *A*) used for 6 months while maintaining alignment; the heel wear is even and heel cups symmetric, positioned in neutral (*vertical*).

3. The shift in weight bearing was no longer evident; both feet were in a neutral position at heel strike and then rolled into a few degrees of supination.
4. He went on to complete his first marathon 6 months later without experiencing any pain in the left hip region. An examination after the race showed no tenderness over the TFL/IT band. After 6 months wear, the heel cups of his new running shoes had maintained a vertical position bilaterally, in keeping with his true weight-bearing pattern: neutral to slight supination (see **Fig. 78**B).

Analysis of case history of runner B

1. On initial examination after his third attempt, there were no findings in keeping with a bursitis. The rapidity of his recovery with rest would also argue against that diagnosis, as did his favorable response to realignment.
2. The malalignment had resulted in the increase in tension in the left TFL/IT band complex, in keeping with the changes noted with a malalignment syndrome:
   a. An automatic increase in tone (facilitation) in the left TFL compared with the right (see **Figs. 59** and **60**Aii); and
   b. Increased tension on the left complex with the shift in weight bearing, increasing supination of the left foot and secondary tendency to left genu varum (see **Fig. 55**).
3. Asymmetry of strength, with relative weakness of left TFL and hip abductors, resulting in earlier fatiguing of these muscles with prolonged exertion.
4. The resulting pain would have caused a further, reactive tensing of these muscles.

SORTING OUT COMBINATIONS OF THE 3 COMMON PRESENTATIONS

As indicated, the 3 common presentations can occur in isolation or with 2 or all 3 together at any time. Supposing that a runner who, in fact, has equal leg length, presented with a 'right anterior, left posterior rotational malalignment' combined with a 'right outflare/left inflare' and also a right 'upslip':

1. On initial examination there would be:
   a. Pelvic obliquity noted in all positions of examination.

b. In keeping with the right anterior rotation: asymmetry of all pelvic landmarks on side-to-side and front-to-back comparison (see **Fig. 13**) and a lengthening of the right leg, shortening of the left, when lying down on the sitting–lying test (see **Figs. 16** and **25**).

c. In keeping with the flare noted: the right ASIS further out from midline (see **Fig. 14**Ai) and lower than the left one when observed with the runner lying supine (see **Fig. 18**A, B).

2. The outflare/inflare is corrected successfully by blocking attempted movement of the knees (**o**utward on the l**o**w right, **i**nward on the h**i**gh left side; see **Figs. 20** and **22**). The right and left ASIS and PSIS will now be equidistant from midline and level with each other (see **Fig. 14**Aii, Bii and 18C).

3. In 90%, correction of an outflare/inflare simultaneously corrects a coexisting rotational malalignment. If that has not happened, there would be persistence of the asymmetry of the landmarks, the apparent leg length difference and the relative lengthening of the right leg that was noted on the initial sitting–lying test on lying down (see **Figs. 16** and **25**).

4. Correction of the rotational malalignment using MET—blocking right hip extension, left hip flexion (see **Figs. 28–34**)—uncovers the underlying right upslip with persistence of the pelvic obliquity, upward displacement of all the right landmarks, and a relative shortening of the right leg but both legs now moving together on the sitting–lying test (see **Fig. 40**). Successful correction by using repeated gentle traction on the right leg (see **Fig. 41**) will result in a level pelvis and symmetric landmarks, including matching malleoli that move together.

IMPLICATIONS FOR THE TREATING PHYSICIAN

The signs and symptoms seen in association with pelvic malalignment and the malalignment syndrome may cause confusion that can result in misdiagnosis, inappropriate and possibly harmful investigation and treatment and failure to provide the treatment indicated. Recognition of malalignment is of significance because it can aggravate, mimic, overlap with or precipitate another medical disorder. The following discussion describes problems typically seen in runners presenting with an upslip or rotational malalignment and associated malalignment syndrome. Given the tendency to right pronation, left supination, a number of the abnormal forces are accentuated by running on a road sloping down to the left; that is, against the traffic in North America (see **Fig. 58**).

Aggravation or Precipitation of Another Medical Disorder

In the runner with an upslip or rotational malalignment, these disorders primarily involve the neuromusculoskeletal system and problems are in large part the result of the associated shift in weight bearing, instability of the pelvic ring, and asymmetric muscle strength and tension. Typical examples include the following.

Back pain arising from conditions of the pelvis or spine

The runner may have a known condition of the spine, such as a bulging or protruding disc, facet joint degeneration, spondylolisthesis, progressive idiopathic scoliosis, and yet remain asymptomatic.[52,53] Superimposing the stresses attributable to malalignment, with pelvic obliquity and compensatory curves, can tip the balance and cause these conditions to become symptomatic. Superimposing these stresses on a normal pelvis and spine can also result in back pain eventually.[39,54–57] For example, the rotation of the L1-L4 vertebrae into a compensatory right lumbar convexity closes the left and opens the right facet joints (see **Fig. 26**; see also **Fig. 46**). Either facet joint can eventually become symptomatic; for example, with irritation of the approximated surfaces and/or nerve fibers lying in the vicinity of the joint or within ligaments/capsules that end up elongating on being put under increased tension with any separation of the surfaces. Simply realigning the pelvis to remove these additional stresses may resolve the discomfort.

Hip and knee joint osteoarthritis
Pelvic malalignment that results in a functional leg length difference and asymmetric weight-bearing changes the loading pattern on the hip and knee joint surfaces. Leg length difference, whether anatomic or functional, has been implicated in the acceleration of hip and knee osteoarthritis. Degeneration and pain are more likely to involve the hip joint on the long leg side and the knee on the short leg side.[33] With the malalignment, the problem is compounded by 1 lower extremity turning outward, the other inward (see **Figs. 42** and **47**), also by the tendency toward genu valgum on 1 side and genu varum on the other (see **Figs. 42**, **55** and **56**).

Iliotibial band friction syndrome
As part of the TFL/IT band complex, the left IT band in particular is at risk of becoming irritated and inflamed, sometimes coupled with an underlying bursitis, where:

1. The TFL/IT band runs across the greater trochanter, and
2. The lateral IT band crosses the lateral femoral condyle.

The problem is more likely to occur on the left side and there may be snapping over either prominence, with tension increased in the complex on this side as a result of:

1. Facilitation of the left TFL (see **Figs. 59** and **60**Aii); and
2. Separation of its origin and insertion with the tendency to supination/secondary genu varum, also with a left innominate posterior rotation (see **Figs. 55** and **61**).

Patellofemoral compartment syndrome
The malalignment can trigger or aggravate a patellofemoral syndrome, more likely to affect the right patella and its lateral facet owing to a combination of factors:

1. Lateral displacement of the patella with:
   a. The increase in the Q-angle, as the right foot pronates and the knee tends toward genu valgum (see **Figs. 42** and **55**).
2. Outward rotation of the right femur (see **Fig. 42**A).
3. Functional weakness, reorientation, and early fatiguing of the right quadriceps affecting especially vastus medialis (see **Figs. 62** and **63**).

Plantar fasciitis and achilles tendonitis
These issues are more likely to occur on the side that pronates, given the increased tension in both structures caused by the foot rolling inward (see **Figs. 47**Aii and **49**; **Fig. 79**) as a result of:

1. A separation of the origin and insertion:
   a. Of the fascia, as the longitudinal and transverse arches of the foot progressively collapse through the initial part of stance phase (see **Fig. 79**B) or
   b. Of triceps surae as the calcaneus everts (see **Figs. 47**Aii and **49**).
2. Earlier activation of the windlass mechanism on progressing through foot-flat and in anticipation of push-off from the forefoot (see **Figs. 49** and **79**).[46]
3. The increased dorsiflexion possible on that side (see **Fig. 71**).

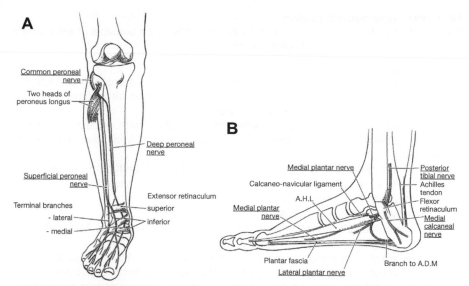

Fig. 79. Structures put under tension by pronation. (*A*) The medial terminal branches of the superficial and the distal part of the deep peroneal nerve. (*B*) On the medial side of the ankle: posterior tibial and medial calcaneal nerve; plantar nerves (in particular, the medial one); plantar fascia, flexor retinaculum and Achilles tendon. ADM, abductor digiti minimi; AHL, abductor hallucis longus. (Schamberger 1987).

Stress fracture

The runner is at increased risk of suffering a stress fracture of the tibia/fibula (presenting as shin splints) and lateral metatarsals on the left side, on account of:

1. Decreased ability to absorb shock at the foot/ankle level in stance phase, with:
   a. Increased plantarflexion range available (see **Fig. 71**) and tendency to supination; and
   b. Left calcaneal inversion, limiting transverse tarsal joint motion (see **Fig. 72**B).
2. The lateral shift in weight bearing, onto the fourth and fifth metatarsal heads (see **Fig. 57**Bii).

Compartment syndrome

Running can result in repetitive overloading and swelling of muscles within a specific compartment, exacerbated by running on a sloping road surface (see **Figs. 55** and **58**):

1. Right anterior or medial compartment: right pronation increasing traction forces on the functionally weak tibialis anterior and posterior, respectively, both working hard to control the tendency to pronation (see **Figs. 55** and **56**);
2. Right posterior compartment: right pronation and increased ankle dorsiflexion range augmenting traction forces on triceps surae[46]; and
3. Left lateral compartment syndrome, with left supination increasing traction forces on the functionally weak left peroneus longus/brevis, both working hard to control the tendency to supination (see **Figs. 55** and **56**).

Tibial stress syndrome/shin splints

Shin splints may be medial, lateral or anterior. In addition to a possible stress fracture or compartment syndrome, differential diagnoses include:

1. Periostalgia:
   Tenderness typically noted along the origin of the right tibialis posterior and left peroneus longus (subjected to pronation and supination forces, respectively).
2. Asymmetrical stresses caused by the malalignment.
   The resulting shin splints are usually activity-related, with excessive traction on the periosteal origins, exacerbated by any functional weakness and ease of fatigability:
   a. Given the tendency to increased right pronation and shift to medial bearing, more likely to occur on the right side (or right worse than left):
      i. Medially: involving tibialis posterior;
      ii. Anteriorly: involving tibialis anterior;
   b. Laterally: typically involving left peroneus and brevis (see **Figs. 55** and **56**).
3. Referred pain triggered by the malalignment.
   If trigger points, periostalgia, stress fracture, and compartment syndrome have been ruled out, the shin splints may be on the basis of referral, especially if:
   a. They are not necessarily activity- related, vary in the shape or area involved depending on which structures are being irritated at any given time, and
   b. The discomfort is not confined to the area supplied by a specific nerve and is relieved by realignment (see Case History: Runner A).

   In that case, they may be felt:

   a. Anteriorly: in the tibial sclerotome with irritation of the sciatic nerve (**Fig. 80**); or
   b. Anterolaterally: from the upper parts of the posterior SI joint ligaments (see **Fig. 77**) or the ligaments of the hip joint (see **Figs. 1**A and **73**).

Metatarsalgia, hallux valgus, and medial bunion formation

The tendency to right pronation and medial weight-bearing increase pressure on the medial aspect of the first toe, predisposing to formation of a medial bunion, hallux valgus and, eventually, formation of a secondary Morton's toe (see **Fig. 57**A, Bi). The shift also increases weight bearing on the sesamoids and medial metatarsal heads, with callus formation (typically noted under the second and third). The runner is at increased risk of experiencing pain from overloading of the right sesamoids and medial metatarsals. Increased left supination predisposes to lateral metatarsalgia and callus formation (see **Fig. 57**Bii).

Peripheral nerve involvement

1. Nerves affected by right medial shift and tendency to pronation:
   a. Right saphenous and posterior tibial nerve (see **Figs. 55** and **56**A). Both are put under tension along their length and the saphenous also where it runs under the distal fibula. The posterior tibial is at risk of entrapment and compression within the posterior tarsal tunnel as the overlying flexor retinaculum is also subjected to these medial traction forces (see **Fig. 79**).[58]
   b. Peroneal nerve: deep branch distal to ankle; medial terminals of superficial branch.
   c. Left sural nerve (see **Fig. 56**A). Excessive ankle eversion with pronation approximates the distal fibula, talus, and calcaneus, narrowing the space available for the nerve as it traverses this area.[58]

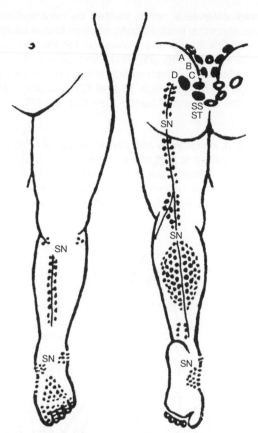

Fig. 80. Pattern of sciatica caused by sciatic nerve (SN) irritation that can occur with sacro-iliac joint instability from relaxation (laxity) of the posterior sacroiliac (A, B, C, D), sacrospi-nous (SS), and sacrotuberous (ST) ligaments. (*Adapted from* Hackett GS. Ligament and tendon relaxation (skeletal disability) treated by prolotherapy (fibro-osseous proliferation). 3rd ed. Charles C. Thomas, Springfield, IL 1958.)

2. Nerves affected by left lateral shift and tendency to supination:
   a. Left distal plantar nerves (see **Fig. 79**B). These forces can activate a latent Mor-ton's neuroma by narrowing the space between the third and fourth metatarsal heads, irritating the natural thickening formed here by the junction of a branch from the medial and lateral plantar nerves.
   b. Left peroneal nerve (see **Figs. 56**B and **79**A):
      i. Proximally, where it winds around the fibula and lies between the 2 heads of peroneus longus, with any excessive traction on the nerve and muscle; or
      ii. Distally, if a deviant superficial branch ends up winding around the distal fibula.
   c. Posterior tibial nerve (see **Figs. 56**B and **79**B). Excessive ankle inversion with supination can approximate the distal tibia, talus, and calcaneus to the point of irritating or even compressing this distal branch of the tibial nerve within the posterior tarsal tunnel.[58]
3. Meralgia paresthetica.

The lateral femoral cutaneous nerve, formed by contributions from L2 and L3, can be subjected to abnormal traction/compression forces caused by the malalignment as it runs between iliacus and psoas, under the inguinal ligament and to the lateral thigh (see **Fig. 21; Fig. 81**). Resulting pain and/or paresthesias in the anterolateral and posterolateral thigh region may overlap with symptoms referred to the lateral hip/thigh region (see **Figs. 73** and **77**) or arising from underlying structures; for example, the greater trochanter (see **Fig. 2**); TFL/IT band (see **Figs. 55** and **59–61**).

Pelvic floor dysfunction, coccydynia, and sacroccoccygeal junction pain

The pelvic floor musculature is part of the "inner core" that, along with the "outer core" muscles, help to stabilize the pelvis and trunk in anticipation of carrying out activities such as walking, running or standing on one leg while maintaining balance (see **Fig. 23**).[3,4,6] Pelvic floor dysfunction for whatever reason (eg, pressure on

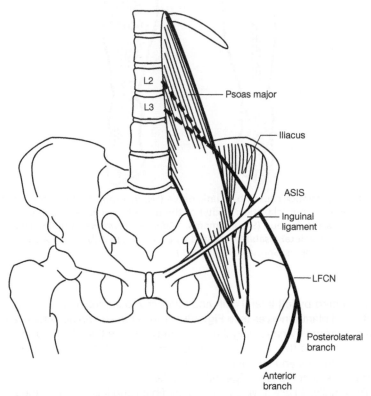

Fig. 81. Course of the lateral femoral cutaneous nerve (LFCN), which supplies sensation to the skin of the anterolateral thigh region (see also **Fig. 21**). Irritation/injury can occur at a number of points. On the left side (shown), malalignment-related causes include (1) compression (a) with any excessive/persistent increase in tension in left psoas major and iliacus, as it runs between them, (b) with a left innominate inflare, as it runs under the inguinal ligament (c) at both sites with a left innominate anterior rotation; (2) lateral traction forces caused by (a) a left innominate outflare, (b) excessive left supination, affecting it at the anterior superior iliac spine (ASIS)–inguinal ligament junction and also at the distal point where it is still relatively fixed as it penetrates the subcutaneous layers to reach the skin.

these muscles from an abdominal mass, fibroid, cyst, visceral adhesions/scars) and/or associated sacrococcygeal joint dysfunction can be a cause of instability of the pelvic ring and recurrent malalignment (**Fig. 82**).[40] Alternately, the pelvic floor dysfunction may be a complication of malalignment, triggered by changes such as chronic asymmetric tension in pelvic muscles and ligaments. Either way, the pelvic floor dysfunction may complicate the malalignment because it can be associated with coccydynia and visceral symptoms including dysmenorrhea, urinary frequency/urgency/nocturia, stress incontinence, dyspareunia, and vaginal wall pain.[16,59–61]

Mimicking Another Medical Disorder

Piriformis syndrome and sciatica

Piriformis syndrome, as originally described by Yeomans in 1928, implies:

1. Compromise of the sciatic nerve where it exits through the greater sciatic notch or subsequently, as it or its tibial and peroneal components pass below, through, or above piriformis on their way to the leg (see **Fig. 2**), with a sharp, lancinating or burning pain felt in the buttock and radiating below the knee, possibly also dermatomal numbness or paresthesias;
2. Positive straight leg raising and Lasegue's sign; and
3. Increased pain in the distribution of the sciatic nerve or its components on being stressed further by bending/lifting or passively increasing tension in piriformis; for example, passive flexion, abduction and internal rotation (the FAIR maneuver).[62]

A bona fide piriformis syndrome very likely exists.[63–65] However, the 3 common presentations of pelvic malalignment can all affect piriformis (eg, increased tension with facilitation or reaction to a painful or unstable SI joint; chronic tension myalgia and trigger point formation) to the point of compromising the sciatic nerve or its branches and evoking symptoms and signs that may be similar to those noted

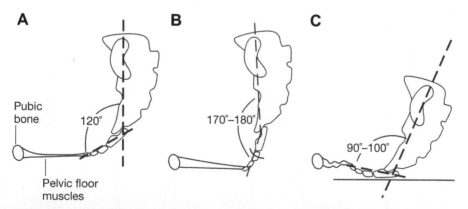

Fig. 82. Effect of angulation of the coccyx on the inserting ligaments and pelvic floor muscles. (*A*) Normal angulation of 120° relative to the sacrum, with a 30° range of motion; there is normal pelvic floor tone. (*B*) Excessive extension angulation resulting in hypertonus of the pelvic floor. (*C*) Excessive flexion angulation resulting in hypotonus of the pelvic floor (eg, passively on sitting in a slouched position); however, this angulation may also result with a chronic increase in tension in pelvic floor muscles from whatever cause (eg, irritation by a fibroid, cyst, or other pelvic mass; malalignment of the pelvic ring).

with a "piriformis syndrome". However, pain/paresthesias in the buttock, possibly with radiation to the posterior thigh and calf, that tend to come and go and vary from day to day in intensity and location are often more a reflection of irritation of the SI joint ligaments, which are primarily supplied by S1/S2 (see **Fig. 76**), and the SI joint itself. These symptoms usually decrease or resolve completely with realignment. The 2 disorders can coexist and symptoms may overlap. A bona fide piriformis syndrome may become apparent on realignment, in which case specific treatments (eg, physiotherapy, medication, possibly injections, or even decompression) may be indicated to resolve the problem.

Mid back pain and thoracolumbar syndrome

The thoracolumbar junction area is put under stress when malalignment results in pelvic obliquity and a compensatory curve that reverses in the thoracolumbar region (see **Figs. 17, 24, 59** and **70**B). These changes, superimposed on the reversal from a lumbar lordosis to thoracic kyphosis and reorientation of the facet joint surfaces between L1 and T11, are capable of triggering mid back pain from discs and facet joints (see **Fig. 45**). The combination can also precipitate a "thoracolumbar syndrome", with irritation of cutaneous perforating branches originating from the posterior roots of T11, T12 and L1.[66] Although there may be tenderness elicited with pressure applied to the spine and adjacent muscles in the T11-L1 region, the runner will note pain and/or paresthesias distal to the site of origin, that is, in the distribution of one or more of the 3 branches (**Fig. 83**):

1. Anterior: to the inner upper thigh, abdomen and groin (close to McBurney's point and capable of mimicking appendicitis and other problems of the appendix);
2. Lateral: over the lateral hip region (mimicking pain from the hip and trochanter); and
3. Posterior: over the buttocks area (simulating low back/SI joint pain).

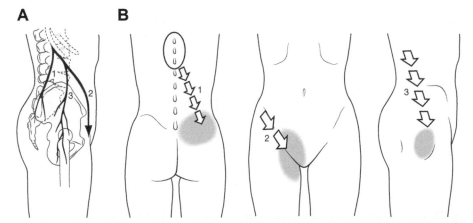

Fig. 83. Problems relating to the T12 and L1 cutaneous branches. (*A1, B1*) Posterior branch, low back pain. (*A2, B2*) anterior branch, pseudovisceral pain. (*A3, B3*) lateral perforating branch, pseudohip pain. (*From* Schamberger W. The malalignment syndrome: Diagnosing and treating a common cause of acute and chronic pelvic, limb and back pain. Edinburgh (UK): Churchill Livingstone; 2013. *Adapted from* Maigne R. Thoracolumbar junction syndrome: a source of diagnostic error. J Orthoped Med 1995; 17: 84–9.)

Symptoms usually respond to manipulation/mobilization of the T11-L1 or to pelvic realignment when malalignment is responsible for the stress on the junction.

Osteitis condensans ilii, sacroiliitis, spondyloarthropathy

Degeneration of the SI joint may become evident starting in the 30s or 40s but most people show some mobility and space between the surfaces of the joint well into their 70s and 80s.[67,68] The intricate configuration of the joint (see **Fig. 8**) combined with any osteoarthritic changes and the effects of joint malalignment—overlapping of joint edges, asymmetrical approximation and separation of surfaces (see **Figs. 8–10, 19,** and **26**)—can easily lead to misinterpretation of findings on radiography, computed tomography scans, or MRI and the clinical examination. As a result, degeneration and inflammatory conditions of the joint are probably overdiagnosed. If there is any concern, a trial of realignment, appropriate laboratory tests, selective joint injection and bone scans are indicated. Malalignment causes asymmetrical stresses on the symphysis pubis (see "osteitis pubis"), facet and SI joints that can result in increased bone turn over. Any SI joint changes seen on a bone scan tend to be asymmetrical, often localized to a small area(s); comparatively higher tracer concentration on one side may result in an SIS ratio that is asymmetric but usually still within normal limits.

Osteitis pubis

The runner presenting with pelvic malalignment may report pain from the central pubic or groin region which may arise locally or be on a referred basis (see **Figs. 77** and **83**A2, B2). The pubic bones are displaced relative to each other, stressing the symphysis pubis, which may be painful on direct palpation if not outright symptomatic (see **Figs. 10, 13, 24** and **38**). Pain on joint distraction would be in keeping with a ligamentous, capsular, or disc problem as these are stressed by the malalignment (see **Figs. 1, 2** and **24**), whereas pain caused by joint compression is more likely to indicate joint pathology. Degenerative changes on radiographs and a positive bone scan could be consistent with such pathology. However, findings suggestive of osteitis pubis can result with the increased stress on the pubic symphysis caused by malalignment and hip/SI joint dysfunction.[69]

Post-realignment pain and paresthesias

In the first 2 to 4 weeks after the initial realignment, some runners may experience pain or paresthesias in places that were never a problem while malalignment was present. Typically these symptoms, which may be mistakenly thought to be an entirely new problem affecting some part of the neuromusculoskeletal system, can arise from ligaments, muscles, or joint capsules that have undergone shortening and are now suddenly subjected to tension on realignment. Symptoms, which may remain localized to the contracted structures or be referred to a distant site(s), usually abate spontaneously as normal length is gradually regained.

Iliolumbar ligament pain

These ligaments, which originate from the transverse process of L4 and L5 and have both a "superficial" and a "deep" insertion onto the iliac crest, help maintain lumbosacral and SI joint stability (see **Fig. 1A**).[70] They can be subjected to increased tension with pelvic or spine malalignment that causes, for example, separation of their origins and insertions. The ligaments need to be considered in the differential diagnosis of pain around the greater trochanter, lateral thigh and groin, on the basis of referral to their sclerotomal and dermatomal distributions (see **Fig. 77**).

Overlap with Findings Attributable to a Coexisting Medical Disorder

The following case histories serve as typical examples that illustrate this point.

Case history: runner C—central disc protrusion

A 45-year-old runner presented with back pain localized just below the thoracolumbar junction. Full neurologic assessment revealed only a questionable root stretch test and an asymmetric weakness in lower extremity muscles, the latter in keeping with the pattern typically associated with the rotational malalignment found on examination. Repeated attempts by a manual therapist and self-corrections he carried out between visits failed to achieve lasting alignment and had no effect on his back pain. Subsequent computed tomography scans showed an L3-L4 central disc protrusion that likely caused irritation of the dura and secondary changes (eg, asymmetrical muscle tension or spasm) capable of causing the malalignment. Surgical resection relieved his pain and postoperative attempts at realignment were eventually successful.

Case history: runner D—radiculopathy

A runner complained of a feeling of weakness in the left lower leg and paresthesias felt intermittently over parts of the posterior thigh and calf, also a more consistent patch of numbness along the lateral aspect of the left foot. Findings were limited to a rotational malalignment, asymmetric weakness of bilateral lower extremity muscles, and decreased touch and pin prick appreciation over the sole of the left foot. Repeat left bowstring/straight leg raising root stretch tests elicited a somewhat variable report of left buttock/posterior thigh discomfort, but Maitland's slump test was negative and Lasegue's sign absent. Radiographs showed some degenerative changes in the lower lumbar levels.

Whenever treatment allowed him to maintain alignment for a few days in a row:

1. He reported having only the feeling of weakness and a numbness in the sole;
2. Clinical findings were limited to 4/5 weakness of left peroneus longus, a decreased left ankle reflex, the questionable left stretch test and decreased sensation not just over the sole of the foot but also along the posterior calf region.

MRI showed a large L5-S1 posterolateral disc protrusion that impinged on the S1 root. Findings relating to the left S1 radiculopathy (confirmed on electrodiagnostic studies) were hidden intermittently by the overlapping with symptoms attributable to a recurrence of the malalignment, coupled with referral from the irritated sacrospinous and sacrotuberous ligaments (see **Figs. 76** and **77**).

Comments on case histories C and D

1. When attempts at realignment fail repeatedly, ensure that an underlying problem that may be causing malalignment to recur has been ruled out. Typical causes to consider include disc protrusions, radiculopathies, and abdominal masses (eg, uterine fibroids, ovarian cysts, aneurysms).
2. A radiculopathy results in a relatively consistent pattern of pain, sensory changes, weakness, and reflex changes. In contrast, pelvic malalignment can cause pain and paresthesias that may be localized or referred, can vary in terms of when and where they are felt and also in intensity, and may mimic a root or nerve lesion; however, weakness is not myotomal, reflexes remain intact, and the root stretch test is negative.

TREATMENT

Correction of the 3 most common presentations of pelvic malalignment can be achieved in most runners, even those of advanced age.[26,27,67,68] However, the aim should be to get to the stage where alignment is being maintained most of the time and the runner can return to a normal lifestyle that hopefully includes being able to resume training. Although most will respond to appropriate treatment within 3 to 4 months, others may take up to 1 to 2 years for symptoms to resolve and for the body tissues and the mind to adjust fully to the new state of being in alignment.[19,48] Hence, achieving this goal requires a commitment on the part of the runner and adherence to a treatment approach that includes not just realignment, but that also focuses on all the factors that can affect the long-term outcome of the therapy.

A Comprehensive Treatment Program

A progressive treatment program that includes participation by the runner is most likely to achieve lasting realignment and resolution of symptoms. The program should have the following components.

1. Supervision by someone trained in manual therapy.

   The therapist should be skilled in the use of manipulation, mobilization, MET, and other manual therapy techniques, as indicated by the presentation at hand. Complementary treatment measures, such as acupuncture or massage, may be indicated for decreasing persistent pain and relaxing tight tissues to help achieve and maintain alignment. However, although these modalities may sometimes achieve realignment by relaxing muscles and allowing pelvic bones to slot back into their normal position, manual therapy approaches remain the key to achieving long-term results.

2. Instruction of the runner, including the following.

   a. How to carry out self-assessment and self-treatment.

      Being able to do the sitting–lying test and assessment of pelvic landmarks allows the runner to detect any recurrences of malalignment on a day-to-day basis. He or she may be able to achieve correction using self-treatment techniques or opt to see the therapist before the next scheduled appointment. This approach increases the chances of maintaining alignment for increasing periods of time and getting symptoms to settle down more quickly.

   b. What activities to avoid.

      Sitting for longer periods of time (especially in a slouched position), lifting heavy weights, and running and carrying out maneuvers with a torsion component (eg, twisting the pelvis and trunk when reaching up/downward or to 1 side) all predispose to recurrence of malalignment especially during the initial stage.

   c. The basics of a graduated exercise program.

      Initial strengthening of the inner and outer core muscles is essential for regaining stability of the pelvis and spine; emphasis is also on ensuring that muscles are contracting in the first place and in proper sequence/coordination with other muscles in their own and other, interacting slings.[42,71–74] Once alignment is starting to be maintained, and at the therapist's discretion, the runner may gradually get back to improving overall strength and cardiovascular fitness. Concentrating on a graduated walking program is indicated if attempts at running continue to cause recurrences of malalignment; running in a pool may be an option to consider at that stage.

3. Return to a normal lifestyle.

The final stage of treatment is aimed at regaining normal movement patterns, balance, and proprioception, to enable the runner to carry out activities of daily living and, hopefully, start back on a regular training program. Techniques aimed at achieving this stage may include yoga exercises, the use of biofeedback and enrollment in a structured program such as Rehabilitation Pilates.[75,76]

Shoes

If daytime and training shoes show any of the typical changes caused by malalignment (see **Figs. 51–54**), the runner should be advised to:

1. Discontinue their use immediately and replace them with walking/running shoes that are relatively neutral; that is, not intended to counter pronation or supination.
2. Delay purchase of new shoes specific for a pronator or supinator until alignment is being maintained and the true weight-bearing pattern has been determined.

Orthotics

The runner should be advised as follows:

1. He or she should discontinue use of any orthotics that were provided before the diagnosis of the pelvic malalignment. These were most likely made from a cast taken when the runner was out of alignment, in which case they may incorporate unwanted changes relating to any previous shift in weight bearing and asymmetries of joint ranges of motion. If that is the case, they pose a risk of perpetuating abnormal forces at the foot level that could predispose to recurrences of malalignment once correction has been achieved (see **Fig. 75**).
2. If orthotics are felt to be indicated (eg, to provide more cushioning and/or some support for the medial longitudinal arch), then off-the-shelf orthotics are an adequate interim measure because they will provide not only symmetric support but also more symmetric proprioceptive input from the sole that may increase the chance of maintaining realignment (see **Fig. 50**).
3. If orthotics are felt indicated once the runner is starting to maintain alignment and his or her true weight-bearing pattern has become evident, the new orthotics:
   a. Should preferably be constructed using data obtained while:
      i. The runner is known to be in alignment and
      ii. Weight bearing; for example, walking across a computerized sensory pad.
   b. May incorporate:
      i. Posting to counter residual excessive pronation or supination, especially if there are ongoing problems caused by these forces; for example, a TFL/IT band complex that continues to be painful after realignment in someone who turns out to be a supinator;
      ii. A heel lift to make up for a true leg length difference that has been revealed on realignment and could predispose to recurrence of the malalignment.

Sacroiliac Belt and Compression Shorts

An SI belt, compression shorts, or a combination of these may help to decrease pain and maintain realignment; however, their use should be limited to the initial treatment period when recurrences are more likely to occur. In someone with ongoing instability of the pelvis for whatever reason, addition of figure-of-8 hip and thigh straps provide adjustable compressive forces. Belts may also be placed so as to apply pressure to a specific tender point or other areas in the pelvic region (eg, a specific ligament or muscle) when simple manual pressure exerted on these sites is noted to decrease the runner's pain and/or reinforce contraction in some of the core muscles.[40]

Injections

Prolotherapy
Prolotherapy is indicated when failure to maintain alignment is attributable to laxity of a joint capsule and ligaments.[43,77,78] Injection of an irritant, such as hyperosmolar glucose, causes inflammation and triggers a natural response leading to new collagen formation and eventual strengthening of these supportive structures. Growth factor, platelet-rich plasma, and a number of other derivatives have also proven useful for stimulating collagen formation.[79] Prolotherapy may also prove helpful in decreasing pain from persistently tender tendon or ligament insertions following realignment, probably by strengthening the fibro-osseous junction and settling down any irritated or hypersensitive nerve fibers.

Cortisone
The use of cortisone should be limited given the risk of infection, weakening, and even rupture of the connective tissue being injected. However, a restricted number of spaced injections of cortisone combined with a local anesthetic may prove helpful to settle down any residual inflammation and pain in ligaments and tendons that:

1. Is aggravating to the point of causing muscles to tense up, recurrences of malalignment and generally interfering with the runner's treatment and recovery; and
2. Persists even though the runner has been maintaining alignment; this tends to be a problem particularly involving the posterior SI joint and iliolumbar ligaments.

Surgery

Surgery may play a role when:

1. The runner's recurrent malalignment can be attributed to:
   a. Joint laxity resulting with joint degeneration and/or laxity/tearing of the supporting ligaments (see Fig. 11B);
   b. Ongoing pain definitely arising from the structure considered for resection or fusion; for example, pain localized by selective blocks to an abnormal disc, facet or SI joint; or
   c. Asymmetrical forces are acting on a joint; for example, the hingelike motion around the facet joint contralateral to a unilateral sacral lumbarization or L5 sacralization.
2. The runner has complied fully with all recommendations and the conservative approach has definitely failed.

For example, in the case of instability of one or both SI joints, this may be as a result of joint degeneration, laxity of the supporting ligaments, or a combination of these. If all treatment measures, including prolotherapy injections, have failed and progress is stalled because of the pain and an inability to achieve or maintain alignment, surgery may be indicated.[80] The procedure of choice is:

1. A bilateral SI joint fusion with a bone plug and fixation with 2 screws on each side.
2. To have the procedure carried out with:

a. A manual therapist in attendance, to ensure the bones of the pelvic ring are in alignment throughout the procedure; and

b. Simultaneous electrodiagnostic monitoring (eg, ongoing side-to-side comparison of L5 and S1 sensory latency) to allow for quick detection of any compromise of the lumbosacral plexus or a root and appropriate modification of the surgical technique.

When Malalignment Fails to Respond to a Course of Treatment

In the runner who may or may not derive temporary benefit with realignment but fails to maintain alignment, the following possibilities should be considered:

1. The treatment program:
   a. Has failed to address some of the issues that can be responsible for recurrences; for example, wearing the wrong type of shoes, or orthotics cast while out of alignment); and
   b. Has not considered the use of other techniques that may help to achieve lasting alignment; for example, acupuncture or dry-needling to resolve residual muscle spasm; a trial of other manual therapy techniques, such as craniosacral release[20,81] or ones that concentrate on alignment at the occipitocervical junction[22-24]; these techniques are worth considering because they may prove successful when other approaches aimed mainly at the pelvis or lower spine have failed.
2. The malalignment may be a manifestation of an underlying medical problem that has so far escaped detection (see "Implications for the treating physicians").
3. The runner has actually not adhered fully to the treatment program. Athletes in general are more likely to abandon formal treatment at the first sign of any improvement and go back to their sport. Returning to running before having achieved adequate stability of the pelvis and spine only invites recurrence of a problem that is unlikely to resolve completely with just intermittent therapy.

Summary

1. More than 80% of runners, like the general population, are likely to be out of alignment.
2. The standard back examination should include assessment of pelvic alignment to avoid misdiagnosis and inappropriate investigations and treatment.
3. An awareness of pelvic malalignment and the phenomenon of the malalignment syndrome is essential to allow one to provide proper care of a runner because:
   a. The abnormal biomechanics and any associated discomfort result in compensatory measures that are usually less efficient in terms of biodynamics and energy requirements and can set back the runner's training.
   b. Failure to achieve alignment may impair the runner's:
      i. Recovery from specific problems that are the result of the malalignment; and
      ii. Ability to advance and achieve his or her maximum performance.
4. The 3 most common presentations usually respond to a supervised, progressive treatment program that includes a teaching component, including instruction in self-assessment and self-treatment techniques that the runner can use effectively on a day-to-day basis to maintain alignment and improve his or her chances of recovery.
5. The validity of any research into the biomechanics of running (eg, assessing the effect of various types of orthotics) should be questioned if the study has failed to look at whether pelvic malalignment was present and whether the altered,

asymmetrical biomechanical changes attributable to the malalignment itself could have affected the results of the study.

REFERENCES

1. Mann R. Biomechanics of running. In: Mack RP, editor. American Academy of Orthopedic Surgeons: symposium on the foot and leg in running sports. St Louis (MO): CV Mosby; 1982. p. 1–29.
2. Snijders CJ, Vleeming A, Stoeckart R. Transfer of lumbosacral load to iliac bones and legs. I. Biomechanics of self-bracing of the sacroiliac joints and its significance for treatment and exercise. Clin Biomech (Bristol, Avon) 1993;8(6):285–95.
3. Vleeming A, Snijders CJ, Stoeckart R, et al. The role of the sacroiliac joint in coupling between the spine, pelvis, legs and arms. In: Vleeming A, Mooney V, Dorman T, et al, editors. Movement, stability and low back pain. Edinburgh (United Kindom): Churchill Livingstone; 1997. p. 53–71.
4. Hungerford BA, Gilliard W. The pattern of intrapelvic motion and lumbopelvic muscle recruitment alters in the presence of pelvic girdle pain. In: Vleeming A, Mooney V, Stoeckart R, editors. Movement, stability and lumbopelvic pain. Integration of research and therapy. 2nd edition. Edinburgh (United Kingdom): Churchill Livingstone; 2007. p. 361–76.
5. DonTigny RL. Critical analysis of the functional dynamics of the sacroiliac joint as they pertain to normal gait. J Orthop Med 2005;27:3–10.
6. Porterfield JA, DeRosa C. Conditions of weight bearing: asymmetrical overload syndrome (AOS). In: Vleeming A, Mooney V, Stoeckart R, editors. Churchill Livingstone; 2007. p. 391–403.
7. Hodges PW, Richardson CA. Inefficient muscular stabilization in the lumbar spine associated with low back pain. A motor control evaluation of transversus abdominis. Spine 1996;21(22):2640–60.
8. DonTigny RL. Function and pathomechanics of the sacroiliac joint. A review. Phys Ther 1985;65:35–44.
9. Greenman PE. Clinical aspects of sacroiliac joint in walking. In: Vleeming A, Mooney V, Dorman TA, et al, editors. Movement, stability and low back pain. Edinburgh (United Kingdom): Churchill Livingstone; 1997. p. 235–42.
10. Sturesson B, Uden A, Vleeming A. A radiostereometric analysis of movements of the sacroiliac joints during the standing hip flexion tests. Spine 2000;25(3):364–8.
11. Resnick D. Ankylosing spondylitis. In: Resnick D, editor. Diagnosis of bone and joint disorders. 4th edition. Philadelphia: WB Saunders; 1975. p. 1023–81.
12. Masi AT, Benjamin M, Vleeming A. Anatomical, biomechanical and clinical perspectives on sacroiliac joints: an integrative synthesis of biodynamic mechanisms related to ankylosing spondylitis. In: Vleeming A, Mooney V, Stoeckart R, editors. Movement, stability and lumbopelvic pain. Integration of research and therapy. 2nd edition. Edinburgh (United Kingdom): Churchill Livingstone; 2007. p. 205–27.
13. Vleeming A, Stoeckart R, Volkers ACW, et al. Relation between form and function in the sacroiliac joint. I. Clinical anatomical aspects. Spine 1990;15(2):130–2.
14. Vleeming A, Stoeckart R, Volkers ACW, et al. Relation between form and function in the sacroiliac joint. II. Biomechanical aspects. Spine 1990;15(2):133–6.
15. Gracovetsky S. Stability or controlled instability. In: Vleeming A, Mooney V, Stoeckart R, editors. Movement, stability and pelvic pain. Integration of research and therapy. 2nd edition. Edinburgh (United Kingdom): Churchill Livingstone; 2007. p. 279–94.

16. DonTigny RL. A detailed and critical biomechanical analysis of the sacroiliac joints and relevant kinesiology: the implications for lumbopelvic function and dysfunction. In: Vleeming A, Mooney V, Stoeckart R, editors. Movement, stability and pelvic pain. Integration of research and therapy. 2nd edition. Edinburgh (United Kingdom): Churchill Livingstone; 2007. p. 265–78.
17. Lee DG. The evolution of myths and facts regarding function of the pelvic girdle. In: Vleeming A, Mooney V, Stoeckart R, editors. Movement, stability & lumbopelvic pain: integration of research and therapy. 2nd edition. Edinburgh (United Kingdom): Churchill Livingstone; 2007. p. 191–200.
18. Sahrmann SA. Diagnosis and treatment of movement impairment syndromes. St Louis (MO): Mosby; 2002.
19. Bray H, Moseley GI. Disrupted working body schema of the trunk in people with back pain. Br J Sports Med 2011;45(3):168–73.
20. Upledger JE, Larni Z. Somatoemotional release and beyond. Palm Beach Gardens (FL): U1 Publishing; 1990.
21. Stevens S, Steinberg K. Treatment: manual therapy modes. In: Schamberger W, editor. The malalignment syndrome. 2nd edition. Edinburgh (United Kingdom): Churchill Livingstone; 2013. p. 523–42.
22. Foran P. NUCCA technique. Can Chiropract 1999;4:6–8.
23. Sterling M, Jull GA, Wright A. Cervical mobilization: concurrent effects on pain, sympathetic nervous system and motor activity. Man Ther 2001;6: 72–81.
24. Dunn J, Glymph ID. Investigating the effect of upper cervical adjustments on cycling performance. Vector 1999;2(4):6.
25. Klein KK. Progression of pelvic tilt in adolescent boys from elementary through high school. Arch Phys Med Rehabil 1973;54:57–9.
26. Schamberger W. The malalignment syndrome: Implications for medicine and sport. Edinburgh (United Kingdom): Churchill Livingstone; 2002.
27. Schamberger W. The malalignment syndrome: Diagnosing and treating a common cause of acute and chronic pelvic, limb and back pain. Edinburgh (United Kingdom): Churchill Livingstone; 2013.
28. Chaitow I. Muscle energy techniques. 3rd edition. Edinburgh (United Kingdom): Churchill Livingstone; 2007.
29. Lee DC, Walsh MC. Workbook of manual therapy techniques for the vertebral column and pelvic girdle. 2nd edition. Altona (Canada): Friesen Printers; 1996.
30. Mitchell FL Jr, Mitchell PKG. The muscle energy manual, vol I: concepts and mechanisms of the musculoskeletal screen, cervical region evaluation and treatment. East Lansing (MI): MET Press; 2005.
31. Kassarjian A, Brisson M, Palmer WE. Femeroacetabular impingement. Eur J Radiol 2007;63:29.
32. Lee DG. Instability of the sacroiliac joint and the consequences for gait. In: Vleeming A, Mooney V, Dorman TA, et al, editors. Movement, stability and low back pain. The essential role of the pelvis. Edinburgh (United Kingdom): Churchill Livingstone; 1997. p. 231–3.
33. Campbell-Smith S. Long-leg arthropathy. Ann Rheum Dis 1964;28:359–65.
34. Dorman TA, Brierly S, Fray J, et al. Muscles and pelvic gears: hip abductor inhibition in anterior rotation of the ilium. J Orthop Med 1995;17:96–100.
35. Korr IM. Somatic dysfunction, osteopathic manipulative treatment and the nervous system: a few facts, some theories, many questions. J Am Osteopath Assoc 1986;86:109–14.

36. Guymer AJ. Proprioceptive neuromuscular facilitation for vertebral joint conditions. In: Grieve GP, editor. Modern manual therapy of the vertebral column. Edinburgh (United Kingdom): Churchill Livingstone; 1986. p. 622–39.
37. Janda V. Muscle weakness and inhibition (pseudoparesis) in back pain syndromes. In: Grieve GP, editor. Modern manual therapy of the vertebral column. Edinburgh (United Kingdom): Churchill Livingstone; 1986. p. 197–201.
38. Vleeming A, Stoeckart R. The role of the pelvic girdle in coupling the spine and the legs: a clinical-anatomical perspective on pelvic stability. In: Vleeming A, Mooney V, Stoeckart R, editors. Movement, stability & lumbopelvic pain: integration of research and therapy. 2nd edition. Edinburgh (United Kingdom): Churchill Livingstone; 2007. p. 113–37.
39. Willard FH. The muscular, ligamentous and neural structure of the lumbosacrum and its relationship to low back pain. In: Vleeming A, Mooney V, Stoeckart R, editors. Movement, stability & lumbopelvic pain: integration of research and therapy. 2nd edition. Edinburgh (United Kingdom): Churchill Livingstone; 2007. p. 5–45.
40. Lee DG. The pelvic girdle, 4th edition. An integration of clinical expertise and research. Edinburgh (United Kingdom): Churchill Livingstone; 2011.
41. Sweeting R. Dynamometer detection of unilateral weakness in those with malalignment and seemingly strong muscles on manual testing. Unpublished; personal communication. In: Schamberger W, editor. The malalignment syndrome. Edinburgh (United Kingdom): Churchill Livingstone; 2002. p. 2012.
42. Hides JA, Belavy DL, Cassar L, et al. Altered response of the anterolateral abdominal muscles to simulated weight-bearing in subjects with low back pain. Eur Spine J 2009;18(3):410–8.
43. Hackett GS. Ligament and tendon relaxation (skeletal disability) treated by prolotherapy (fibro-osseous proliferation). 3rd edition. Springfield (IL): Charles C. Thomas; 1958.
44. Sunderland S. Nerves and nerve injuries. 3rd edition. Melbourne (Australia): Churchill Livingstone; 1978.
45. Dahlen LB, McLean WG. Effects of graded experimental compression on slow and fast axonal transport in rabbit vagus nerve. J Neurol Sci 1986;72: 19–30.
46. Fraser S. Comparison of a physiotherapy program versus dexamethasone injections for plantar fasciopathy in prolonged standing work. Clin J Sport Med 2014; 24(3):211–7.
47. Armour PC, Scott JH. Equalization of limb length. J Bone Joint Surg 1981;63B: 587–92.
48. Tsao H, Galea MP, Hodges PW. Reorganization of the motor cortex is associated with postural control deficits in recurrent low back pain. Brain 2008;131(8): 2161–71.
49. Dorman TA. Failure of self-bracing at the sacroiliac joint: the slipping clutch syndrome. J Orthop Med 1994;16:49–51.
50. Lentell GL, Katzman LL, Walters MR. The relationship between muscle function and ankle stability. J Orthop Med 1992;14:85–90.
51. Garn SN, Newton RA. Kinesthetic awareness in subjects with multiple ankle sprains. Phys Ther 1988;68:1667–71.
52. Magora A, Schwartz A. Relation between the low back pain syndrome and X-ray findings. 1. Degenerative arthritis. Scand J Rehabil Med 1976;8:115–25.
53. Jensen MC, Brant-Zawadski MN, Obuchowski N, et al. Magnetic resonance imaging of the lumbar spine in people without back pain. N Engl J Med 1994; 331:69–73.

54. Adams MA, Bogduk N, Burton B, et al. The biomechanics of low back pain. 2nd edition. Edinburgh (United Kingdom): Churchill Livingstone; 2006.
55. Vleeming A, Pool-Goudzwaard AL, Hammudoghlu D, et al. The function of the long dorsal sacroiliac ligament: its implication for understanding low back pain. Spine 1996;21(5):556.
56. DonTigny RL. Anterior dysfunction of the sacroiliac joint as a major factor in the etiology of idiopathic low back pain syndrome. Phys Ther 1990;70:250–65.
57. Paris SV, Viti J. Differential diagnosis of low back pain. In: Vleeeming A, Mooney V, Stoeckart R, editors. Movement, stability & lumbopelvic pain: integration of research and therapy. 2nd edition. Edinburgh (United Kingdom): Churchill Livingstone; 2007. p. 381–90.
58. Schamberger W. Nerve injuries around the foot and ankle. Med Sci Sports 1987; 23:105–20.
59. Barral J-P, Mercier P. Visceral manipulation. Seattle (WA): Eastland Press; 1988.
60. Barral J-P. Visceral manipulation II. Seattle (WA): Eastland Press; 1989.
61. Barrall J-P. Urogenital manipulation. Seattle (WA): Eastland Press; 1993.
62. Beatty RA. The piriformis muscle syndrome: a simple diagnostic manoeuvre. Neurosurgery 1994;34:512–4.
63. Kirschner JS, Foye PM, Cole JL. Piriformis syndrome: diagnosis and treatment. Muscle Nerve 2009;40:10–8.
64. Papadopoulos EC, Khan SN. Piriformis syndrome and low back pain: a new classification and review of the literature. Orthop Clin North Am 2004;35: 65–71.
65. Stewart JD. The piriformis syndrome is overdiagnosed. Muscle Nerve 2003;28: 644–6.
66. Maigne R. Thoraco-lumbar junction syndrome: a source of diagnostic error. J Orthop Med 1995;17:84–9.
67. Vleeming A, Van Wingerden JP, Dikstra PF. Mobility of the sacroiliac joints in the elderly: a kinematic and radiological study. Clin Biomech 1992;7:170–6.
68. Walker JM. The sacroiliac joint: a critical review. Phys Ther 1992;72:903–16.
69. Walheim GG, Selvic G. Mobility of the pubic symphysis. Clin Orthop Relat Res 1984;191:129–35.
70. Pool-Goudzwaard A, Hoek van Dijke G, Mulder P, et al. The iliolumbar ligament: its influence on stability of the sacroiliac joint. Clin Biomech (Bristol, Avon) 2004; 18(2):99–105.
71. Hodges PW. Core stability exercise in chronic low back pain. Orthop Clin North Am 2003;34:245–54.
72. Hodges PW, Cholewicki J. Functional control of the spine. In: Vleeming A, Mooney V, Stoeckart R, editors. Movement, stability & lumbopelvic pain: integration of research and therapy. 2nd edition. Edinburgh (United Kingdom): Churchill Livingstone; 2007. p. 489–512.
73. McGill SM, Grenier S, Kavcic N, et al. Coordination of muscle activity to assure stability of the lumbar spine. J Electromyogr Kinesiol 2003;13:353.
74. Richardson CA. Impairment in muscles controlling pelvic orientation and weight-bearing. In: Richardson CA, Hodges PW, Hides JA, editors. Therapeutic exercise for lumbopelvic stabilization. Edinburgh (United Kingdom): Churchill Livingstone; 2004. p. 3–7.
75. Menezes A. The complete guide to Joseph H. Pilates techniques of physical conditioning. Alameda (CA): Hunter House; 2000.
76. LaTouche R, Escalante K, Linares M. Treating non-specific chronic low back pain through the Pilates method. J Body Mov Ther 2008;12(4):364–70.

77. Dorman TA. Pelvic mechanics and prolotherapy. In: Vleeming A, Mooney V, Dorman TA, et al, editors. Movement, stability and low back pain. The essential role of the pelvis. Edinburgh (United Kingdom): Churchill Livingstone; 1997. p. 501–22.
78. Hauser RA, Hauser MA. Dextrose prolotherapy for unresolved low back pain: a retrospective case series study. J Prolother 2009;3:145–55.
79. Crane D, Everts P. Platelet rich plasma (PRP) matrix grafts: PRP application in musculoskeletal medicine. Pract Pain Manage 2008.
80. Lippitt AB. Recurrent subluxation of the sacroiliac joint: diagnosis and treatment. Bull Hosp Joint Dis 1995;54:94–102.
81. Upledger JE. Craniosacral therapy II: beyond the dura. Seattle (WA): Eastland Press; 1987.

Core and Lumbopelvic Stabilization in Runners

Carlos E. Rivera, MD

KEYWORDS

- Core stability • Runners • Lumbopelvic control • Core muscles • Core rehabilitation
- Core strengthening

KEY POINTS

- Core muscles provide stability that allows generation of force and motion in the lower extremities, distributes impact forces, and allows controlled and efficient body movements.
- Imbalances or deficiencies in the core muscles can result in increased fatigue, decreased endurance, and injury in runners.
- Core strengthening should incorporate the intrinsic needs of the core for flexibility, strength, balance, and endurance, and the function of the core in relation to its role in extremity function and dysfunction.
- Specific exercises are effective in strengthening the core muscles.

WHAT IS THE CORE?

- A common view of the core or lumbopelvic hip complex of the body includes the spine, hips and pelvis, proximal lower limbs, and abdominal structures. The principal function of this complex is to create stability for the generation of force and motion in the distal joints.
- When the system works efficiently, the result is appropriate distribution of forces, optimal control and efficiency of movement, and functional movement through the kinetic chain.[1]
- Core stability has been defined as "the ability to control the position and motion of the trunk over the pelvis and leg to allow optimum production, transfer and control of force and motion to the terminal segment in integrated kinetic chain activities."[2]
- McKeon and colleagues[3] proposed a foot-core paradigm that describes the importance of base of support in running. This article focuses on the

Funding sources: No funding was received in support of this study.
Conflict of interest: Nil.
Campbell Clinic Orthopaedics, 1211 Union Avenue, Suite 510, Memphis, TN 38104, USA
E-mail address: crivera@campbellclinic.com

Phys Med Rehabil Clin N Am 27 (2016) 319–337
http://dx.doi.org/10.1016/j.pmr.2015.09.003
1047-9651/16/$ – see front matter © 2016 Elsevier Inc. All rights reserved.

lumbopelvic control as it relates to running injuries, acknowledging that the full kinetic chain is critical to evaluate because it relates to running mechanics and injury prevention.

ANATOMY

The core is composed of multiple muscles groups. These muscles can be divided into a local system and global system.[4]

LOCAL SYSTEM

- Defined as muscles that originate and/or insert on the lumbar vertebrae, with the exception of the psoas. Includes multifidus, transverse abdominals (TA), internal obliques, and the pelvic floor muscles.
- Position dependent and acts locally.
- Controls curvature, stiffness, and stability of the lumbar spine.

GLOBAL SYSTEM

- Muscles that originate from the pelvis and insert on the thoracic cage, including rectus abdominis, quadratus lumborum, erector spinae, and external obliques.
- Distributes outer forces acting on the body.
- Transfers load between pelvis and thoracic cage.

PHYSIOLOGY/BIOMECHANICS

Several mechanisms influence spine stability and maintenance of a neutral spine.

- Increasing intra-abdominal pressure contributes to spine stability. One way to stimulate this is by contracting the TA,[5] but it has been shown that to maintain a neutral spine, cocontraction of muscles is of foremost importance and that no 1 muscle is more important than others for this.[6]
- Spinal stability is required before limb movement.[7–9]
- Because running is an endurance event, core stability must include endurance training of the core musculature to maintain stability.
- To create a stable base we recommend starting with exercises that can promote cocontraction while maintaining low compression loads in the spine (Figs. 1–7). A solid base will later allow for control movements.
- Isometric exercises should be held for no more than 8 seconds, then relax and repeat. This technique allows adequate oxygenation of the muscles, avoiding the buildup of harmful lactic acid.[10]

Panjabi[11,12] suggested that 3 subsystems work together to provide stability:

- Passive subsystem
  - Ligaments, vertebral bodies, and intervertebral discs: do not produce force or motion, mainly provide for position/motion sense and communicate with neural system.
- Active subsystem
  - Muscles and tendons: generate forces.
- Neural subsystem
  - Nerves and the central nervous system: determines stability requirements and makes the active system achieve the stability goals.

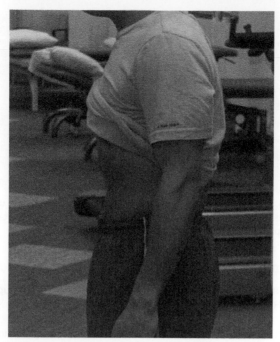

Fig. 1. Abdominal hollowing. Involves drawing in the abdominal wall while the shoulders, ribs, and pelvis remain still and normal breathing is maintained. Coactivates the transverse abdominis and multifidus. This technique was designed to regroove motor control patterns, not to provide stability.

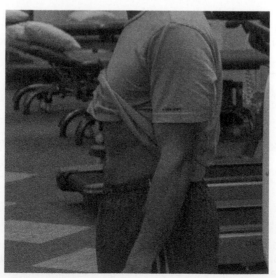

Fig. 2. Abdominal bracing. Submaximal isometric contraction of the 3 layers of the abdominal wall (rectus, obliques, and transverse) produces a muscular girdle; 10% of the maximal voluntary contraction provides enough stability.

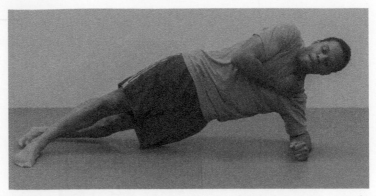

Fig. 3. Side bridge. Lie on your side with your elbow underneath you; rise up so that you are resting 1 forearm/elbow and foot on same side. Place the top foot in front of the lower foot on the mat for support. The test ends when the hips return to floor.

BASIC RUNNING BIOMECHANICS

- Running at any speed can be defined as loss of double-leg support during the gait cycle. Running generally is divided into a stance phase, swing phase, and float phase.
- The pelvis, sacrum, and lumbar vertebrae provide stability to allow the lower extremities to move effectively while running. The pelvis relies on symmetry to function during the running cycle. The planes of motion of the pelvis are rotational, anterior-posterior, and mediolateral. Pelvic biomechanical abnormalities that lead to the most injuries in runners include excessive anterior pelvic tilt, excessive lateral tilt, and asymmetric hip movement.[13] This abnormal pelvic orientation also can lead to excessive strain on the hamstrings, which can increase the risk of injury.[14]
- The core muscles help absorb and distribute impact forces and allow body movements in a controlled and efficient manner. When optimized in function, muscles work in unison to allow breathing during running and the twisting motion

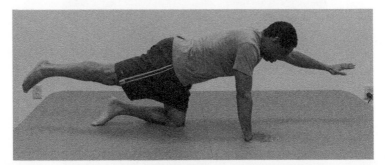

Fig. 4. Bird dog. Get down on your hands and knees with your palms flat on the floor and shoulder width apart. Your knees should be hip width apart and bent 90°. Brace your core and, maintaining a neutral spine (no deviation of spine or hips), raise the opposite arm and leg simultaneously, holding for 6 to 8 seconds, and alternate. Avoid raising the extremities past horizontal. To increase challenge do not return knee or hand to floor when coming back to starting position and repeat same side (like sweeping the floor).

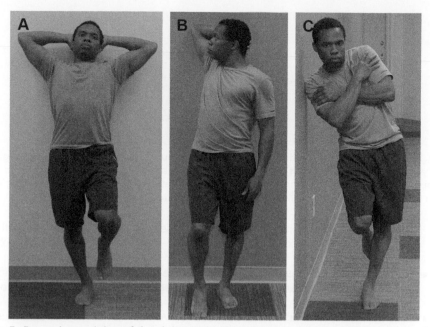

Fig. 5. Eccentric retraining of the abdominals. (*A*) Sagittal. Standing approximately 3 inches away from a wall, try to slowly move the body backwards, keeping feet flat on the floor, to just barely touch the head against the wall. Initially, this can be done with both legs on the ground, then progressed to toe-touch weight bearing on each side and ultimately to single-leg standing. Sagittal plane core strength testing creates eccentric activation in the abdominals, the quadriceps, and hip flexor muscles, and concentric activation in the hip and spine extensors. (*B*) Transverse. Stand about 3 inches away from the wall, and progress as for the sagittal plane test from bilateral weight bearing to single-leg stance and alternately touch 1 shoulder then the other just barely against the wall. Quality of motion and speed can be assessed. This test evaluates transverse plane motions that incorporate abdominal muscles, hip rotators, and spine extensors. (*C*) Frontal. Standing with one side against the wall, brace your core and keep a neutral spine. Toe touching on the inside leg, barely touch the inside shoulder to the wall. This test evaluates eccentric strength of the quadratus lumborum, hip abductors, and some long spinal muscles that are working in a frontal plane. Can progress to single leg for more challenge.

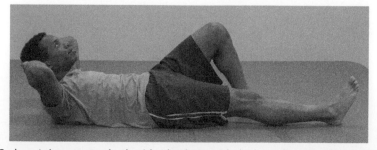

Fig. 6. Curl up. Lying on your back with 1 leg bent with the knee flexed and the other on the floor, brace the abdominals. Elevate the head and shoulders a short distance off the floor. Focus on midthoracic flexion while the head and neck remain locked. To increase the challenge, hold the contraction and take a deep breath before relaxing.

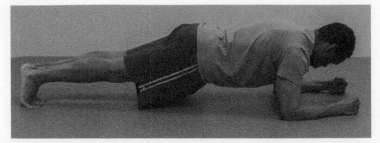

Fig. 7. Planks. In push-up position on the floor, bend your elbows 90° and rest your weight on your forearms. Your elbows should be directly beneath your shoulders, and your body should form a straight line from your head to your feet. Hold the position for as long as you can (at least 8–10 seconds), go to the original position, and repeat.

required during the running cycle. As the pelvis rotates during each stride, the muscles of the thorax keep the spine and the abdomen stable about the axis of the vertebrae.[13]

- The float phase includes forward rotation of the ipsilateral pelvis and hip flexion caused by the psoas and other pelvic muscles, along with the core, to allow twisting of the pelvis.[13]
- Abnormal pelvic mechanics that can lead to overuse injuries include tight muscles that attach to the pelvis, including tensor fascia latae, hamstring, adductors, quadratus lumborum, piriformis, weak muscles like gluteus medius (GMed), gluteus maximus (GMax), and structural deformities like scoliosis or leg length discrepancy.[13]
- The hip flexes (starting with the psoas) and abducts during the swing phase and extends and adducts during stance.
  - Hamstring and the hip extensors start activating in the second half of swing and reach maximal power at beginning of stance.
  - Abductors and adductors provide cocontraction stability for the stance leg.
  - To train this, it is necessary first to "wake up/regroove" the hip musculature. The exercises shown in **Figs. 8–12** can be helpful.

EVALUATION

A complete evaluation of the muscular system should include an assessment of the muscles for overactivity, tightness, weakness, inhibition, and quality of motion.[1]

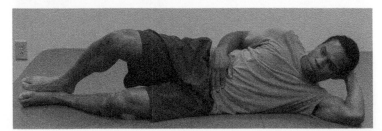

Fig. 8. Glut side-lying snaps. Lie on one side with a thumb on the anterior superior iliac spine. With the hips and knees flexed, spread the knees apart keeping the feet together. This movement activates the gluteus medius (GMed). The purpose is to start "waking up" the muscle that is inhibited. Some recruitment of the hip extensors occurs.

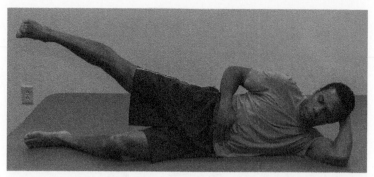

Fig. 9. Lateral leg raises. Lie on one side with hips and knees extended, brace the abdominals, and elevate the upper leg while keeping a neutral position. This movement activates the GMed more and also works the tensor fascia latae. Resistance can be added to the distal leg/ankle.

- Postural muscles, used mainly for standing and walking, tend to get short and tight because they are used frequently and also work against gravity constantly. These muscles include the gastrocsoleus, rectus femoris, iliopsoas, tensor fascia latae, hamstrings, adductors, quadratus lumborum, piriformis, and sartorius.[1] These muscles usually cross 2 joints.
- Phasic muscles, used to propel during running, stay elongated longer and therefore tend to get weak. Muscles that commonly become weak and inhibited are the tibialis anterior, the peroneals, vastus medialis, GMed and GMax, transverse abdominal, and obliques.[1]
- Crossed-pelvic syndrome (CPS).[15]
  ○ In CPS, tightness of the thoracolumbar extensors on the dorsal side crosses with tightness of the iliopsoas and rectus femoris. Weakness of the deep abdominal muscles ventrally crosses with weakness of the GMax and GMed. This pattern of imbalance creates joint dysfunction, particularly at the L4-L5 and L5-S1 segments, sacroiliac joint, and hip joint.

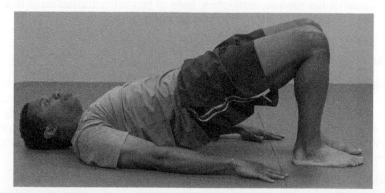

Fig. 10. Back bridge. Lie on your back with your knees bent. Squeeze your buttocks and abdominals, and then raise your buttocks and hips as high as you can while keeping your shoulders on the ground. Hold for 8 to 10 seconds, then lower the body back to the mat. Make sure there is gluteus activation (squeezing your buttocks) before hamstring activation. To inhibit hamstring activation, do mild quadriceps stimulation.

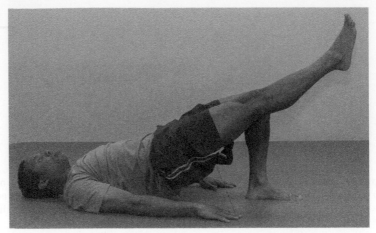

Fig. 11. Single-leg back bridge. Start in the back bridge position and, while keeping abdominals braced and the buttocks tight, extend 1 knee. Make sure to keep your pelvis/hip even.

- o Specific postural changes seen in CPS include anterior pelvic tilt, increased lumbar lordosis, lateral lumbar shift, lateral leg rotation, and knee hyperextension. If the lordosis is deep and short, then imbalance is predominantly in the pelvic muscles; if the lordosis is shallow and extends into the thoracic area, then imbalance predominates in the trunk muscles.
- Test endurance of spine extensors (**Fig. 13**), lateral core (see **Fig. 3**), and anterior core (**Fig. 14**).
  - o McGill[16] described several ratio discrepancies that suggest muscle imbalances. Most relevant probably are:
    - ▪ Flexion/extension greater than 1.
    - ▪ Side bridge (SB)/extension greater than 0.75.
  - o Single-leg squat (**Fig. 15**).
    - ▪ Allows quick evaluation of tightness of the gastrocsoleus and hip flexors/anterior hip capsule, adductors, level of pronation/supination of foot/knee, and weakness of GMax and gluteus minimus.

REHABILITATION

Rehabilitation of the core and lumbopelvic stabilization system should concentrate on both the intrinsic needs of the core for flexibility, strength, balance, and endurance, and on the function of the core in relation to its role in extremity function and dysfunction.[2] A strong spine in isolation is not necessarily a stable spine. Core strengthening for injury prevention and performance incorporating isolated core strengthening principles may not cross over to functional changes without gait retraining.[17]

- Safety principles.
  - o Minimizing tissue stress by avoiding the end range of motion keeps stress to a safe level.[18]
  - o Optimal joint positioning.[18]
- Joint position determines the passive tissue forces and subsequent joint loading as well as the muscle and ligament mechanics.

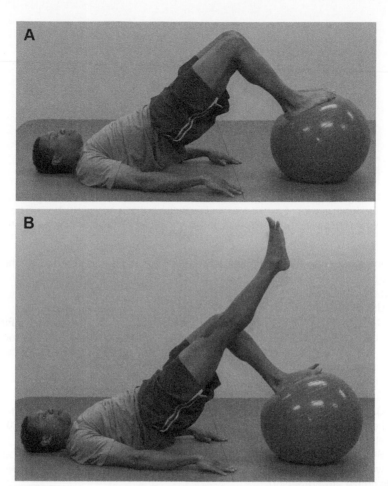

Fig. 12. (*A, B*) Progression of back bridges with feet on labile surface. The purpose is to recruit the hamstrings via hip extension and knee flexion while maintaining dynamic stability of the lumbar spine. In a back bridge position with the feet on the ball, push the ball forward with the feet while maintaining the bridge. The goal is to keep the pelvis elevated (hip extension) as both legs extend and flex at the knees, maintaining a neutral spine while the knees extend and flex from this elevated bridge position.

- Joint position also influences the ability of muscles to generate force.
    - Minimize fatigue. Physiologic fatigue causes poor technique, and poor technique leads to poor performance and increased injury risk. Efficiency of movement and training sessions reduces fatigue.[18]
    - Train to breathe independently of the exertion.
- Tong[19] showed that a high-intensity maximal run may induce core muscle fatigue in runners. Core muscle fatigue, which may be partly attributed to the corresponding respiratory work, may limit running endurance. Inspiratory muscles may share the work of core stabilization during intense exercise, while simultaneously increasing the demand for breathing. Inspiratory muscle training incorporated into a running-specific core training regimen potentially enhances the

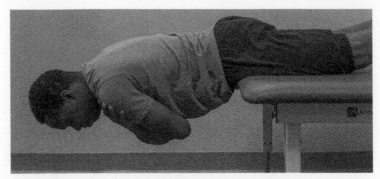

Fig. 13. Biering-Sorensen test. To perform the Sorensen test hold your body horizontally with your weight supported by the hips and legs. Begin timing once the body is horizontal and stop when the upper body descends more than 5° to 10° below the plane of the hips.

training effect on the core muscles in a functional manner to deal with the challenges of intense exercise.

- Maximize flexibility.
  - Use three-dimensional patterns to simulate functional activities.
  - Cat-camel; gentle motion through the full range of motion of the spine (**Fig. 16**).
  - Foam roller to help mobilize soft tissues (emphasis on muscles that tend to be tight: adductors, gastrocsoleus, hip flexors, hamstrings, piriformis, tensor fascia lata, rectus femoris).
  - Three-dimensional Achilles stretch (**Fig. 17**).
  - Gait stretch (**Fig. 18**).
  - Gait stretch with lateral bending and rotation to isolate the psoas (**Fig. 19**).
  - Learn to separate hip flexion (**Fig. 20**) from lumbar flexion (see **Fig. 20**) to be able to maintain a neutral spine.
  - Stretching exercises of the lower extremity (hip/knee/ankle) should be done with emphasis on keeping a neutral spine.
- Maximize strengthening.

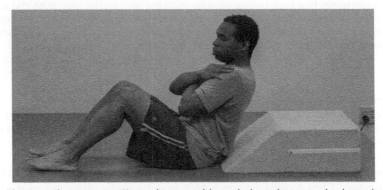

Fig. 14. Flexor endurance test. Sit on the test table and place the upper body against a support with an angle of 60°. Flex both the knees and hips to 90°. Fold the arms across the chest with the hands placed on the opposite shoulders. Maintain the body position while the supporting wedge is pulled back 10 cm to begin the test. The test ends when the upper body descends below the 60° angle.

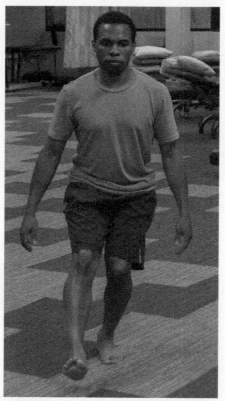

Fig. 15. Single-leg squat. Allows quick evaluation of tightness of the gastrocsoleus and hip flexors/anterior hip capsule, adductors, level of pronation/supination of foot/knee, and weakness of GMax and gluteus minimus.

The creation of a stable base, as well as how to initiate the retraining phase of the hip musculature, was discussed earlier. After achieving this, the next step for the athlete is to maximize strength in order to return to full activity.

All exercises should emphasize conscious bracing of the spine and keeping a neutral spine to allow enough repetitions for it to become a regular brain-ingrained action before movement. For practical application, consider starting a program 2 to 3 times per week, initially with 1 to 2 sets of 15 repetitions and advancing to 3 sets of 15 to 20 repetitions.[20]

In general, we recommend advancing to single-leg exercises as a retraining tool because running is a single-leg activity for loading response.[17] For example, single-leg squats allow GMed activation to control for the hip adduction moment because it results in earlier activation of the GMax than regular squats and better simulates functional activities like running or jumping.[17]

Incorporate training through three-dimensional planes of motion (frontal/sagittal/coronal).

- Squat
  - One-leg squat (see **Fig. 15**).
  - One-leg squat with labile surfaces (BOSU, wobble board) and in multiple planes (**Fig. 21**). This movement requires more motor control with

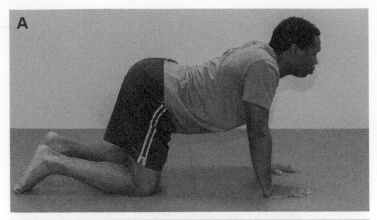

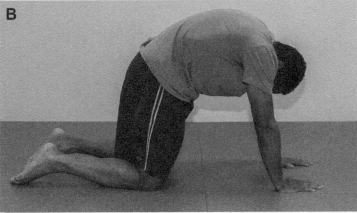

Fig. 16. (*A*, *B*) Cat-camel. Come to a hands and knees position on an exercise mat, positioning your knees underneath your hips and the crease of your wrists directly underneath your shoulders. Your fingers should be pointing forward. Engage your core and abdominal muscles. Imagine you are tightening a corset around your waistline. Keep your spine in a neutral position; avoid any excessive sagging or arching. Pull the shoulder blades toward your hips. Avoid any sagging or arching. Gently exhale. Tuck your tail under and use your abdominal muscles to push your spine upwards toward the ceiling, making the shape of an angry cat. Hold this position for 8 to 10 seconds. Lengthen your neck and allow your head to reach toward your chest, maintaining alignment with the spine. Using the abdominal and low back muscles, tip your tail toward the ceiling, increasing the arch in your mid-back and low back. Allow the abdomen to stretch toward the floor. Pull your shoulder blades down your back. Hold this position for 8 to 10 seconds before returning to the starting position.

higher core muscle activation and helps to stimulate balance and proprioception.
- Lunges
  - Excellent overall exercise for the lower extremity because it requires balance, strength, and flexibility through multiple joints.
  - Can be done in multiple planes and with many different challenges (**Fig. 22**).
- Power runner (**Fig. 23**)
- Step-ups with upper extremity reaches

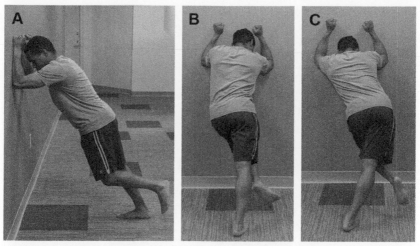

Fig. 17. (*A–C*) Three-dimensional Achilles stretch. Lean against a wall with a split stance with one foot forward and one back. Ensure that the heel of the back leg is kept in contact with the floor at all times. Then bend your front knee and lean forward, bringing your pelvis to the wall until you feel the stretch in the back of your calf. Hold for 8 to 10 seconds, relax, and repeat. In the position of the first stretch bring the front knee across the body. In the position of the first stretch swivel your hips from side to side.

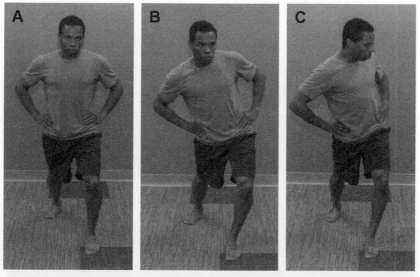

Fig. 18. (*A–C*) Gait stretch. Step 1 leg forward, keeping both feet pointing straight ahead. Keeping your back leg straight and keeping a neutral spine, slowly bend your front leg and push your right buttock forward until you feel a stretch across the front of your right hip joint. Assume the position of the first stretch and rotate your pelvis gently from side to side. Assume the position of the first stretch and swivel your hips gently from side to side.

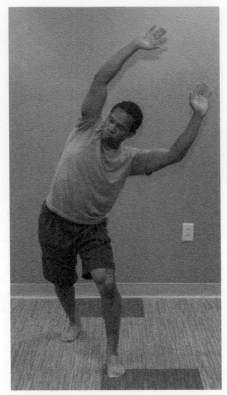

Fig. 19. Psoas stretch. Perform in the same manner as the gait stretch, but add contralateral bending of the torso and slight twisting to isolate the psoas.

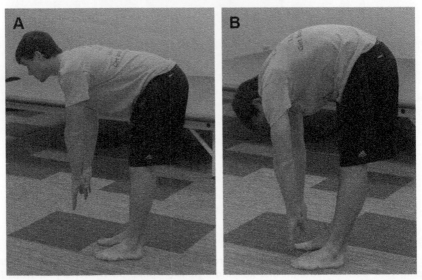

Fig. 20. Practice separating hip flexion (*A*) from lumbar flexion (*B*). Avoiding lumbar flexion and keeping the spine in neutral optimizes hip mobility and takes pressure away from the spine.

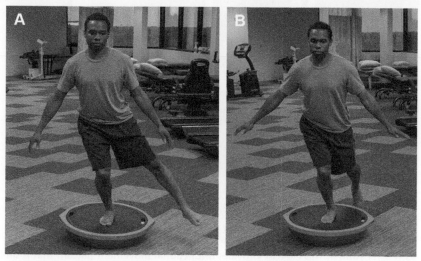

Fig. 21. Squats in 1 leg using balance challenge with lateral (*A*) and posterior reaches (*B*).

- ○ Emphasize neutral spine and hip flexor activity (**Fig. 24**).
- Other challenges, such as straps, balls, and cables, can be used to maximize hip power and core (**Figs. 25** and **26**)
- In addition, exercises that target multiple joints, like kettlebell swings, double-stance squats, and deadlifts, are helpful to develop maximal overall strength. Increases in strength can improve running times and overall performance.[21,22]

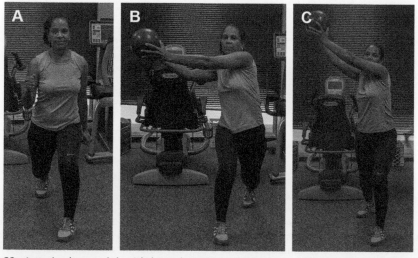

Fig. 22. Anterior lunges (*A*) with lateral reaches with weight challenge (*B*), with diagonal reaches and weight challenge (*C*).

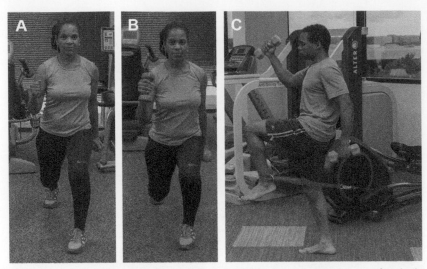

Fig. 23. Power runner. This exercise provides a functional movement pattern that is similar to running. Its purpose is to increase stability of the lower abdominals while using a forward motion at the hip. The exercise is designed to develop sagittal plane control. While balancing on 1 leg, imitate a running motion. As the upper thigh is lifted forward in a running motion, concentrate on maintaining the abdominal brace and lumbopelvic stability while avoiding excessive anterior or posterior pelvic rotation. Raise the opposite arm simultaneously into flexion, while maintaining postural alignment with an erect spine, and allowing only the extremities to move (*A*). Once lumbar spine stability can be maintained without effort, start progressing by adding weight to the hands (*B*) and/or attaching a pulley or resistive cord to the ankle to increase the challenge to the hip flexors (*C*).

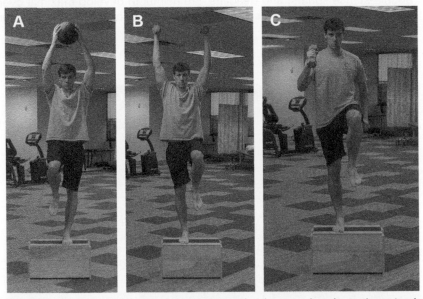

Fig. 24. Step-ups. Start on the ground and step with 1 leg up a bench. As the swing leg is brought up, bring knee at least to 90°. Additional challenges can include an overhead reach with a medicine ball (*A*), dumbbells (*B*), or a power runner motion (*C*). Observe how the spine is always kept neutral and movement always starts with a bracing of the spine that is maintained throughout the exercise.

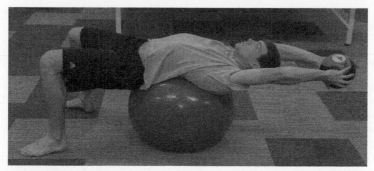

Fig. 25. Abdominal crunch with eccentric overload. Sitting on a Swiss ball (a BOSU ball is also useful) start with arms stretched overhead (by your ears, as in a diving position) and keep arms in this position for the entire exercise. Create an abdominal brace and then slowly lower your trunk, bringing the arms perpendicular to floor and creating an eccentric load in your abdominals. Raise the shoulders by contracting the abdominals as if doing a crunch, and repeat. To add a challenge, hold a medicine ball in your hands. Additional challenges include taking a deep, slow breath while holding the contraction and holding the end positions for 2 to 4 seconds.

SUMMARY

The core muscles are integral to a successful running program. They provide the stability required to allow efficient running, increase endurance, and decrease injury. Core strengthening regimens should consider all facets of core function (flexibility, strength,

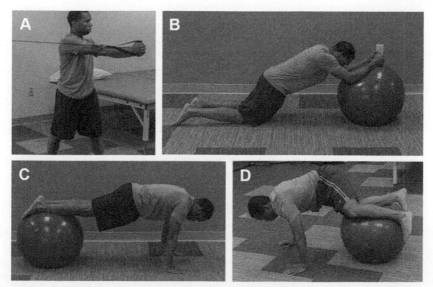

Fig. 26. (A–D) Examples of additional challenges to maximize hip and core strength.

balance, and endurance), and exercises should be chosen with an emphasis on maximizing core efficiency.[23]

REFERENCES

1. Fredericson M, Moore T. Muscular balance, core stability, and injury prevention for middle- and long-distance runners. Phys Med Rehabil Clin N Am 2005;16: 669–89.
2. Kibler WB, Press J, Sciascia A. The role of core stability in athletic function. Sports Med 2006;36(3):189–98.
3. McKeon PO, Hertel J, Bramble D, et al. The foot core system: a new paradigm for understanding intrinsic foot muscle function. Br J Sports Med 2015;49:290.
4. Bergmark A. Stability of the lumbar spine. A study in mechanical engineering. Acta Orthop Scand Suppl 1989;230:1–54.
5. Creswell AG, Oddsson L, Thorstensson A. The influence of sudden perturbations on trunk muscle activity and intra-abdominal pressure while standing. Exp Brain Res 1994;98(2):336–41.
6. Cholewicki J, VanVliet JJ. Relative contribution of trunk muscles to the stability of the lumbar spine during isometric exertions. Clin Biomech 2002;17:99–105.
7. Aruin AS. Directional specificity of postural muscles in feed-forward postural reactions during fast voluntary arm movements. Exp Brain Res 1995;103(2): 323–32.
8. Hodges PW, Richardson CA. Delayed postural contraction of transversus abdominis in low back pain associated with movement of the lower limb. J Spinal Disord 1998;11:46–56.
9. Hodges PW, Richardson CA. Altered trunk muscle recruitment in people with low back pain with upper limb movement at different speeds. Arch Phys Med Rehabil 1999;80:1005–12.
10. McGill SM, Hughson R, Parks K. Lumbar erector spinae oxygenation during prolonged contractions: implication for prolonged work. Ergonomics 2000;43: 486–93.
11. Panjabi MM. The stabilizing system of the spine. Part I. Function, dysfunction, adaptation, and enhancement. J Spinal Disord 1992;5:383–9.
12. Panjabi MM. The stabilizing system of the spine. Part II. Neutral zone and instability hypothesis. J Spinal Disord 1992;5:390–7.
13. Nicola TL, Jewison DJ. The anatomy and biomechanics of running. Clin Sports Med 2012;31:187–201.
14. Opar D, Williams M, Shield A. Hamstring injuries: factors that lead to injury and reinjury. Sports Med 2012;42(3):209–26.
15. Page P, Frank CC, Lardner R. Assessment and treatment of muscle imbalance: the Janda approach. Champaign (IL): Human Kinetics; 2010.
16. McGill SM, Childs A, Liebenson C. Endurance times for low back stabilization exercises: clinical targets for testing and training from a normal database. Arch Phys Med Rehabil 1999;80:941–4.
17. Crowell HP, Davis IS. Gait retraining to reduce lower extremity loading in runners. Clin Biomech 2011;26:78–83.
18. McGill S. Ultimate back fitness and performance. Waterloo (Canada): Waubuno Publishers; 2004. p. 194–5.
19. Tong TK, Wu S, Nie J, et al. The occurrence of core muscle fatigue during high-intensity running exercise and its limitation to performance: the role of respiratory work. J Sports Sci Med 2014;13:244–51.

20. Fredericson M, Harrison C, Tenforde AS, et al. Injury prevention in running sports. In: Liebenson C, editor. Functional training handbook. Philadelphia: Lippincott Williams & Wilkins; 2014.
21. Beattie K, Kenny IC, Lyons M, et al. The effect of strength training on performance in endurance athletes. Sports Med 2014;44(6):845–65.
22. Mikkola J, Vesterinen V, Taipale R, et al. Effect of resistance training regimens on treadmill running and neuromuscular performance in recreational endurance runners. J Sports Sci 2011;29(13):1359–71.
23. Escamilla RF, Lewis C, Bell D, et al. Core muscle activation during Swiss ball and traditional abdominal exercises. J Orthop Sports Phys Ther 2010;40:265–76.

Gait Retraining
Altering the Fingerprint of Gait

Irene S. Davis, PhD, PT[a],*, Erin Futrell, PT, OCS[b]

KEYWORDS

- Running injuries • Gait retraining • Biofeedback • Faded feedback

KEY POINTS

- Evidence links faulty running mechanics with injury and provides a justification and need for altering these mechanics.
- The human body has an amazing ability to adapt and leveraging this ability in order to reduce injury risk is very powerful.
- Altering habitual movement patterns requires practice and adherence to well-established motor control principles.
- More work is needed to determine optimal methods of retraining gait patterns.

INTRODUCTION

Why would it be necessary to alter someone's natural running gait pattern? Running gait patterns are not self-optimized for each individual. Despite Nigg and colleagues'[1] theory of natural movement patterns, individuals often run with patterns that have been shown to be related to injury.[1–4] Some patterns have also been associated with reductions in economy, such as increased vertical oscillation, increased stride length, and excessive arm motion.[5] Although economy is important to overall running performance, this article focuses on the retraining of gait patterns with the goal of reducing the risk of running injuries. Because running injuries result from musculoskeletal overload, the issues contributing to this overload are reviewed first, with a focus on biomechanical factors. The inability of strengthening to alter running mechanics is discussed next. The important components of a retraining program are described,

Disclosures: None.
[a] Department of Physical Medicine and Rehabilitation, Spaulding National Running Center, Spaulding-Cambridge Outpatient Center, Harvard Medical School, 1575 Cambridge Street, Cambridge, MA 02138, USA; [b] Center for Interprofessional Studies and Innovation, MGH Institute of Health Professions, 36, 1st Avenue, Charlestown Navy Yard, MA 02129, USA
* Corresponding author.
E-mail address: ISDAVIS@PARTNERS.ORG

Phys Med Rehabil Clin N Am 27 (2016) 339–355
http://dx.doi.org/10.1016/j.pmr.2015.09.002
1047-9651/16/$ – see front matter © 2016 Elsevier Inc. All rights reserved.

followed by a review of the literature on gait retraining to reduce injury risk in runners. The article concludes with a discussion of the future of conducting gait retraining in runners' natural environments using wearable technology.

FACTORS ASSOCIATED WITH RUNNING INJURIES

Running is a repetitive activity that typically occurs in a linear, forward direction resulting in a fairly invariant load with each foot strike. Because each foot strikes the ground approximately 625 steps per kilometer (1000 steps per mile), musculoskeletal tissues of the lower extremity become susceptible to cumulative overload, leading to overuse injuries. It can be assumed that every runner has a threshold for injury and that this threshold depends on several factors (**Fig. 1**). The runner's overall structure and static alignment plays an important role. For instance, foot structure has been implicated in different types of running injuries.[6] As an example, high-arched runners have been shown to be prone to bony injuries, whereas low-arched runners are prone to soft tissue injuries.[6] Although these structural factors need to be considered, they are effectively nonmodifiable. Dosage is another factor that can influence cumulative load. Training aspects such as how quickly the runner increases mileage, cross-training, and variation of running surfaces all contribute to the overall dosage of running. Dosage is clearly a modifiable risk factor, but there is a subset of runners who, despite reducing their mileage and resting appropriately, are unable to resolve their injuries, and these are the runners who most likely have an underlying mechanical factor that is not being addressed. This observation may explain in large part why the most common risk factor for a running injury is a previous injury.[7] Mechanical factors can be divided into forces (kinetics) and movement patterns (kinematics). A runner showing abnormalities in either of these areas can experience excessive loading in their musculoskeletal systems. Runners experiencing both excessive forces and abnormal movement patterns are likely to have an even greater risk for injury.

The impact transient of the vertical ground reaction force is the immediate increase in force shortly after the foot contacts the ground (**Fig. 2**). A sudden, large impact transient has been associated with injuries. In particular, greater vertical impact peak along with higher vertical average load rates (VALRs) and vertical instantaneous load rates (VILRs) have been linked to tibial stress fractures, plantar fasciitis, and

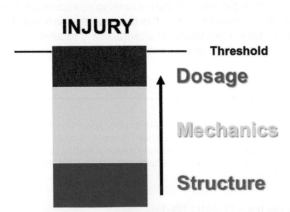

Fig. 1. Basic factors contributing to running injuries. Any 1 or a combination of factors can cause runners to reach their injury thresholds.

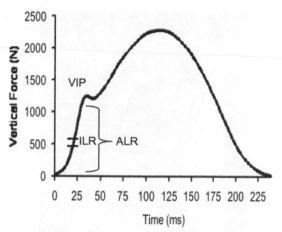

Fig. 2. Calculation of vertical load rates from the vertical ground reaction force during the stance phase of running. The average load rate (ALR) is calculated as the slope of the early impact transient over its most linear portion (20%–80% of the vertical impact peak [VIP]). The instantaneous load rate (ILR) is calculated as the peak slope between any 2 successive points along the same region of interest.

patellofemoral pain.[2–4] A recent prospective study suggests that having a greater VALR increases risk for developing a future running-related injury.[8] Therefore, increased impacts might be considered to be a global indicator for injury, because the musculoskeletal system is composed of viscoelastic structures that are sensitive to rates of loading. It has long been established in animal studies of bone and cartilage that repetitive impulsive loads, even those within physiologic limits, can have damaging effects on musculoskeletal structures.[9–12] As stated by these investigators, joint wear is determined not simply by the total force applied but by the degree and nature of the loading.[10] In terms of movement patterns, there are some common malalignments that clinicians observe in injured runners. At the foot, these include increased stride length, excessive ankle dorsiflexion or inversion at foot strike, excessive foot eversion, and toe-in and toe-out gait (**Fig. 3**). More proximally, increased genu varum and valgum, and anterior pelvic tilt and contralateral pelvic drop, are often seen. However, one of the most common abnormal movement patterns is the combination of excessive hip adduction, internal rotation, and pelvic drop (**Fig. 4**). This particular malalignment has been associated with patellofemoral pain, iliotibial

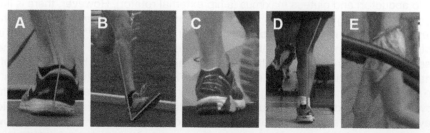

Fig. 3. Malalignments seen in runners. (*A*) Excessive peak rearfoot pronation. (*B*) Excessive ankle dorsiflexion at foot strike. (*C*) Toe-in during stance. (*D*) Genu valgum during stance. (*E*) Excessive anterior tilt of the pelvis.

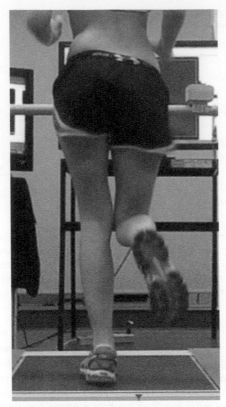

Fig. 4. One of the most common malalignments seen in runners, involving excessive contralateral pelvic drop, hip adduction, and internal rotation.

band syndrome, and tibial stress fractures in runners.[2,4,13] Therefore, this malalignment pattern may be considered another global indicator for injury.

STRENGTHENING ALONE IS NOT ENOUGH

The most common therapeutic approach to altering faulty movement patterns is to strengthen the muscles that control that movement. For example, excessive hip adduction and internal rotation are often treated by strengthening gluteus medius (a hip abductor) and gluteus maximus (a hip external rotator). However, there is little support that strengthening these muscles, without neuromuscular retraining, translates into a change in movement patterns. Snyder and colleagues[14] examined the effects of strengthening the hip abductors and external rotators on hip and knee mechanics during running in healthy active female runners. With the exception of a small increase in hip adduction excursion, the investigators noted no changes in hip and knee kinematics following a strengthening program compared with baseline. However, their study did not focus on individuals with abnormal mechanics, which may have limited its ability to examine potential changes in faulty mechanics. However, Mascal and colleagues[15] reported on a case study involving a female runner with anterior knee pain associated with excessive hip adduction, internal rotation, and contralateral pelvic drop during a step-down maneuver. These abnormal mechanics were significantly reduced following a 14-week strengthening program. Note that the strengthening program focused on the proper mechanics during the single-leg stance and step-down exercises. Therefore, this additional neuromuscular reeducation could have influenced the participants' movement patterns and alignment during this specific dynamic task. Willy and Davis[16] examined the effect of a hip-strengthening program on otherwise healthy runners who showed excessive hip adduction with running. These individuals underwent a typical 6-week strengthening program addressing the hip abductors and external rotators. These runners showed an approximate 40% increase in strength of these muscles compared with a control group who did no strengthening. Despite this increase in strength, these runners showed nearly identical poststrengthening hip mechanics compared with their baseline values (**Fig. 5**). Instruction and practice in proper single-leg stance activities were also included in the strengthening program. Like Mascal and colleagues,[15] Willy and Davis[16] noted significant improvements in the hip mechanics of the single-leg squat. However, these changes did not translate to alterations during the higher-demand activity of running. This finding clearly underscores the need for the retraining to be activity specific.

BRIEF HISTORY OF GAIT RETRAINING

The idea of altering gait patterns using feedback is not novel. The earliest forms of feedback were limb load monitors placed within the shoe of a patient.[17–19] The aim of this type of feedback was to produce an equal load distribution between lower extremities during gait. Electromyography is one of the most widely used forms of feedback reported in the literature. Reports of improvements in gait symmetry in terms

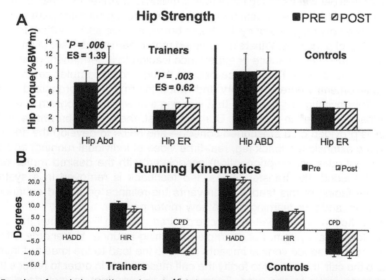

Fig. 5. Results of study by Willy and Davis.[16] (A) Comparison of hip strength values. Note the significant change in the Trainer group. (B) Comparison of prestrengthening and poststrengthening hip kinematics in the Trainer group. Note the lack of change in hip movement patterns, despite the increase in strength noted in this group. ABD, abduction; CPD, contralateral pelvic drop; ER, external Rotation; ES, effect Size; HADD, hip adduction; HIR, hip internal rotation; *, statistically significant (P<.05). (*Data from* Willy RW, Davis IS. The effect of a hip-strengthening program on mechanics during running and during a single-leg squat. J Orthop Sports Phys Ther 2011;41(9):625–32).

of spatiotemporal parameters and joint motion patterns have been reported with the use of electromyogram feedback.[20-24] Feedback on joint angles has been provided through the use of electrogoniometers for patients with genu recurvatum.[25-27] Almost all of these studies have reported successful results. However, none of these assessed the persistence or retention of these gait patterns over time, and most of these studies involved patients with neurologic disorders.

Reports of real-time feedback training then began to emerge in the orthopedic literature. In 2005, White and Lifeso[28] provided real-time force feedback from an instrumented treadmill to patients who walked asymmetrically following a hip replacement. They reported a significant improvement in symmetry of ground reaction forces at weight acceptance following an 8-week (3 times per week) gait retraining program. In a related study, Dingwell and colleagues[29] used an instrumented treadmill to improve the gait patterns of a group of unilateral, transtibial amputees. Before the training, asymmetries in the measured parameters were 4.6 times greater in the amputee group compared with the control group. These asymmetries were significantly reduced following the training. However, the long-term persistence of these changes was not monitored in either study and both investigations focused on walking gait. The physical demands of running are greater than those of walking, thus increasing the challenges of altering habitual running gait patterns.

COMPONENTS OF A RETRAINING PROGRAM

Altering any motor pattern that has become habituated over many years can be difficult, and this is especially true for retraining runners. Runners strike the ground approximately 625 steps per kilometer (1000 steps per mile). An individual who runs 32 km (20 miles) per week can log more than 1 million foot strikes per year, or 10 million foot strikes if they have been running for 10 years. Altering a motor pattern that has been reinforced over millions of cycles takes both guidance and practice. In a review on motor control principles, Winstein[30] defined motor learning as a set of internal processes associated with practice or experience leading to a permanent change in the capability for responding. These processes are thought to be complex central nervous system phenomena whereby sensory and motor information is organized and integrated.[30] This investigator suggests that learning a new motor program is enhanced with feedback provided in 2 phases. During the first, the acquisition phase, extrinsic feedback is provided on a prescribed schedule and helps to develop the connection between the extrinsic feedback (eg, real-time video of individual running) and the internal sensory cues (ie, proprioception) associated with the desired motor pattern. During the second, the transfer phase, the feedback is removed in a systematic fashion. The fading of this feedback prevents the reliance on it, and enhances the internalization, and thus learning, of the new motor pattern.

Although altering a motor pattern may be desired, it is also likely to alter the loads on the musculoskeletal system. For example, retraining a runner to become a forefoot striker in order to reduce vertical impacts reduces the load to the knee but increases the load to the calf. It is critical to fortify the calf musculature in order to reduce the risk of an overuse injury to this area. Therefore, it is important to include a specific strengthening program in any gait retraining intervention to anticipate increased demands to other components of the kinetic chain.

ALTERING MOVEMENT PATTERNS IN RUNNERS

One of the earliest gait retraining studies in runners was conducted by Messier and Cirillo[31] in 1989. Runners were seen 3 times per week for 5 weeks. Before each training session, subjects were shown a videotape of their running and were instructed on the features of gait they were to modify. These mechanics were subject specific and included characteristics such as excessive vertical oscillation, overstriding, excessive trunk lean, and excessive arm motion. This group of runners significantly altered the desired kinematic gait variables compared with a control group of runners who received no feedback before their training sessions. This study shows that runners are able to alter their mechanics with retraining. However, persistence of these changes following training was not examined, and it is therefore unclear whether true motor learning occurred.

With the development of real-time motion analysis systems, gait retraining could be augmented with real-time feedback on specific joint angles. Using this technology, Noehren and colleagues[32] investigated 10 female runners with a history of patellofemoral pain (average duration of 75.7 months) who showed excessive hip adduction. These runners underwent 8 sessions (over 2 weeks) of gait retraining, learning how to activate the gluteal muscles in order to reduce hip adduction. Markers were placed on the lower extremities so that hip adduction could be monitored in real time. The hip adduction angle of the most involved side was displayed on a monitor in front of the runner during the stance phase of each foot strike. This angle was superimposed on a graph of a normal hip adduction trajectory with a shaded region denoting ±1 standard deviation of this mean value (**Fig. 6**). Runners were asked to keep their hip adduction angles within the shaded region by modulating the activation of their gluteal muscles. The investigators were highly interested in the persistence of these changes. Therefore, they used a paradigm that incorporated the concepts of motor learning that were described by Winstein.[30] Subjects gradually increased their run times from 10 to 30 minutes over the 8 sessions. During the first 4 sessions, runners were provided feedback 100% of the time (acquisition phase). During the last 4 sessions, feedback was faded (transfer phase) such that they received only 3 minutes of feedback during the last session (1 in the beginning, 1 in the middle, and 1 in the end) (**Fig. 7**). Their gait data were examined at baseline, immediately posttraining, and at 1-month follow-up. Runners were able to reduce their hip adduction, internal rotation, and contralateral pelvic drop following gait retraining (**Fig. 8**). In addition, they were able to maintain this at

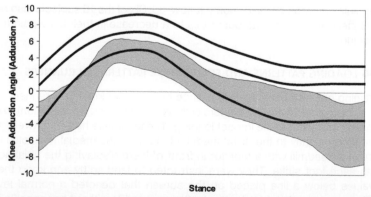

Fig. 6. Real-time feedback of hip adduction angle during a retraining session. The shaded region represents ±1 standard deviation from the mean value of hip adduction based on a healthy population of runners. With each stance, the hip adduction angle is provided on a monitor in front of the runner. Runners are instructed to modulate their gluteal activation until they are able to keep their hip adduction angle within the targeted shaded region.

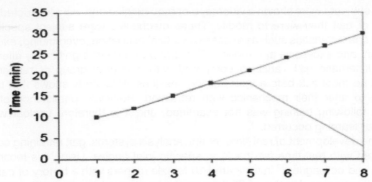

Fig. 7. Faded feedback design used in many of the gait retraining studies. Run time is increased from 10 to 30 minutes over 8 sessions. Feedback is provided 100% of the time over the first 4 sessions and then is gradually removed over the last 4 sessions.

the 1-month follow-up. Controlling their hips better during running also led to reduced vertical load rates, which have been shown to be related to patellofemoral pain.[33] Along with persistency, an indication of learning is the ability to transfer the new motor pattern to an untrained activity.[34–36] These investigators noted that hip alignment also improved during the activity of a single-leg squat. Most important to the patients, there was a complete resolution of pain and significant improvement in overall function.

Although these real-time motion analysis systems can provide powerful feedback, they are unlikely to be readily available in clinical settings. Therefore, Willy and colleagues[32,37] repeated the study of Noehren and colleagues[32] using a similar female patient population with chronic patellofemoral pain (average pain duration, 51 months). However, they simply used a mirror as the real-time feedback. They used an identical faded feedback design, and their subjects' posttraining improvements in hip mechanics were similar to those described by Noehren and colleagues.[32] In addition, the investigators found these changes to persist at both 1-month and 3-month follow-ups. As with Noehren and colleagues,[32] the reductions in hip adduction transferred to other functional activities including a single-leg squat and a step-down maneuver. Again, pain was resolved, function restored, and all runners returned to at least their pretraining mileage by the 3-month follow-up. Six of the 10 subjects also reported running higher mileage, and attributed this to a decrease in their knee pain following gait retraining.

ALTERING LOADING PATTERNS AND FOOT STRIKE PATTERNS IN RUNNERS

Gait retraining has also been used to reduce high-impact loading in runners. Crowell and Davis[38] recruited 10 healthy runners with high tibial shock (acceleration) to engage in a retraining study to reduce impact loading. These runners had a lightweight accelerometer affixed tightly to the distal medial tibia above the medial malleolus (**Fig. 9**). They ran on a treadmill with a monitor in front of them displaying the tibial accelerations with each foot strike. They were instructed to land softly and keep their tibial shock values below a line placed on the screen that denoted a normal level (see **Fig. 9**). They were simply told to land as softly as possible without any specific instruction on how to do so. These investigators used a similar feedback paradigm as Noehren and colleagues[32] and Willy and colleagues.[32,37] All runners reported that the new gait pattern felt natural by the sixth retraining session. In addition, runners were able to reduce their tibial shock, by 48% on average. Vertical instantaneous and average load

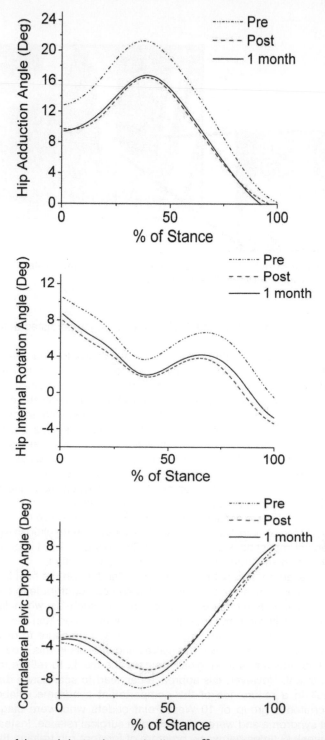

Fig. 8. Results of the study by Noehren and colleagues.[32] Note the reduction in hip adduction, internal rotation, and contralateral pelvic drop, at both 1-month and 3-month follow-ups; *, statistically significant (*P*<.05). (*Data from* Noehren B, Scholz J, Davis I. The effect of real-time gait retraining on hip kinematics, pain and function in subjects with patellofemoral pain syndrome. Br J Sports Med 2011;45(9):691–96).

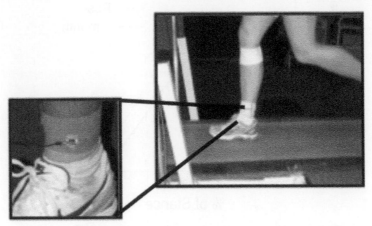

Fig. 9. Measurement of tibial shock while running. A lightweight accelerometer is tightly affixed (and overwrapped) to the distal medial tibia.

rates were also reduced by 34% and 32%. These changes persisted at the 1-month follow-up.

Running with a forefoot strike (FFS) pattern has been shown to reduce impact loading and can be an effective approach to reducing patellofemoral joint pain. Patellofemoral pain is related, in part, to increases in the patellofemoral contact stresses.[39,40] It has been shown that a FFS results in a reduced vertical force at early stance because of lower rates of loading. This reduced vertical force is coupled with an increased knee flexion angle (thus greater patellofemoral contact area) in early stance. These combined biomechanical factors lead to a reduced patellofemoral contact stress and potentially less pain.[41] In a case series of 3 patients with chronic patellofemoral pain, Cheung and Davis[42] transitioned the runners from a rearfoot strike pattern to an FFS pattern. Instrumented insoles were used to provide an audible sound when the runners landed on their heels. Runners underwent 8 sessions of gait retraining using the faded feedback design of others.[32,37] They were able to successfully transition these runners to an FFS pattern that persisted at both 1 and 3 months. This transition resulted in significant reductions in vertical impact peaks, as well as VALRs and VILRs. Most importantly, these runners showed marked improvements in their pain and function.

In addition to exacerbating patellofemoral pain, landing on the heel increases the demand of the anterior muscles of the lower leg and can contribute to compartment syndrome. When the demand becomes excessive, such as when landing with increased ankle dorsiflexion, the muscles hypertrophy faster than the fascial compartments can accommodate, which causes increased pressure to develop in the compartment, potentially damaging the nerves and vessels in this area. A common approach to this problem is to surgically release the fascia to relieve the pressure in the compartment. However, this approach can lead to scar tissue development, and can result in a recurrence of the compartment syndrome. Diebel and colleagues[43] recruited a group of 10 West Point cadets who were diagnosed with compartment syndrome and were indicated for a surgical release. Instead, they underwent a 6-week (3 times per week) program of forefoot run training that included running drills, cadence practice, video recording, metronome feedback, and barefoot running. At the end of 6 weeks, intracompartmental pressures had returned to normal, symptoms had resolved, vertical load rates were reduced, and cadence was significantly improved. All runners were able to return to their preinjury running, all increased their run times, and all were able to avoid a surgical release.

The recent shift toward adopting a more anterior foot strike pattern during running has led to transition studies using healthy individuals. Warne and colleagues[44] conducted a 4-week intervention to gradually transition to a FFS pattern in minimal footwear (Vivo Barefoot Evo, Terra Plana, London, United Kingdom). The program included technique instruction, a prescribed schedule of running progression, as well as a stretching and strengthening component focused on the foot and ankle. At the end of the 4-week program, 8 of the 10 runners had transitioned successfully to a FFS pattern. However, it is unclear whether motor learning occurred, because there were no follow-up assessments to determine persistence. McCarthy and colleagues[45] conducted a similar intervention study. This group of 9 rearfoot strike runners was provided minimal footwear (Vibram FiveFingers Classic). They were instructed in a foot-strengthening program and were then given a prescribed 12-week progressive running program to be conducted independently. A control group of 10 runners continued to run their normal mileages in their standard footwear. At the end of the training, the intervention group showed significantly greater plantarflexed ankles at foot strike, indicating a FFS pattern. However, as with Warne and colleagues,[44] there was no assessment of short-term or long-term persistence of these changes. The persistence and retention of these changes, especially in the long term, must be evaluated in order to establish gait retraining as an effective method to alter foot strike pattern and provide a treatment strategy to reduce running injuries.

CASE STUDY OF TRANSITIONING INTERVENTION WITH LONG-TERM FOLLOW-UP

A 24-year-old female runner had running-related deep knee joint pain and lateral knee pain on the right for approximately 7 months before being seen as a patient at the Spaulding National Running Center (SNRC) in Cambridge, Massachusetts. At the time of her initial evaluation, extended walking, stairs, and squatting were all painful. She had also tried swimming and cycling, and both were painful in the knee. Before her time at the SNRC, she underwent a course of physical therapy that consisted primarily of stretching and strengthening, which did not improve her symptoms. She was referred back to her physician because of lack of progress. She had radiographs and MRI of her knee, which were negative for disorder. She stated that her knee was painful at all times during activities of daily living and reported a verbal analog pain scale of 2 out of 10 at best and 7 out of 10 at worst.

This patient ran with a rearfoot strike (RFS) bilaterally, showing vertical impact peaks (**Fig. 10**). She showed weakness of her foot and ankle muscles bilaterally, only completing 5 heel raises on the left and 2 on the right. When asked to run with an FFS pattern while barefoot, her right deep knee joint pain immediately reduced from 7 out of 10 to 5 out of 10 and her right lateral knee pain reduced from 5 out of 10 to 0 out of 10. Vertical impact peaks were immediately eliminated (see **Fig. 10**) and VILR and VALR were decreased by 36% and 40% on the injured right side, respectively (**Fig. 11**). These reductions are consistent with results we published in a group of 49 patients seen in the SNRC clinic.[46]

This runner underwent a 7-week program consisting of 4 weeks of foot and lower leg progressive strengthening and 8 sessions of gait retraining using a faded feedback design to transition to an FFS pattern. At the end of the sessions, this patient was running for 30 minutes with a consistent FFS pattern and no pain. She was instructed to increase her mileage by 10% per week following discharge.

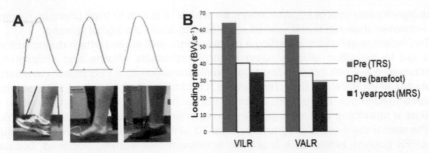

Fig. 10. Long-term follow-up on a patient who underwent a supervised transition to running with a FFS pattern using foot and ankle strengthening and gait retraining. (*A*) Foot strike pattern and associated vertical ground reaction forces: (*left*) baseline with shoes (RFS); (*middle*) baseline, barefoot (FFS); and (*right*) 1-year follow-up, minimal shoes (FFS). (*B*) VILR and VALR at baseline (Pre) when the patient was running with shoes (*red*), barefoot (*white*), and 1-year after, when running in her minimal shoes (*blue*). Note the reduction of her load rates when barefoot at baseline and in her minimal shoes at 1 year after.BW, body weight; MRS, minimal running shoe; TRS, traditional running shoe.

The patient returned for a 1-year follow-up. Since her discharge, she has continued to run in minimal shoes an average of 15 miles per week and she has been pain free. She now runs with an FFS with 10% reduced stride length compared with her baseline at time of injury. Her VILR and VALR in the minimal footwear were reduced by 36% and 52% respectively on the injured right side (see **Fig. 11**). Not noted in the graph is the

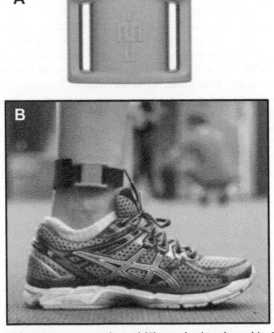

Fig. 11. (*A*) An inertial measurement unit, and (*B*) attached to the ankle. These devices facilitate the measurement of gait in runners in their natural environments.

reduction of her VILR and VALR of 58% and 63% on the left, uninjured side, indicating the transfer of mechanics to the contralateral leg. This case study supports the association of impacts with knee pain, as well as the reduction of knee pain with reduction of the impacts.[33,41,42] It also supports the hypotheses that transitioning to an FFS pattern with minimal footwear resulted in reduction of vertical impact loading in both the short-term and long-term follow-up. This case shows that the transition to an FFS pattern can be accomplished without injury when the runner is adequately prepared. In addition, it signifies that these changes can be maintained in the long term. In addition, it shows that this approach was successful in eliminating injury in a runner who had undergone a previous unsuccessful course of physical therapy.

MONITORING RUNNERS IN THEIR NATURAL ENVIRONMENTS

Most studies of running mechanics and gait retraining have been conducted in the laboratory, which is clearly an artificial setting. Data are typically collected overground, as a runner traverses a runway with a force plate at its center. Depending on the length of the runway, the ability to reach a typical running speed and maintain it for several steps can be limited. In addition, the runner's foot must land fully on the force plate, increasing the chance for targeting. Alternatively, data can be collected on a treadmill. Although kinematics between overground and treadmill running have been deemed similar, the treadmill constrains the runner to a single speed, unlike running outdoors where speed is likely to vary.[47] Both overground and treadmill running do not mimic the natural environment of banked surfaces, hills, and other variations in terrain. In addition, the mechanics of runners who know they are being observed may not be representative of their true mechanics. Therefore, there is great ecologic value in studying runners in their natural environments.

Willy and colleagues[48] showed a simple way to train runners to increase their cadence outside of the laboratory. These investigators used a wireless accelerometer that transmitted data to a computerized watch that displayed running time, distance, and strides/ per minute during a running session. Sixteen runners, screened for high-impact loading, were included in the intervention and 14 runners served as the controls. Following a baseline instrumented gait analysis in the laboratory, runners in the intervention group were instructed to complete 8 typical runs and to aim for increasing their cadence by 7.5%.[49] Subjects were instructed to use the feedback when they thought they needed it, because self-controlled feedback has recently been shown to improve motivation.[30] An intermittent feedback design was incorporated whereby the self-controlled feedback was provided on alternate days.[30] Data were collected in the laboratory at baseline, following the retraining, and at a 1-month follow-up. Runners were able to increase their cadence by approximately 8%. This increase resulted in an approximate 18% reduction in vertical load rates. Although this is a significant decrease, the posttraining values of 83 BW/s are still considered high for the speed they were running.[2] Other measures to reduce impact, such as transitioning to an FFS pattern, may be preferred when aiming to reduce load rates as much as possible in an injured population. In addition, peak hip adduction, a common malalignment in runners, was reduced by 2.5°, or 14% from preintervention values. This finding was consistent with the findings of Heidersheidt and colleagues,[49] who reported similar reductions when running with a higher cadence. The changes these investigators noted persisted at the 1-month follow-up. This study also assessed changes in cumulative load with alterations in gait patterns. Despite the increase in number of steps, the cumulative eccentric knee work over the course of a run was lower with the increased cadence. Note that all gait assessments were conducted in the laboratory under the observation of the investigators. As such, this gait may not be representative of the runners' gaits in their natural environments.

The development of mobile monitoring devices has made it possible to analyze aspects of running mechanics outside of the laboratory environment. Inertial measurement units, allow the study of accelerometry, as well as joint kinematics. In addition, instrumented insoles are emerging in the market to detect foot pressures during running. These devices have Bluetooth capability that can wirelessly monitor, record, and provide feedback on a variety of biomechanical measures in real time and in multiple environments. These developments will help to advance gait retraining research that is more ecologically valid.

SUMMARY

In summary, people have a considerable untapped ability to adapt their own movement patterns. The concept of retraining motor patterns is not new. However, there continues to be some skepticism about the ability to alter the automatic function of both walking and running gaits. In terms of running, there is evidence that links mechanics with injury. This evidence provides the justification for altering these mechanics. Increased hip adduction and vertical impact loading have been most commonly associated with injury. As such, most retraining studies are focused on these issues. However, gait retraining principles can be applied to any gait abnormality that is thought to be related to an overuse musculoskeletal problem. Although all of the retraining studies to date have resulted in improvements in gait mechanics, the optimal retraining paradigms are likely yet to be determined. Studies need to compare the efficacy of different types of feedback (visual, haptic, auditory) as well as different feedback schedules. Most studies involved small subject numbers. It is important to know whether the success of these small studies translates to larger study populations. In addition, long-term follow-ups (ie, 1 year and beyond) are needed to establish the retention and persistence of gait changes. Studies need to include more tests that examine the transfer of new patterns to other untrained activities. In addition, clinicians need to monitor runners and retrain their gait patterns in their natural environments. In conclusion, more work is needed in order to understand the optimal way to retrain gait patterns in runners. To provide individuals with the ability to alter faulty movement patterns in ways that can reduce injury risk is a powerful tool.

REFERENCES

1. Nigg BM, Baltich J, Hoerzer S, et al. Running shoes and running injuries: myth-busting and a proposal for two new paradigms: "preferred movement path" and "comfort filter". Br J Sports Med 2015;49(20):1290–4.
2. Milner CE, Ferber R, Pollard CD, et al. Biomechanical factors associated with tibial stress fracture in female runners. Med Sci Sports Exerc 2006;38(2):323–8.
3. Pohl MB, Hamill J, Davis IS. Biomechanical and anatomic factors associated with a history of plantar fasciitis in female runners. Clin J Sport Med 2009;19(5):372–6.
4. Noehren B, Hamill J, Davis I. Prospective evidence for a hip etiology in patellofemoral pain. Med Sci Sports Exerc 2013;45(6):1120–4.
5. Williams KR, Cavanagh PR. Relationship between distance running mechanics, running economy, and performance. J Appl Physiol (1985) 1987;63(3):1236–45.
6. Williams DS 3rd, McClay IS, Hamill J. Arch structure and injury patterns in runners. Clin Biomech (Bristol, Avon) 2001;16(4):341–7.

7. Saragiotto BT, Yamato TP, Hespanhol LC Jr, et al. What are the main risk factors for running-related injuries? Sports Med 2014;44(8):1153–63.
8. Zadpoor AA, Nikooyan AA. The relationship between lower-extremity stress fractures and the ground reaction force: a systematic review. Clin Biomech 2011; 26(1):23–8.
9. Radin EL, Paul IL. Response of joints to impact loading. I. In vitro wear. Arthritis Rheum 1971;14(3):356–62.
10. Radin EL, Parker HG, Pugh JW, et al. Response of joints to impact loading – III: relationship between trabecular microfractures and cartilage degeneration. J Biomech 1973;6:51–7.
11. Burr DB, Milgrom C, Boyd RD, et al. Experimental stress fractures of the tibia. Biological and mechanical aetiology in rabbits. J Bone Joint Surg Br 1990;72(3): 370–5.
12. Schaffler MB, Radin EL, Burr DB. Mechanical and morphological effects of strain rate on fatigue of compact bone. Bone 1989;10(3):207–14.
13. Ferber R, Noehren B, Hamill J, et al. Competitive female runners with a history of iliotibial band syndrome demonstrate atypical hip and knee kinematics. J Orthop Sports Phys Ther 2010;40(2):52–8.
14. Snyder KR, Earl JE, O'Connor KM, et al. Resistance training is accompanied by increases in hip strength and changes in lower extremity biomechanics during running. Clin Biomech 2009;24(1):26–34.
15. Mascal CL, Landel R, Powers C. Management of patellofemoral pain targeting hip, pelvis, and trunk muscle function: 2 case reports. J Orthop Sports Phys Ther 2003;33(11):647–60.
16. Willy RW, Davis IS. The effect of a hip-strengthening program on mechanics during running and during a single-leg squat. J Orthop Sports Phys Ther 2011;41(9): 625–32.
17. Wannstedt GT, Herman RM. Use of augmented sensory feedback to achieve symmetrical standing. Phys Ther 1978;58(5):553–9.
18. Seeger BR, Caudrey DJ. Biofeedback therapy to achieve symmetrical gait in children with hemiplegic cerebral palsy: long-term efficacy. Arch Phys Med Rehabil 1983;64(4):160–2.
19. Seeger BR, Caudrey DJ, Scholes JR. Biofeedback therapy to achieve symmetrical gait in hemiplegic cerebral palsied children. Arch Phys Med Rehabil 1981; 62(8):364–8.
20. Burnside I, Tobias H, Bursill D. Electromyographic feedback in the remobilization of stroke patients: a controlled trial. Arch Phys Med Rehabil 1982;63(5):217–22.
21. Colborne GR, Olney SJ, Griffin MP. Feedback of ankle joint angle and soleus electromyography in the rehabilitation of hemiplegic gait. Arch Phys Med Rehabil 1993;74(10):1100–6.
22. Colborne G, Wright F, Naumann S. Feedback of triceps surae EMG in gait of children with cerebral palsy: a controlled study. Arch Phys Med Rehabil 1994;75(1):40–5.
23. Petrofsky JS. The use of electromyogram biofeedback to reduce Trendelenburg gait. Eur J Appl Physiol 2001;85:491–5.
24. Intiso D, Santilli V, Grasso MG, et al. Rehabilitation of walking with electromyographic biofeedback in foot-drop after stroke. Stroke 1994;25(6):1189–92.
25. Hogue R, McCandless S. Genu recurvatum: auditory biofeedback treatment for adult patients with stroke or head injuries. Arch Phys Med Rehabil 1983;64(8): 368–70.
26. Morris M, Matyas T, Bach TM, et al. Electrogoniometric feedback: its effect on genu recurvatum in stroke. Arch Phys Med Rehabil 1992;73(12):1147–54.

27. Olney SJ, Colborne GR, Martin CS. Joint angle feedback and biomechanical gait analysis in stroke patients: a case report. Phys Ther 1989;69(10):863–70.
28. White SC, Lifeso RM. Altering asymmetric limb loading after hip arthroplasty using real-time dynamic feedback when walking. Arch Phys Med Rehabil 2005; 86(10):1958–63.
29. Dingwell JB, Davis BL, Frazder DM. Use of an instrumental treadmill for real-time gait symmetry evaluation and feedback in normal and trans-tibial amputee subjects. Prosthet Orthot Int 1996;20(2):101–10.
30. Winstein CJ. Knowledge of results and motor learning–implications for physical therapy. Phys Ther 1991;71(2):140–9.
31. Messier SP, Cirillo KJ. Effects of a verbal and visual feedback system on running technique, perceived exertion and running economy in female novice runners. J Sports Sci 1989;7:113–26.
32. Noehren B, Scholz J, Davis I. The effect of real-time gait retraining on hip kinematics, pain and function in subjects with patellofemoral pain syndrome. Br J Sports Med 2011;45(9):691–6.
33. Davis IS, Bowser BJ, Hamill J. Vertical impact loading in runners with a history of patellofemoral pain syndrome. Med Sci Sports Exerc 2010;42(5):682.
34. Salmoni AW, Schmidt RA, Walter CB. Knowledge of results and motor learning: a review and critical reappraisal. Psychol Bull 1984;95(3):355–86.
35. Schmidt RA, White JL. Evidence for an error detection mechanism in motor skills. J Mot Behav 1972;4(3):143–53.
36. Sherwood DE, Lee TD. Schema theory: critical review and implications for the role of cognition in a new theory of motor learning. Res Q Exerc Sport 2003;74(4): 376–82.
37. Willy RW, Scholz JP, Davis IS. Mirror gait retraining for the treatment of patellofemoral pain in female runners. Clin Biomech (Bristol, Avon) 2012;27(10):1045–51.
38. Crowell HP, Davis IS. Gait retraining to reduce lower extremity loading in runners. Clin Biomech (Bristol, Avon) 2011;26(1):78–83.
39. Farrokhi S, Keyak JH, Powers CM. Individuals with patellofemoral pain exhibit greater patellofemoral joint stress: a finite element analysis study. Osteoarthritis Cartilage 2011;19(3):287–94.
40. Heino Brechter J, Powers C. Patellofemoral stress during walking in persons with and without patellofemoral pain. Med Sci Sports Exerc 2002;34(10):1582–93.
41. Bonacci J, Vicenzino B, Spratford W, et al. Take your shoes off to reduce patellofemoral joint stress during running. Br J Sports Med 2013;48(6):425–8.
42. Cheung RTH, Davis IS. Landing pattern modification to improve patellofemoral pain in runners: a case series. J Orthop Sports Phys Ther 2011;41(12):914–9.
43. Diebal AR, Gregory R, Alitz C, et al. Forefoot running improves pain and disability associated with chronic exertional compartment syndrome. Am J Sports Med 2012;40(5):1060–7.
44. Warne JP, Kilduff SM, Gregan BC, et al. A 4-week instructed minimalist running transition and gait-retraining changes plantar pressure and force. Scand J Med Sci Sports 2013;24(6):964–73.
45. McCarthy C, Fleming N, Donne B, et al. 12 weeks of simulated barefoot running changes foot-strike patterns in female runners. Int J Sports Med 2014;35(5): 443–50.
46. Samaan CD, Rainbow MJ, Davis IS. Reduction in ground reaction force variables with instructed barefoot running. J Sport Health Sci 2014;3(2):143–51.
47. Fellin RE, Manal K, Davis IS. Comparison of lower extremity kinematic curves during overground and treadmill running. J Appl Biomech 2010;26(4):407–14.

48. Willy RW, Buchenic L, Rogacki K, et al. In-field gait retraining and mobile monitoring to address running biomechanics associated with tibial stress fracture. Scand J Med Sci Sports 2015. [Epub ahead of print].
49. Heiderscheit BC, Chumanov ES, Michalski MP, et al. Effects of step rate manipulation on joint mechanics during running. Med Sci Sports Exerc 2011;43(2):296–302.

Index

Note: Page numbers of article titles are in **boldface** type.

A

Achilles tendinopathy, 122–124
Achilles tendonitis
  malalignment syndrome in runners aggravating or precipitating, 300
Adolescence
  of female athletes
    health considerations related to growth spurt in, 153
    as vulnerable time, 154
  growth during
    unique considerations for athlete, 180–182
  running injuries during, **179–202**
    apophyseal injuries, 182–186
    epidemiology of, 180
    introduction, 179–180
    JOCD, 189–190
    lower extremity tendon injuries, 183, 187–188
    MTSS, 183, 189
    prevention of, 194–196
    treatment of, 190–194
Anemia
  iron deficiency with and without
    in female runners, 165
Ankle injuries
  in runners, **121–137** (See also specific types and Foot and ankle injuries, in runners)
Ankle sprains, 126–127
Anterior tibial tendinopathy, 131
Apophyseal injuries
  during adolescence and childhood, 182–186
Asymmetrical ligament tension
  malalignment syndrome in runners and, 284–286
Asymmetrical lower extremity range of motion
  malalignment syndrome in runners and, 286–290
Asymmetrical muscle tone
  malalignment syndrome in runners and, 273–281
Asymmetrical weight bearing and pattern of shoe wear
  malalignment syndrome in runners and, 268–272
Asymmetry of muscle strength and bulk
  malalignment syndrome in runners and, 281–284

B

Back pain
  mid

Phys Med Rehabil Clin N Am 27 (2016) 357–371
http://dx.doi.org/10.1016/S1047-9651(15)00105-9
1047-9651/16/$ – see front matter © 2016 Elsevier Inc. All rights reserved.

Moving?

Make sure your subscription moves with you!

To notify us of your new address, find your **Clinics Account Number** (located on your mailing label above your name), and contact customer service at:

Email: **journalscustomerservice-usa@elsevier.com**

800-654-2452 (subscribers in the U.S. & Canada)
314-447-8871 (subscribers outside of the U.S. & Canada)

Fax number: 314-447-8029

Elsevier Health Sciences Division
Subscription Customer Service
3251 Riverport Lane
Maryland Heights, MO 63043

*To ensure uninterrupted delivery of your subscription, please notify us at least 4 weeks in advance of move.